L9D9M

ENABLING AMERICA

Assessing the Role of
Rehabilitation Science and Engineering

Edward N. Brandt, Jr., and Andrew M. Pope, *Editors*

Committee on Assessing Rehabilitation Science and Engineering

Division of Health Sciences Policy

INSTITUTE OF MEDICINE

NATIONAL ACADEMY PRESS
Washington, D.C. 1997

National Academy Press • 2101 Constitution Avenue, N.W. • Washington, D.C. 20418

NOTICE: The project that is the subject of this report was approved by the Governing Board of the National Research Council, whose members are drawn from the councils of the National Academy of Sciences, the National Academy of Engineering, and the Institute of Medicine. The members of the committee responsible for the report were chosen for their special competences and with regard for appropriate balance.

This report has been reviewed by a group other than the authors according to procedures approved by a Report Review Committee consisting of members of the National Academy of Sciences, the National Academy of Engineering, and the Institute of Medicine.

The Institute of Medicine was chartered in 1970 by the National Academy of Sciences to enlist distinguished members of the appropriate professions in the examination of policy matters pertaining to the health of the public. In this, the Institute acts under both the Academy's 1863 congressional charter responsibility to be an adviser to the federal government and its own initiative in identifying issues of medical care, research, and education. Dr. Kenneth I. Shine is president of the Institute of Medicine.

Support for this project was provided by funds from the U.S. Department of Health and Human Services (Contract No. 282-95-0035). Additional funding to support the publication and dissemination of the report was provided by the J. W. Kieckhefer Foundation, the American Physical Therapy Association, and the U.S. Department of Veterans Affairs, the Centers for Disease Control and Prevention, and the National Institutes of Health. The opinions expressed in this publication are those of the Committee on Assessing Rehabilitation Science and Engineering and do not necessarily reflect the views of the sponsors.

Library of Congress Cataloging-in-Publication Data

Enabling America : assessing the role of rehabilitation science and
    engineering / Edward N. Brandt, Jr., and Andrew M. Pope, editors ;
    Committee on Assessing Rehabilitation Science and Engineering,
    Division of Health Sciences Policy, Institute of Medicine.
        p. cm.
    Includes bibliographical references (p.   ) and index.
    ISBN 0-309-06374-4 (cloth)
        1. Rehabilitation technology—United States. 2. Medical
    rehabilitation—United States.   I. Brandt, Edward N. (Edward
    Newman), 1933- . II. Pope, Andrew MacPherson, 1950- .
    III. Institute of Medicine (U.S.). Committee on Assessing
    Rehabilitation Science and Engineering.
    RM950.E53 1997
    362.1'786'0973—dc21   97-21183

Additional copies of this report are available from the National Academy Press, 2101 Constitution Avenue, N.W., Lock Box 285, Washington, D.C. 20055. Call (800) 624-6242 or (202) 334-3313 (in the Washington Metropolitan Area). Internet **http://www.nap.edu.**

For more information about the Institute of Medicine, visit the IOM home page at **http://www2. nas.edu/iom.**

Cover art: Will Mason, National Academy Press

The serpent has been a symbol of long life, healing, and knowledge among almost all cultures and religions since the beginning of recorded history. The image adopted as a logotype by the Institute of Medicine is based on a relief carving from ancient Greece, now held by the Staatliche Museen in Berlin.

COMMITTEE ON ASSESSING REHABILITATION SCIENCE AND ENGINEERING

EDWARD N. BRANDT, JR. (*Chair*), Regents Professor and Director, Center for Health Policy, College of Public Health, University of Oklahoma Health Sciences Center, Oklahoma City

SHARON BARNARTT, Professor and Chair, Department of Sociology, Gallaudet University

CAROLYN BAUM, Assistant Professor of Occupational Therapy and Neurology and Director, Department of Occupational Therapy, Washington University School of Medicine

FAYE BELGRAVE, Associate Professor of Psychology, Director of Applied Social Program, Department of Psychology, George Washington University

CLIFFORD BRUBAKER, Professor and Dean, School of Health and Rehabilitation Sciences, University of Pittsburgh

DIANA CARDENAS, Professor, University of Washington School of Medicine, Department of Rehabilitation Medicine, University of Washington Medical Center, Seattle

DUDLEY S. CHILDRESS, Professor of Biomedical Engineering and Orthopedic Surgery and Director, Prosthetics Research Laboratory and Rehabilitation Engineering Research Program, Northwestern University

DONALD L. CUSTIS, Director (Retired) for Medical Affairs and Associate Executive Director for Health Policy, Paralyzed Veterans of America, Potomac, Md.

SUE K. DONALDSON, Professor of Physiology, School of Medicine, and Professor and Dean, School of Nursing, Johns Hopkins University

DAVID GRAY, Professor of Health Sciences Program in Occupational Therapy, Washington University School of Medicine

DAVID E. KREBS, Professor and Interim Director, Graduate Program in Clinical Investigation, Massachusetts General Hospital Institute of Health Professions, and Director, Massachusetts General Hospital Biomotion Laboratory, Boston

ELLEN J. MACKENZIE, Professor, Department of Health Policy and Management; Senior Associate Dean for Academic Affairs; and Director, Center for Injury Research and Policy, Johns Hopkins University School of Hygiene and Public Health

MARGARET TURK, Associate Professor, Department of Physical Medicine and Rehabilitation and Pediatrics, State University of New York Health Sciences Center at Syracuse

iii

GLEN WHITE, Assistant Professor, Department of Human Development and Family Life, University of Kansas, Lawrence

SAVIO L.-Y. WOO, Ferguson Professor and Vice Chairman for Research, Department of Orthopaedic Surgery, School of Medicine, University of Pittsburgh

EDWARD YELIN, Professor of Medicine and Health Policy, University of California, San Francisco

WISE YOUNG, Professor, Department of Neurosurgery, New York University Medical Center, New York City

IOM Health Sciences Policy Board Member/Committee Liaison

RICHARD JOHNS, Distinguished Service Professor of Biomedical Engineering and Professor of Medicine, Johns Hopkins University School of Medicine

Study Staff

ANDREW M. POPE, Study Director
GEOFFREY S. FRENCH, Research Assistant
THELMA M. COX, Project Assistant

Division Staff

VALERIE PETIT SETLOW, Director, Division of Health Sciences Policy
JAMAINE TINKER, Financial Associate
LINDA DePUGH, Administrative Assistant

Preface

In my career as an academician, political appointee (Assistant Secretary for Health, 1981–1984), and health policy maker, I have rarely, if ever, been involved in an activity of such magnitude as the one that resulted in this report. The range of issues was broad, deep, and complex, spanning from subcellular biochemistry and genetics to human behavior, health, and public policy. Moreover, the recommendations that emanated from our assessment of the research (and the programs that support it) have the potential to directly affect the health, productivity, and quality of life of millions of Americans.

The assessment of rehabilitation science and engineering that was conducted by the committee required different methods of data collection and analysis. Partly as a consequence of the breadth, depth, and complexity of our task, but also out of a desire to be as comprehensive as possible, the committee cast a broad net for the collection of information. Data on current federal research projects were important, of course, but so were informed opinions regarding needs, priorities, and the relative effectiveness of federal research programs. Thus, the committee polled consumers through various means, held focus groups with professional associations, interviewed federal agency officials (past and present), and reviewed current federal research activities. Collecting, organizing, and processing this information was a formidable task in itself, and the Institute of Medicine staff is to be commended for their efforts in supporting the committee's work in this regard. The committee is also indebted to numerous other individuals and organizations who generously provided us with information and assistance during our deliberations. Appendix A of this report contains the names of those who wrote background papers, participated in our meetings, made presentations, or otherwise assisted us in our work. Special recognition for the fundamental roles that they played in the initiation of this activity should be given to Senator Robert Dole, R. Alexander Vachon, Philip Lee, Suzanne Stoiber, and Lynn Gerber.

As the committee began to draw conclusions, there was a general sense of agreement on the shortcomings in the organization and administration of federal research programs in disability and rehabilitation-related research. In summary, these were as follows: a need for improved coordination, a need for more research, and a need for enhanced visibility of rehabilitation-related research within the federal research programs. Although I suspect that few will argue with the needs that are identified and described in this report, I am sure that some will disagree with the proposed solutions.

In developing these solutions, the committee's calls for more research and improved coordination were not made reflexively or out of mere self-interest, but rather resulted from rather extensive debate and deliberation. Coming to agreement on the recommendation for changes in the organization and administration of the major programs was perhaps the most difficult challenge. Developing a solution that would help ensure both scientific rigor in research and responsiveness to consumers was the priority, but political sensitivities could not be ignored. There was general consensus that the federal government needed a strong coordinating body, but the size, powers, and location of that body were all open to debate. In this regard, as the largest and most visible of federal programs supporting rehabilitation-related research, the National Institute on Disability and Rehabilitation Research (NIDRR) program received much attention, and it is not without careful consideration that the committee makes its recommendation to move the NIDRR program from the U.S. Department of Education to the U.S. Department of Health and Human Services. The committee considered and discussed many options in great depth; disability and rehabilitation, after all, are education issues to many people, but they are also labor issues and health issues. In the end it was decided that placement at a higher administrative level within an agency that could nurture its growth, help ensure its scientific development, and facilitate its interaction with other related programs that proved to be the winning argument.

In any event, it seems clear that although current efforts are generally of high quality, they are nonetheless inadequate in the face of the needs of the millions of Americans with potentially disabling conditions and the annual costs that range in the neighborhood of $300 billion annually, to say nothing of the emotional costs and the associated issues of quality of life. What is needed is an expanded and improved federal effort that will enhance the visibility of disability and rehabilitation science, expand research, and do both in a more coordinated fashion.

Finally, the committee feels strongly about the importance of enhancing the federal effort in rehabilitation science and engineering, and about the recommendations that are made in this report for accomplishing this objective. Implementing our recommendations for improving coordination, expanding research, and enhancing visibility will not only improve the health and quality of life of millions of Americans, it is quite simply the right thing to do. Such an enhanced effort will help ensure that the best science is brought to bear on these issues in a well-coordinated and efficient manner, with the ultimate result of *Enabling America*.

Edward N. Brandt, Jr., *Chair*
Committee on Assessing Rehabilitation
Science and Engineering

Acronyms

AAP	Association of Academic Physiatrists
AAPM&R	American Academy of Physical Medicine and Rehabilitation
ACRM	American Congress of Rehabilitation Medicine
ADA	Americans with Disabilities Act of 1990
ADL	activities of daily living
ADRR	Agency on Disability and Rehabilitation Research
AHCPR	Agency for Health Care Policy and Research
AOA	Administration on Aging
AOTA	American Occupational Therapy Association
APTA	American Physical Therapy Association
ASHA	American Speech-Language-Hearing Association
ASPE	Assistant Secretary for Planning and Evaluation
CAPTE	Commission on Accreditation in Physical Therapy Education
CATN	Consumer Assistive Technology Transfer Network
CbD	cerebellar disorders
CCOP	Community Clinical Oncology Program
CDC	Centers for Disease Control and Prevention
CG	Center of Gravity
CHAMPUS	Civilian Health and Medical Program of the Uniformed Services
CHQ	Child Health Questionnaire
CMA	Community Medical Alliance

CP	Center of Pressure
CPRD	Committee on Prosthetics Research and Development
CRISP	Computer Retrieval of Information on Scientific Projects
CRRN	Certified Rehabilitation Registered Nurse
DDP	Disabilities Prevention Program
DHHS	U.S. Department of Health and Human Services
DOD	U.S. Department of Defense
DOE	U.S. Department of Energy
EIS	Epidemiology Intelligence Service
FIM	Functional Independence Measure
FSQ	Functional Status Questionnaire
GDP	Gross Domestic Product
HMO	health maintenance organization
HRQL	health-related quality of life
HSR&D	health services research and development
HUD	U.S. Department of Housing and Urban Development
IADL	instrumental activities of daily living
ICD	institutes, centers, and divisions, National Institutes of Health
ICDR	Interagency Committee on Disability Research
IOM	Institute of Medicine, National Academy of Sciences
I-QOL	quality-of-life measure specific to urinary incontinence
MCO	managed care organization
MIP	managed indemnity plan
MRCC	Medical Rehabilitation Coordinating Committee, National Institutes of Health
MRS	Medical Research Service
NARIC	National Rehabilitation Information Center
NCEH	National Center for Environmental Health
NCI	National Cancer Institute
NCIPC	National Center for Injury Prevention and Control
NCMRR	National Center for Medical Rehabilitation Research
NHIS	National Health Interview Survey
NHP	Neighborhood Health Plan
NICHD	National Institute of Child Health and Human Development

NIDRR	National Institute on Disability and Rehabilitation Research
NIH	National Institutes of Health
NRTA	Postdoctoral Individual National Research Training Award
NSF	National Science Foundation
OMAR	Office of Medical Applications of Research
OSERS	Office of Special Education and Rehabilitative Services
OT	occupational therapy
OTT	Office of Technology Transfer
OVR	Office of Vocational Rehabilitation
PT	physical therapy
PVA	Paralyzed Veterans of America
QWB	Quality of Well-Being Scale
RAPD	Research Aiding Persons with Disabilities
RCT	randomized controlled trial
RESNA	Rehabilitation Engineering and Assistive Technology of North America
RRAC	Research Realignment Advisory Committee
RR&D	Rehabilitation Research and Development
RRTC	Rehabilitation Research and Training Centers
RSA	Rehabilitation Services Administration
SBIR	Small Business Innovative Research
SF-36	Standard Form of the Health Status Questionnaire
SHMO	social health maintenance organizations
SIPP	Survey of Income and Program Participation
SSA	Social Security Administration
SSDI	Social Security Disability Income
TDD	telecommunications device for the deaf
TT	technology transfer
UDS	Uniform Data System for Medical Rehabilitation
UI	urinary incontinence
VA	U.S. Department of Veterans Affairs
VHA	Veterans Health Administration
WHO	World Health Organization

Contents

xiii

ENABLING AMERICA

Executive Summary

ABSTRACT

In response to a request from the U.S. Congress, the Institute of Medicine prepared a report that (1) assesses the current knowledge base in rehabilitation science and engineering; (2) evaluates the utility of current rehabilitation models; (3) describes and recommends mechanisms for the effective transfer and clinical translation of scientific findings that will promote health and health care for people with disabling conditions; and (4) critically evaluates the current federal programmatic efforts in rehabilitation science and engineering.

The report describes general priorities for rehabilitation science and engineering as (1) strengthening the science, (2) focusing on the enabling–disabling process, and (3) transferring technology. The report also describes a new model of the enabling–disabling process, including clear reference to the importance of the environment in causing, preventing, and reducing disability.

Limited visibility, support, and coordination of existing federal research programs are described as major issues of concern. Moreover, the large annual costs (approximately $300 billion—more than 4 percent of the gross domestic product) associated with disability and rehabilitation are in stark contrast to the relatively small amount of funding ($133 million) that supports the major federal programs of research in rehabilitation science and engineering.

To address these concerns, the report recommends that the National Institute on Disability and Rehabilitation Research program be relocated from the U.S. Department of Education to the U.S. Department of Health and Human Services, where it would more effectively serve as the foundation of a new Agency on Disability and Rehabilitation Research that would have enhanced authority for coordinating federal research programs.

1

The United States has long judged the success of its efforts to improve the health of its citizens on the basis of mortality statistics. Gains in human longevity, however, have been accompanied by increases in the incidence and prevalence of disabling conditions. At this point in the evolution of the nation's health care system, emphasis has begun to shift from the quantity of life to the quality of life. As a result, attention is now being focused not only on the prevention and treatment of disease and injury but also on rehabilitation and health promotion for people with disabling conditions.

The population of people with disabilities is sizable in the United States—49 million Americans or about one of every seven citizens has some type of disabling condition. Approximately one third of these people have a disabling condition so severe that they are unable to carry out the major activities of their age group, such as attending school, working, or providing self-care. About another third are restricted in their major activities, and the remaining third are limited in other types of activities. In 1992, about one quarter of all disabling conditions stemmed from impairments such as sensory impairments, paralysis, or mental retardation, and the remaining three quarters were due to diseases or disorders such as emphysema, heart disease, or arthritis.

The economic costs associated with disability are enormous. Expressed in 1994 terms, the medical care expenditures (direct costs) amount to approximately $160 billion, and the indirect costs (lost productivity) amount to approximately $155 billion, for a grand total of over $300 billion annually—more than 4 percent of the gross domestic product. Cost savings, as well as clinical benefit, however, are clearly associated with early, aggressive intervention, vigilant and knowledgeable monitoring of chronic conditions, and appropriate use of assistive technology.

With a clear understanding of the importance of effective rehabilitation and an appreciation of the advances in rehabilitation science, Senator Dole (1995) stated the following in requesting an Institute of Medicine (IOM) study of federal programs in rehabilitation research:

> Advances in rehabilitation science are essential to realizing the Nation's commitment to equal opportunity, economic self-sufficiency, and full participation of Americans with disabilities. There are important questions of the adequacy of Federal efforts in both meeting the needs of the rapidly growing number of Americans with disabilities, and in realizing the new opportunities of science and technology on behalf of people with disabilities. The committee believes an independent assessment of the current Federal efforts in rehabilitation science and engineering is warranted and requests that the Secretary [of Health and Human Services] make appropriate arrangements with the Institute of Medicine . . . to undertake such a review.

In response to this request, the Institute of Medicine assembled this committee to address the following questions:

- What is the current content, quality, and adequacy of the knowledge base in rehabilitation science and engineering?
- How useful are current disability models, and do they reflect the interdisciplinary and multidisciplinary nature of rehabilitation and the importance of environmental factors in mediating disability?
- What is the best way to effectively translate scientific findings into clinical benefits for people with disabilities and disabling conditions?
- How productive, relevant, and well-coordinated are current federal research efforts in rehabilitation science and engineering?

Following a brief description of concepts and definitions, the remainder of this summary presents an overview of the committee's responses to these questions and a summary of the committee's conclusions and recommendations.

CONCEPTS, DEFINITIONS, AND MODELS

Rehabilitation is the process by which physical, sensory, or mental capacities are restored or developed. This is achieved not only through functional change in the person, such as strengthening injured limbs, but also through changes in the physical and social environments, such as making buildings accessible to wheelchairs. Rehabilitation strives to reverse what has been called the disabling process, and may therefore be called the *enabling process*.

An overview of the enabling and disabling processes, and how disabling conditions affect a person's access to the environment is shown in Figure 1. Access to the environment, depicted as a square, represents both physical space and social structures (family, community, society). The person's degree of physical access to and social integration into the generalized environment is shown as degree of overlap of the symbolic person and the environmental square. A person who does not manifest disability (Figure 1a) is fully integrated into society and has full access to both: (1) social opportunities (e.g., employment, education, parenthood, leadership roles) and (2) physical space (e.g., housing, workplaces, transportation). A person with disabling conditions has increased needs (shown as the increased size of the individual) and is dislocated from their prior integration into the environment (Figure 1b).

The enabling (or rehabilitative) process attempts to rectify this displacement, either by restoring function in the individual (Figure 1c) or by expanding access to the environment (Figure 1d) (e.g., building ramps).

4

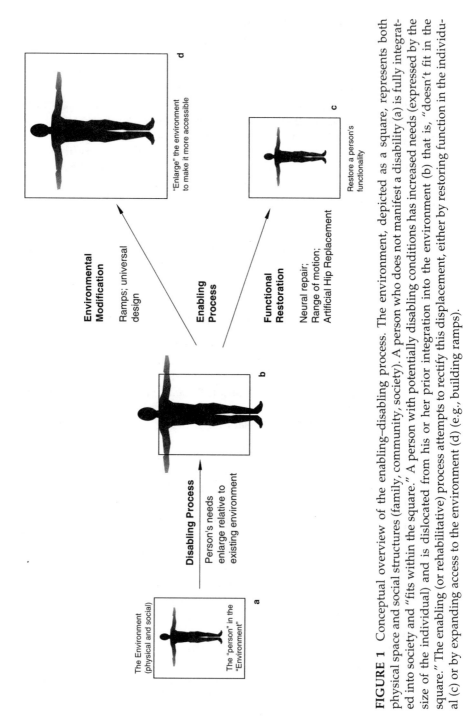

FIGURE 1 Conceptual overview of the enabling–disabling process. The environment, depicted as a square, represents both physical space and social structures (family, community, society). A person who does not manifest a disability (a) is fully integrated into society and "fits within the square." A person with potentially disabling conditions has increased needs (expressed by the size of the individual) and is dislocated from his or her prior integration into the environment (b) that is, "doesn't fit in the square." The enabling (or rehabilitative) process attempts to rectify this displacement, either by restoring function in the individual (c) or by expanding access to the environment (d) (e.g., building ramps).

This does not mean to imply that functional restoration and environmental modification (sometimes characterized as cure and care) are mutually exclusive. Indeed, the most effective rehabilitation programs include both. This overview model separates the two only to illustrate that disability is the interaction between the disabling conditions of an individual and the environment, and therefore strategies that affect either the environment or the disabling conditions can affect disability.

Rehabilitation science and engineering, as defined in this report, is the field of study that encompasses basic and applied aspects of the health sciences, social sciences, and engineering related to restoring functional capacity in a person and improving their interactions with the surrounding environment. This term reflects the synergistic importance of both science and engineering in advancing rehabilitation efforts and addressing the needs of people with disabling conditions. What is unique about rehabilitation science and engineering is the melding of knowledge from several disciplines to understand the fundamental nature of the *enabling–disabling processes*, that is, how disabling conditions develop, progress, and reverse, and how biological, behavioral, and environmental factors can affect these transitions.

Disability Models

As originally described by Saad Nagi in the 1950s and refined most recently in the 1991 IOM report *Disability in America*, the disabling process has four major components: pathology, impairment, functional limitation, and disability (see Table 1). *Pathology* refers to molecular, cellular, or tissue changes caused by disease, infection, trauma, congenital conditions, or other factors. An example is the death of spinal cord neurons following injury. *Impairment* occurs at the organ or organ systems level and results in an individual's loss of a mental, physiological, or biochemical function, or abnormalities in these functions. *Functional limitation* is an inability or hampered ability to perform a specific task, such as climb a flight of stairs.

A *disability* is defined as a limitation in performing certain roles and tasks that society expects of an individual. It is the expression of the gap between a person's capabilities and the demands of the environment— the interaction of a person's limitations with social and physical environmental factors. Many disabling conditions are thus preventable or reversible with proper and adequate rehabilitation, including environmental modification. A *secondary condition* is any additional physical or mental health condition that occurs as a result of having a primary disabling condition. Secondary conditions quite often increase the severity of an individual's disability and are also highly preventable.

TABLE 1 Concepts of Pathology, Impairment, Functional Limitation, and Disability (IOM, 1991)

Pathology	Impairment	Functional Limitation	Disability
Definition			
Interruption or interference of normal bodily processes or structures	Loss and/or abnormality of mental, emotional, physiological, or anatomical structure or function: includes all losses or abnormalities, not just those attributable to active pathology; also includes pain	Restriction or lack of ability to perform an action or activity in the manner or within the range considered normal that results from impairment	Inability or limitation in performing socially defined activities and roles expected of individuals within a social and physical environment
Level of Reference			
Cells and tissues	Organs and organ systems	Organism— action or activity performance (consistent with the purpose or function of the organ or organ system)	Society— task performance within the social and cultural context
Example			
Denervated muscle in arm due to trauma	Atrophy of muscle	Cannot pull with arm	Change of job; can no longer swim recreationally

With this in mind, the committee enhanced the 1991 IOM model to show more clearly how biological, environmental (physical and social), and lifestyle/behavioral factors are involved in reversing the disabling process, i.e., rehabilitation, or the enabling process. The enhancements include bidirectional arrows between the various states of the enabling–disabling process to indicate that the disabling process (described in the 1991 IOM model) can be reversed with proper interventions (i.e., the enabling process; see Figure 2). The model also

The Enabling–Disabling Process

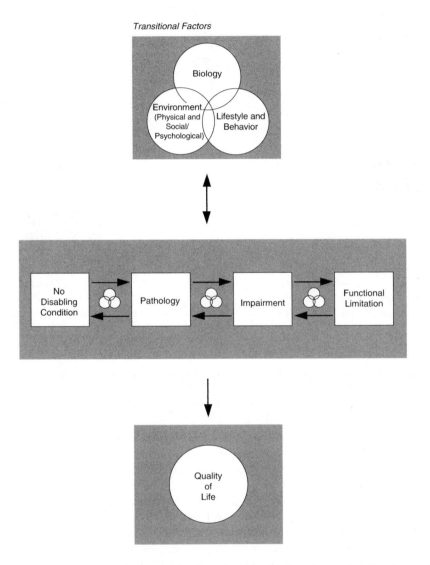

FIGURE 2 Modified IOM model. The *Disability in America* model (Institute of Medicine, 1991) is revised to include bidirectional arrows and a state of "no disabling condition," and to show transitional factors and quality of life interacting as part of the enabling–disabling process. The state of "disability" does not appear in this model since it is not inherent in the individual but, rather, a function of the interaction of the individual and the environment.

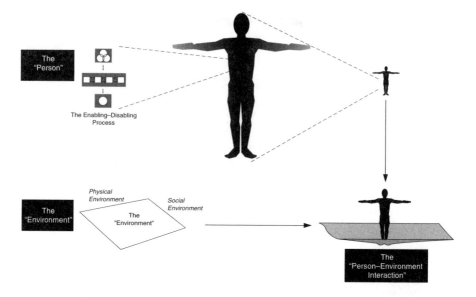

FIGURE 3 The person–environment interaction. The enabling–disabling process is depicted as being an active part of the individual person. The physical and social environments are depicted as a three-dimensional mat, with social factors on one side and physical factors on the other. The interaction of the person and the "environmental mat" is depicted as a deflection in the mat.

includes a new category—no disabling conditions—to indicate that complete rehabilitation is feasible.

To help clarify the fact that disability is not inherent in the individual, but rather is a product of the interaction of the individual with the environment, disability does not appear in Figure 2. Figures 3 and 4 show more accurately the committee's interpretation of disability as a function of the interaction of the person with the environment. More specifically, the fact that the amount of disability that an individual experiences results in large part from the quality of the surrounding environment—for example, whether appropriate and adequate care is accessible and whether a social support network is in place. Thus, for any given limitation in function, the amount of disability that one experiences will depend on the quality of the social and physical environment.

REHABILITATION SCIENCE AND ENGINEERING RESEARCH

As defined and described in this report, the major realms of knowledge and research within rehabilitation science and engineering are pa-

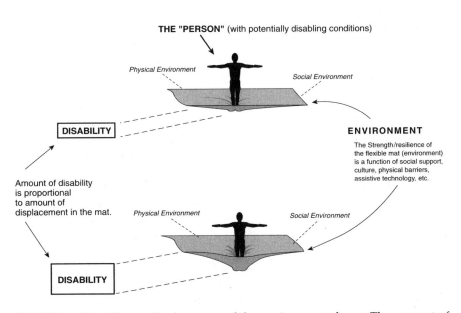

Disability is a function of the interaction between the person and the environment

THE "PERSON" (with potentially disabling conditions)

Physical Environment

Social Environment

DISABILITY

ENVIRONMENT

The Strength/resilience of the flexible mat (environment) is a function of social support, culture, physical barriers, assistive technology, etc.

Amount of disability is proportional to amount of displacement in the mat.

Physical Environment

Social Environment

DISABILITY

FIGURE 4 Disability as displacement of the environmental mat. The amount of disability that a person experiences is a function of the interaction between the person and the environment. The amount of displacement in the environmental mat is a function of the strength of the physical and social environments that support an individual and the magnitude of the potentially disabling condition. The amount of displacement represents the amount of disability that is experienced by the individual.

thology, impairment, functional limitation, and disability. Rehabilitation-related research in these areas are summarized below, followed by a section on health services research.

Pathology and Impairment Research

Rehabilitation-related research in pathology and impairment focuses on the altered function of molecules, cells, organs, and organ systems as it relates to human functional limitations and disabilities, including mechanisms for the recovery of, or compensation for, such altered function. A number of sciences contribute to this research, including medicine, physiology, cell biology, neuroscience, developmental biology, gerontology, biochemistry, genetics, molecular biology, pharmacology, engineering and physical sciences, social and behavioral sciences, and health sciences. Genetics and molecular biology, for example, offer powerful investigative techniques that can be used to provide an understanding of the causes and nature of some inherited disabling diseases. This area of research also holds promise for generating biological markers and animal models for these diseases, as well as the means for replacing or restoring the functions of defective or missing genes. Genetics research may also lead to the development of the capacity for regrowth of cells, organs, or limbs.

One of the contributions of engineering to rehabilitation science and engineering is within the realm of creating altered, supportive environments (external or internal) for people with disabling conditions. These engineered environments limit or reverse the functional manifestations of pathology and organ impairment by compensating for or replacing the altered or lost function with engineered structures and devices. The majority of current rehabilitation engineering research is in the fields of material sciences, biomedical engineering, and engineering technology development. Research in the development of prosthetics and orthotics, implantable lenses and pacemakers, and implantable drug delivery systems are some examples of engineered devices that reduce or eliminate impairment and improve function.

Recent findings in neuroscience and medicine hold promise for helping prevent and reverse neurological impairments, which are major causes of disabling conditions. Many of the therapeutic advances in this area have centered on preventive, regenerative, and restorative therapies for spinal cord and brain injuries. For example, a number of drugs given shortly after traumatic brain or spinal cord injury can significantly improve neurological recovery. Other compounds have been shown in laboratory and animal studies to foster the regeneration of severed spinal cord tissue and restore lost motor functions. An understanding of the neuronal control of skeletal muscle contractions should also prove to be useful to researchers trying to artificially mimic that control with electrical devices for individuals with paralysis. Pharmacological and physical therapies for relaxation of skeletal muscles also are being developed and show promise for relieving the prolonged and often painful muscle contractions associated with various disabling conditions. In addition, recent studies with animals suggest that recovery of function of muscles atrophied as a result of a lack of use due to injury or illness is possible with appropriate exercise.

Functional Limitation Research

Functional limitation is the expression of a potentially disabling condition at the level of the whole organism, and functional limitation research focuses on limiting or preventing disability by improving the capacity to perform specific activities.

Spinal dysfunction in general and back pain in particular, because they limit the ability to lift and to be generally active, are leading causes of functional limitation and potential disability. Among the research efforts that hold promise in this area are those that seek to determine the most mechanically efficient and least impairment-provoking means of lifting. The engineering of orthotic support structures, for example, offers potential assistance in this area.

Another important area of functional limitations research focuses on elimination in people who lack bladder and bowel control due to spinal cord injury, stroke, multiple sclerosis, prostate cancer, or other causes. New biomedical engineering approaches offer promising means of controlling micturition and defecation through implanted stimulators with external controls that can markedly reduce the limitations placed on individuals who sometimes find it difficult to work or travel because of continence problems.

Other common functional limitations include those associated with hearing and vision loss. Although research has defined many of the pathologies and impairments associated with many of these limitations, important research remains in understanding how damage to the visual pathways affects functional limitations. This may lead to the development of visual training programs, behavioral strategies, and environmental adaptations that can contribute to the optimal functioning of individuals with such disabling conditions. Science and engineering has developed low-vision aids, text-to-speech reading machines, advanced mobility and guidance aids, and other assistive devices for those with vision loss.

Another important research area centers on improvements to hearing aid devices and the rehabilitation strategies that put them to optimal use. Research in this area focuses on several levels, including the cellular level (e.g., improved electrodes for cochlear implants), signal processing level (e.g., improved digital processing software for enhancing speech perception with computer-based hearing aids), assessment level (e.g., physiologically based techniques for detecting and quantifying hearing impairments in neonates), and behavioral level (e.g., alternative communication skills).

Disability Research

Whether or not a particular physical condition is disabling to a particular individual depends on the natural and built environments, the culture of a society or the subculture of a group, the political, economic, or familial structures of a society, and the intrapersonal processes of an individual. Providing the physical and social environmental adaptations and supports that a person with a potentially disabling condition needs can often ameliorate those conditions and facilitate full participation in society. Universal design and universal engineering of environments and equipment to meet the physical needs of a wide range of abilities clearly has many advantages. Social and behavioral sciences provide an understanding of the social variables that affect disability. Designing rehabilitation programs so that they maximize the consumer's psychological control can be an important step in preventing disability and facilitating rehabilitation.

Despite the growing recognition of the importance of the environment in determining the prevalence and severity of disability, the committee could find relatively little research that explicitly focused on the effects of the environment in producing or reducing disability.

Health Services Research

Health services research, with respect to rehabilitation, focuses on how best to organize, deliver, and finance interventions for people with disabling conditions. In general, there has been little interaction between the fields of health services research and rehabilitation science and engineering. However, to the extent that health services research has included disability and rehabilitation in its agenda, it has focused primarily on issues regarding the care of children and elderly people; few studies have focused on the needs of working-age adults. Yet the number of working-age adults is growing faster than any other segment of the population of people with disabling conditions.

The development of a more comprehensive health services research agenda in rehabilitation science and engineering is particularly important and timely because of the growing demand for rehabilitation services, the changing expectations of both providers and consumers, and the continued interest in health care reform with an emphasis on cost-containment and value. New approaches to the organization, financing, and delivery of health services are being proposed. The potential impacts of these changes on access, quality, and outcomes of services for people with disabling conditions need to be evaluated.

The committee identified three areas in which more research is particularly important if the field is to better ensure that people with disabilities have access to the best possible care at costs that are affordable to the individual consumer and to society as a whole. The three areas are: (1) evaluate the cost-effectiveness of specific interventions as well as new and existing approaches to the organization and delivery of services; (2) understand better the primary health-care and long-term support needs of people with disabling conditions; and (3) evaluate the potential impact of alternative models of managed care on access to and use of services, quality of care, costs, and outcomes.

TECHNOLOGY TRANSFER

Technology transfer is the transmittal of developed ideas, products, and techniques from a research environment to one of practical application, and as such it is an important component of rehabilitation science and engineering. Opportunities for initiating effective technology transfer activities occur both at the beginning stages of a research project, and at its end. The former involves bringing academic and industrial participants into a research program as partners who then have a stake in the research and who are free to use or market the findings. The latter depends on disseminating the findings of research to the greater industrial or medical communities. Implementation usually consists of conferences, publications, easily accessed databases, and other means of publicizing the conclusions of research.

Many government agencies have programs that are designed to facilitate technology transfer. There is, however, no well-organized mechanism for distributing research findings in rehabilitation science and engineering to those providing services.

An important barrier to translating research into clinical practice is simply the paucity of relevant research. In addition, little formal theory exists in rehabilitation to guide researchers; practitioners' clinical decision "knowledge" is often obtained from experience. Finally, the mechanisms for effectively transferring the evidence that does exist to the practicing clinician and to the rehabilitation consumer are scarce.

REHABILITATION SCIENCE AND
ENGINEERING AS A FIELD OF STUDY

Rehabilitation science and engineering, defined in this report as encompassing basic and applied aspects of the health sciences, social sciences, and engineering as they relate to restoring human functional capacity and improving a person's interactions with the surrounding environment, is beginning to emerge as an organized, multidisciplinary field of study. Three observations led to this conclusion. First, rehabilitation science and engineering research is currently conducted within a variety of health professional, basic science, and engineering disciplines. Second, the multidisciplinary understanding of the enabling–disabling process represents the overlap between the various and unique disciplines in rehabilitation science, each with a distinct perspective on disability and rehabilitation. This common area of knowledge is the essence of the field of rehabilitation science and engineering. Finally, the research in the separate health, basic science, and engineering disciplines, although complementary, is not comprehensive or rigorously focused; each has more to give and more to learn from a well-developed confluence of knowledge. The organization of rehabilitation science and engineering as a field of study will help to stimulate innovations and coordinate the growth of knowledge from rehabilitation research.

As a field of study, rehabilitation science and engineering will not replace any existing discipline or necessitate the removal of content or research from the existing disciplines. It will, however, create new opportunities to coalesce the knowledge that is necessary to improve research and be more responsive to the needs of people with disabling conditions. By its nature, the emerging field of rehabilitation science and engineering is both scientific and academic, but not professional, and does not require the creation of a new category of health care professional. Its scientific strength comes from its use of rigorous, objective methods to determine acceptable knowledge and operation within the context of contemporary empiricism (i.e., using deductive reasoning, objectivity, and theoretical models). Likewise, rehabilitation science and engineering is a field of study whose primary aim is to elucidate and understand phenomena. With academic and scientific structure, rehabilitation science and engineering will provide a focus for multidisciplinary research and generate a common knowledge base for individuals working in a rehabilitation team.

ORGANIZATION AND ADMINISTRATION

For the purpose of assessing the combined adequacy of federal efforts in addressing the health needs of people with disabling conditions, the committee reviewed the five major federal programs that focus on rehabilitation-related research and the overall organization and administration of these programs. Currently, the spectrum of federal programs that support research in rehabilitation science and engineering is such that each program has a unique, worthwhile, and complementary mission. The Centers for Disease Control and Prevention (CDC) investigates prevention and secondary conditions, the National Science Foundation and the National Center for Medical Rehabilitation Research (NCMRR) research basic engineering and medical rehabilitation, respectively, the National Institute for Disability and Rehabilitation Research (NIDRR) focuses on disability and the whole person in the environment, and the U.S. Department of Veterans Affairs is able to tailor its research agenda to the needs of its constituents. This represents a broad spectrum of rehabilita-

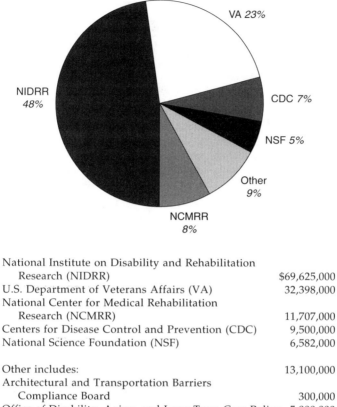

National Institute on Disability and Rehabilitation
  Research (NIDRR) $69,625,000
U.S. Department of Veterans Affairs (VA)   32,398,000
National Center for Medical Rehabilitation
  Research (NCMRR)   11,707,000
Centers for Disease Control and Prevention (CDC)   9,500,000
National Science Foundation (NSF)   6,582,000

Other includes: 13,100,000
Architectural and Transportation Barriers
  Compliance Board   300,000
Office of Disability, Aging, and Long-Term Care Policy   5,000,000
Social Security Administration   5,000,000
U.S. Department of Housing and Urban
  Development, Office of Policy Development
  and Research   100,000
U.S. Department of Transportation   2,700,000

FIGURE 5 Traditional view of federal spending in rehabilitation-related research.

tion research, with NIDRR representing 48 percent of the appropriated funding (see Figure 5).

Further analysis of these programs—including the related efforts outside NCMRR at NIH—revealed certain trends in the overall federal research effort in rehabilitation science and engineering (see Figures 6 and 7). Given the current constraints and limitations of funding, these findings show a generally good balance of effort, but with most of the research focusing on pathology and impairment, and a relatively smaller proportion of research focusing on disability per se.

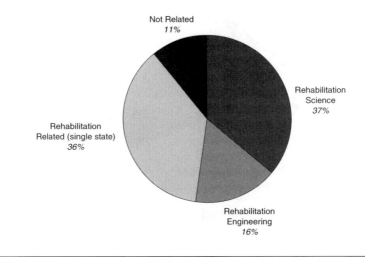

Relevance Category	Amount Funded	Number of Projects	Percent Funding
Rehabilitation science	$101,105,292	543	37
Rehabilitation engineering	$44,129,995	293	16
Rehabilitation related (single state)	$100,540,664	540	36
Not related	$30,207,510	193	11
Totals	$275,983,461	1,569	100

FIGURE 6 Percentage of overall research funding (not including center grants) in four categories of relevance to rehabilitation research for the Fiscal Year 1995 program. Rehabilitation science: Projects that address movement among states in the enabling–disabling process. Rehabilitation engineering: Projects that address devices or technologies applicable to one of the rehabilitation states. Rehabilitation related (single state): Projects that address one rehabilitation state exclusively. Not related: Projects that do not clearly address any rehabilitation state. For additional information, see Appendix A in the full report.

In assessing a constellation of programs of this size and complexity, with the overall mission of addressing health needs of such magnitude, it is not surprising to find some apparent problems. Foremost among these are the need for improved coordination among the various and numerous federal research programs and the need for additional research in rehabilitation science and engineering that will help to improve the health, quality of life, and productivity of the millions of Americans with disabling conditions.

A series of options was considered for addressing the identified issues and problems. Of prime interest was a strategy to improve what is presently the largest program that focuses on disability and rehabilitation-related re-

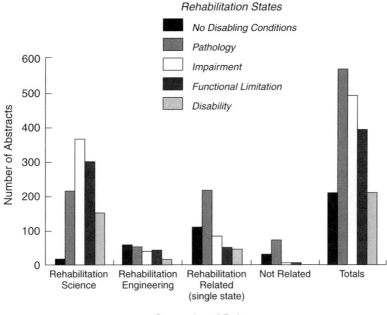

FIGURE 7 Number of abstracts within each category of relevance[a] that address the specific states of the enabling–disabling process[b] for Fiscal Year 1995. NOTE: Many abstracts address multiple states. For additional information, see Appendix A in the full report.

[a]Rehabilitation science: Projects that address movement among states in the enabling–disabling process. Rehabilitation engineering: Projects that address devices or technologies applicable to one of the rehabilitation states. Rehabilitation-related (single state): Projects that address one rehabilitation state exclusively. Not related: Projects that do not clearly address any rehabilitation state.

[b]No disabling conditions: Research that addresses the state of function or use of subjects with no disabling conditions to investigate mechanisms that are potentially relevant to assessing and treating disabling conditions. Pathology: Research that examines changes of molecules, cells, and tissues that may lead to impairment, functional limitation, or disability, distinguished from pathology by manifestation at organ or system level. Impairment: Research that analyzes changes in particular organs, systems, or parts of the body. Impairment is distinguished from functional limitation due to emphasis on organ and components instead of whole body. Functional limitation: Research that examines functional changes involving the entire subject, manifested by task performance. Disability: Research that focuses on the interaction of the subject with and in the larger context of the physical and social environment.

search: NIDRR. The committee's recommendation for how to accomplish this is one of the three overarching recommendations that follow.

CONCLUSIONS AND OVERARCHING RECOMMENDATIONS

The committee concludes that, given the large potential for improving the health, productivity, and quality of life for 49 million Americans, the field of rehabilitation science and engineering receives disproportionately inadequate attention from the federal government. The large annual cost estimates (approximately $300 billion—more than 4 percent of the gross domestic product) for disability and rehabilitation are in stark contrast to the relatively small amount of funding that is directed toward research in rehabilitation science and engineering. Current expenditures amount to less than $7 in research per year for each person with a disabling condition, whereas the costs of disability due to expenditures for health care and lost productivity are more than 1,000 times greater (approximately $7,500 per capita). Most importantly, however, significant savings in health care costs, lost wages, and reduced emotional costs could be realized by enhancing research in rehabilitation science and engineering and improving the health, productivity, and quality of life of people with disabling conditions.

With this in mind, three fundamental needs emerged from the committee's assessment and deliberations. The first is a need to recognize rehabilitation science and engineering as an academic and scientific field of study, the continued development of which will result in significant contributions to the science and ultimately to consumers. The second is a need to focus on a set of priorities for research that will advance the field of study and improve the health, productivity, and quality of life for people with disabling conditions. Perhaps most importantly, the third need is to enhance the federal effort in rehabilitation science and engineering by expanding research, raising visibility, and improving coordination. Three overarching recommendations on how to address these needs are described below.

Recognize the Field of Study

Rehabilitation science and engineering is the body of knowledge that exists at the confluence of multiple disciplines, drawing from and contributing to each one. At this point in the evolution of the science, there is a sufficient knowledge base and level of research to organize a rigorous scientific structure for the field. Such organization would facilitate accelerations in multidisciplinary education, training, and research, all of which would combine to advance the field of rehabilitation science and engineering and more effectively address the needs of people with disabling conditions. Thus, the committee's first overarching recommendation is as follows:

> *Overarching Recommendation 1. Rehabilitation science and engineering should be more widely recognized and accepted as an academic and scientific field of study. As such, the field should receive greater financial support, serve as the basis for developing new opportunities in multidisciplinary research and education, and ultimately improve the health and quality of life of people with disabling conditions. This new field should be consistent with the model of the enabling–disabling process that is defined and described in this report.*

Emphasize Priorities

Many topics and areas require investigation, and identifying priorities is not simple. The process cannot be based on prevalence alone or simply on cost. Recommendations for specific rehabilitation science and engineering research efforts are detailed in the individual chapters of this report. In addition, Appendix A contains suggested research priorities from various professional associations and other sources. Acknowledging the limited ability of any assembly of individuals to identify research priorities with great acuity and detail, the committee chose instead to describe general priorities that should be fundamentally important to any research and to the advancement of rehabilitation science and engineering as a whole. Thus, the committee's second overarching recommendation is as follows:

> *Overarching Recommendation 2. As the field of rehabilitation science and engineering continues to evolve and gain recognition as an academic and scientific field of study, three general priorities will and should be of fundamental importance to its growth and to the ultimate improvement of health, productivity, and quality of life for people with disabling conditions: strengthen the science, focus on the enabling–disabling process, and transfer the technology. (See Box 1.)*

Enhance the Federal Effort

In general, weaknesses in the current spectrum of federal programs in disability and rehabilitation-related research are not due to inappropriate priorities or other problems within the programs themselves, but rather to a general insufficiency in the magnitude of the overall program of

BOX 1
General Priorities for Rehabilitation Science and Engineering

As the field of rehabilitation science and engineering continues to evolve and gain recognition as an academic and scientific field of study, there are three general priorities that will and should be of fundamental importance to its growth and to the ultimate improvement of health, productivity, and quality of life for people with disabling conditions.

1. Strengthen the science. Develop and validate accurate tools for measuring and predicting functional limitations, disability, and outcomes.
2. Focus on the enabling–disabling process. Investigate critical factors in the physical, social, and psychological environments that can affect transitions in the enabling–disabling process over the lifecourse.
3. Transfer the technology. Develop and implement effective linkages between research and practice that will involve consumers, assure quality, and enhance service delivery.

research, its limited visibility, and a lack of effective coordination of the overall constellation of programs. Thus, the constellation of federal research programs in rehabilitation science and engineering needs to be reorganized and administered in a fashion that will improve interagency coordination, enhance visibility, and expand research for the purposes of improving the health, independence, productivity, and quality of life for people with disabling conditions.

As the largest federal program with a focus on disability and rehabilitation-related research, NIDRR's program was of major interest to the committee. The NIDRR mission and its constituency of people with disabling conditions are fundamentally important to the research agenda of rehabilitation science and engineering espoused by this committee. The committee concluded, however, that despite vigorous pursuit of its mission, NIDRR has been restricted in its ability to fully execute its mission primarily by virtue of its administrative position within the U.S. Department of Education and the Interagency Committee on Disability Research's lack of real authority. An important example of the former is the need for improved peer review processes that are unobtainable in the present administrative location.

For the purpose of improving the overall federal effort and addressing the priorities described in Overarching Recommendation 2 above, the committee makes the following overarching recommendation.

Overarching Recommendation 3. The committee recommends that the NIDRR program of activities and its annual appropriation of approxi-

mately $70 million be moved from the U.S. Department of Education to the U.S. Department of Health and Human Services and that it serve as the foundation for the creation of a new Agency on Disability and Rehabilitation Research (ADRR). ADRR would assume the tasks that were formerly assigned to the Interagency Committee on Disability Research and be given enhanced authority through review of disability and rehabilitation-related research plans and control of funding for interagency collaboration. To further support and enhance the overall federal effort, all major programs in disability and rehabilitation-related research should be elevated within their respective agencies or departments. (Recommendation 10.1)

There are several advantages and benefits to be gained from moving NIDRR to DHHS. First of all, the move would be an opportunity to review the program's mission and personnel, and make appropriate changes to the program's structure. Secondly, it would move NIDRR closer administratively to NIH and CDC, which should facilitate coordination among the agencies. Finally, it would allow improvements in the peer review process, including larger, more permanent peer review panels that could be formed to allow for the review of a more heterogeneous mix of applications, and broader representation (including people with disabling conditions) on the review panels. In addition, moving NIDRR from the U.S. Department of Education to the U.S. Department of Health and Human Services would provide the program with a more nurturing and supportive environment, raise the visibility of disability and rehabilitation as an important health issue, and perhaps most importantly, allow it to serve more effectively as the core of an interagency coordinating body for disability and rehabilitation-related research.

One of the most important activities of ADRR would be the coordination of federal research on rehabilitation science and engineering. To help achieve this objective, ADRR would annually review plans for research in the following year submitted by all relevant agencies and would also have the ability both to fund interagency research and to enhance funding in areas of identified need. To help ensure participation in the coordinating activities, ADRR could be supported in part by a set-aside fund from the major agencies and by direct appropriation.

In keeping with the committee's task of making recommendations within differing levels of fiscal expenditure, Table 2 presents guidance on how funds could be distributed in a configuration of programs consistent with this committee's recommendations. The table shows the present funding levels and two options for expanded programs of research at a cost of $100 million and $200 millon.

TABLE 2 Major Federal Programs in Disability and Rehabilitation-Related Research Showing the Organization of the Proposed New ADRR in DHHS and Two Levels of Funding to Enhance the Overall Federal Effort

Agency	Current Funds	$100 Million of Additional Funds		$200 Million of Additional Funds	
		New Funds	New Totals	New Funds	New Totals
U.S. DEPARTMENT OF HEALTH AND HUMAN SERVICES					
Administration on Disability and Rehabilitation Research (new agency)	**$70***	**$52.5**	**$123**	**$105**	**$175**
I. Coordination-Linkage Division	0	25	25	35	35
a. Interagency committee and subcommittee					
b. Multiple agency projects					
c. Rehabilitation resource support centers					
II. Disability and Rehabilitation Research Division	39	15	54	39	78
a. Rehabilitation research, including centers and field-initiated research of issues such as employment, education, personal assistance services, parenting, policy, independent living.					
b. Disability studies					
III. Engineering and Environmental Research Division	22	7	29	22	44
a. Assistive technology and engineering, including centers and field-initiated research					
b. Universal design, including mass transportation and Americans with Disabilities Act compliance					
IV. Training and Career Development Division	3	2.5	5.5	3	6
a. Allied health and engineering					
b. Services training					
c. Recruitment of scientists with disabling conditions					

V. Information Integration and Dissemination Division	6	3	9	6	12
a. Information integration					
b. Dissemination					
National Institutes of Health (NCMRR)	$15	$11.3	$26	$23	$38
Thematic program projects for six priority areas					
Develop clinical trials of new therapies (not cures) that improve health status and reduce secondary conditions, and coordinate with that of ADRR Centers program					
Centers for Disease Control and Prevention	$9	$6.8	$16	$14	$23
Current programs					
Establish population-based studies of people with disabling conditions, their needs for services and assistive technologies, and the effects of changing national, state, and local policies on participation by people with disabilities in major life activities, including their health costs and demographics					
Establish population-based surveillance systems for monitoring the incidence and impact of secondary conditions					
Develop and evaluate community-based interventions to reduce the incidence and impact of secondary conditions and promote the independence and productivity of people with disabling conditions.					
Fund longitudinal studies on disability (e.g., National Health Interview Survey-Disability Supplement expanded)					
Fund the development of a common terminology for the field					
U.S. DEPARTMENT OF VETERAN AFFAIRS	$32	$24	$56	$48	$80
NATIONAL SCIENCE FOUNDATION	$7	$5.3	$12	$11	$18
TOTAL	$133	$100	$233	$200	$333

*Current NIDRR funding.

1

Introduction

Advances in rehabilitation science are essential to realizing the Nation's commitment to equal opportunity, economic self-sufficiency, and full participation of Americans with disabilities. There are important questions of the adequacy of Federal efforts in both meeting the needs of the rapidly growing number of Americans with disabilities, and in realizing the new opportunities of science and technology on behalf of people with disabilities.

—Senator Robert Dole, 1995

The United States has long judged the success of its efforts to improve the health of its citizens on the basis of mortality statistics. However, gains in human longevity have been accompanied by increases in the incidence and prevalence of chronic impairments, functional limitations, and disabilities. At this point in the evolution of the nation's health care system, emphasis has begun to shift from the quantity of life to the quality of life. As a result, attention is now being focused not only on the prevention and treatment of disease and injury but also on rehabilitation.

REHABILITATION: CONCEPTS AND DEFINITIONS

At its simplest, rehabilitation is the process of recovery from an injury. At its most complex, it is the lifelong process of obtaining "optimal function despite residual disability" (DeLisa et al., 1993, p. 3). The range between these two extremes encompasses a wide variety of disabilities, specialties, and potential interventions. Regardless of the specific setting or circumstances, however, *rehabilitation* is the process by which physical, sensory, and mental capacities are restored or developed in (and for) people with disabling conditions—reversing what has been called the disabling process, and may therefore be called the *enabling process*. This is achieved not only through functional changes in the person (e.g., development of compensatory muscular strength, use of prosthetic limbs, and treatment of posttraumatic behavioral disturbances) but also through changes in the physical and

24

social environments that surround them (e.g., reductions in architectural and attitudinal barriers).

Three other terms and concepts require definition at the outset. *Rehabilitation science*, as defined in this report for the first time, is the study of movement among states[1] in the enabling–disabling process. This involves the fundamental, basic, and applied aspects of the health sciences, social sciences, and engineering as they relate to (1) the restoration of functional capacity in a person and (2) the interaction of that person with the surrounding environment. *Engineering* is the application of science and mathematics by which the properties of matter and the sources of energy in nature are made useful to people in machines, products, systems, and processes. (Rehabilitation engineering is a field of engineering that is of fundamental importance to both the restoration of function and the interaction of people with the environment.) Because of the importance of both science and engineering in advancing rehabilitation efforts and addressing the needs of people with disabling conditions, the committee uses the term *rehabilitation science and engineering* throughout this report to emphasize the importance of both and their synergistic contributions in the process of achieving optimal function.

As originally described by Saad Nagi in the 1950s and refined most recently in the 1991 Institute of Medicine (IOM) report *Disability in America*, the disabling process has four major components: pathology, impairment, functional limitation, and disability (see Table 1-1). *Pathology* refers to molecular, cellular, or tissue changes caused by disease, infection, trauma, congenital conditions, or other factors. An example is the death of spinal cord neurons following injury. *Impairment* occurs at the organ or organ systems level and results in an individual's loss of a mental, physiological, or biochemical function, or abnormalities in these functions. *Functional limitation* is an inability or hampered ability to perform a specific task, such as climb a flight of stairs.

A *disability* is defined as a limitation in performing certain roles and tasks that society expects an individual to perform. Disability is the expression of the gap between a person's capabilities and the demands of the environment—the interaction of a person's limitations with social and physical environmental factors. Many disabling conditions are thus preventable or reversible with proper and adequate rehabilitation, including environmental modification. A *secondary condition* is any additional physical or mental health condition that occurs as a result of having a primary disabling condition. Secondary conditions quite often increase the severity of an individual's disability and are also highly preventable.

---

[1]The states in the enabling–disabling process (pathology, impairment, functional limitation, and disability) are defined below.

TABLE 1-1 Concepts of Pathology, Impairment, Functional Limitation, and Disability (IOM, 1991)

Pathology	Impairment	Functional Limitation	Disability
Definition			
Interruption or interference of normal bodily processes or structures	Loss and/or abnormality of mental, emotional, physiological, or anatomical structure or function: includes all losses or abnormalities, not just those attributable to active pathology; also includes pain	Restriction or lack of ability to perform an action or activity in the manner or within the range considered normal that results from impairment	Inability or limitation in performing socially defined activities and roles expected of individuals within a social and physical environment
Level of Reference			
Cells and tissues	Organs and organ systems	Organism— action or activity performance (consistent with the purpose or function of the organ or organ system)	Society— task performance within the social and cultural context
Example			
Denervated muscle in arm due to trauma	Atrophy of muscle	Cannot pull with arm	Change of job; can no longer swim recreationally

Importance of Team Approach

Effective rehabilitation addresses an individual's physical, psychological, and environmental needs in an organized and personalized manner and is not limited in the case of chronic conditions to some finite period of time following the initiation of a disabling condition. It is only appropriate, then, that an effective rehabilitation program would incorporate the views and skills of many specialists and experts working together for a common goal. Indeed, fundamental to the character and success of rehabilitation is the rehabilitation team, which often includes nurses, engineers, physicians, occupational therapists, physical therapists, physiatrists, speech-language pathologists and audiologists, psychologists, orthotists and prosthetists, and vocational counselors, among others.

The rehabilitative process reflects not only the intricacies of the human but also the complex nature of disability. Rehabilitation includes both basic and applied science; it integrates human behavior and biology, medicine, health sciences and engineering; and it subsumes many disciplines in the coordination of treatment for each person. Likewise, the disabling condition rarely involves a single physiological system or falls entirely in the realm of biology. The treatment must therefore similarly affect the many facets of recovery, influencing the disabling condition, the person, and the surrounding environment. Thus, the full course of rehabilitation ideally involves a team that is simultaneously multidisciplinary, interdisciplinary, and transdisciplinary. Traditionally, these traits have defined exclusive models for team interaction. In multidisciplinary teams, for example, members work essentially singly and each participant acts as an individual consultant, evaluating the individual and providing the discipline-specific treatment recommendations. Interdisciplinary teams feature free communication between the team members to provide integrated care oriented toward the individual, and transdisciplinary teams encourage members to cross over into the traditional treatment areas of other disciplines. A fully integrated model combines each concept, drawing on many specific fields of knowledge as a single unit and synergistically producing an outcome that holistically addresses the person and the disability.

The team approach is important not only in practice but also in rehabilitation research, where much of the focus is turning to disability as the result of the interaction between the characteristics of an individual with disabling conditions and the characteristics of that person's environment. Rehabilitation programs and research are beginning to emphasize the role of the environment in determining disability. As the understanding of disability changes, the rehabilitation strategies have also begun to shift toward environmental interventions. Although this concept of disability is still developing, the team approach to rehabilitation has been a part of the science since its origins.

ORIGINS OF SCIENCE AND ENGINEERING IN REHABILITATION

Origins are almost always difficult to pinpoint. They depend on where one looks, and people looking for them often look within their own areas of expertise and within their own country of origin. French and English people may view the origin of photography differently. Similarly, French and American people may argue about the origins of cinematography. These arguments over origins appear frequently because discoveries and developments often happened in parallel in different countries, but before recent advances in travel and communications, the coincidence of these events was not known.

The Beginnings

Egyptian stelae and Roman mosaics have shown that technology has been used in rehabilitation since antiquity, especially by people who had undergone amputations and people who had had polio. Paintings by Brueghel the Elder show the use of a number of simple technologies in the 16th century by people with disabling conditions.

Wars and conflicts have been primary stimuli for technological innovations in the rehabilitation of people with disabling injuries. The armor makers of the medieval era were skilled at making functionally effective artificial hands and leg prostheses of metal and were probably early forerunners of today's prosthetists and orthotists. In Goethe's play *The Iron Hand*, the noble German knight Götz von Berlichingen remarks that his iron hand had served him better in the fight than ever did the original of flesh.

The Napoleonic wars fostered some technical innovations in rehabilitation, and the enormous number of amputations resulting from the U.S. Civil War more or less created the prosthetics industry in the United States. It was at that time that President Abraham Lincoln established the Veterans Administration (VA; now the U.S. Department of Veterans Affairs). At the same time, the federal government recognized the value of science to the nation, and in 1863, the National Academy of Sciences was established to be an independent, nonprofit adviser to the federal government. However, it was World War I that set the stage for the modern rehabilitation movement. Of particular note were the advances made in Germany during and following that war.

Ferdinand Sauerbruch was one of the first surgeons to recommend multidisciplinary scientific and engineering endeavors in rehabilitation. In Zurich, in 1915, he worked together with Aurel Stodola, a professor of mechanics at the Polytechnical Institute of Zurich, to produce a hand prosthesis that was controlled and powered through muscle cineplasty. Sauerbruch relied heavily on muscle physiologists and anatomists to assist him with decisions about how to successfully bring muscle forces outside the body using the surgical procedure of tunnel cineplasty, a technique that he advanced at an army hospital in Germany. Sauerbruch attributed his successful implementation of this technique to the multidisciplinary approach. Speaking of this development, he said: "Henceforth, surgeon, physiologist, and technician will have to work together" (Sauerbruch, 1916).

Subsequently, at the Charity Hospital in Berlin, Sauerbruch worked together with Konrad Biesalski of the Oscar Helene Heim Hospital to devise better hand replacement techniques. Biesalski developed muscle exercise and stretching equipment, which may have been some of the first physical therapy equipment, for use in training and strengthening an amputee's muscles during the period following Sauerbruch's tunnel cineplasty surgical procedures. Max Biedermann, a well-known German prosthetist, worked with them on designing and fitting arm and hand prostheses. This group worked together after World War I and was likely one of the first rehabilitation teams to work cooperatively on limb replacement. Sauerbruch considered the team approach key to his successes, which were considerable, not only with limb prostheses and rehabilitation but also open-chest surgery, which he pioneered. In addition to providing therapeutic devices, Biesalski reportedly developed the first statistics on people with disabling conditions in Germany. Consequently, Sauerbruch and Biesalski are among the earliest medical pioneers of rehabilitation science and engineering.

In the United States, World War I also created a large demand for rehabilitation services as veterans with disabilities needed to be reintegrated into society and the workforce. As a result, U.S. surgeons studied surgical and prosthetic rehabilitation methods in Europe, which influenced U.S. amputation surgery practices and resulted in the greater provision of artificial limbs. Henry Kessler, an important early figure in the U.S. rehabilitation field, for example, was a proponent of Sauerbruch's methods of cineplasty.

The needs of the veterans with disabilities provided fertile ground on which many different rehabilitation specialties could take root. During this period, occupational and physical therapists contributed not only to the rehabilitation of veterans with disabilities but also to the growing science underlying rehabilitation. Devices designed to measure range of motion and strength, for example, made scientific recording of specific activities possible (Hopkins, 1988). Thus, it is noteworthy that the archetypical attributes of rehabilitation science and engineering were forming simultaneously with the individual disciplines and that early rehabilitation, closely connected with surgery and physical technologies, was characterized by the use of the interdisciplinary team.

The rehabilitation needs of veterans following World War I (and the need for treatment of poliomyelitis) served to stimulate the development of the field of rehabilitation as a whole. Addressing these national needs laid the groundwork for the development of many of the specialties that serve people with disabilities today. The forerunner of the American Orthotic and Prosthetic Association, for example, was formed in 1920 and the American Congress of Physical Therapy was founded the following year. This period in American history also saw the American Speech-Language-Hearing Association founded in 1925, American Congress of Rehabilitation Medicine formed in 1933, American Academy of Orthopaedic Surgery founded in 1935, and American Academy of Physical Medicine and Rehabilitation established in 1938. Box 1-1 shows a timeline for the establishment of many of the rehabilitation professional associations.

Birth of Rehabilitation Science and Engineering in the United States

Modalities such as heat, cold, light, water, massage, and exercise have long been used in medicine, and their use, and like that of prostheses, can be traced to antiquity. As technologies have changed new techniques and apparatuses have been added, such as electrotherapeutics, hydrotherapy, diathermy, topical application of substances, and continuous-range-of-motion machines. Through the years these modalities have been applied by different kinds of physicians, health professionals, and other people. Besides the use of physical modality therapeutic treatments, physical therapists train people to use prosthetics and orthotics to assist them with ambulation. Physical therapy originated to some extent out of physical education and gained considerable status during World War I. At that time there were physical therapy physicians, and physical therapy technicians. John Stanley Coulter, a physical therapy physician had considerable impact on the practice and professional development of the field of physical therapy and on what was ultimately to become physiatry (the name was formally recognized in 1946). The field of physical therapy grew rapidly as a result of World War I and as a result of polio treatment centers. It reached maturity during World War II. Its development paralleled the development of occupational therapy, prosthetics and orthotics, and the field of physical medicine and rehabilitation.

Polio had a dramatic impact on rehabilitation in the United States, and engineering was involved with polio in an interesting way. A physical therapist, Alice Lou Plastridge, who had given President Franklin Delano Roosevelt muscle reeducation treatment, had a practice in Chicago. One of her clients who had had polio was Margaret Pope, the daughter of a wealthy Chicago hosiery manufacturer. Henry Pope was dissatisfied with the braces prescribed for his daughter and had an engineer with his company design new braces for her using aircraft construction techniques. These braces were made available to others through the Pope

---

BOX 1-1
Establishment of Rehabilitation-Related Professional Associations

1890   American Electrotherapeutic Association
1917   American Occupational Therapy Association
1921   American Physical Therapy Association (later, the American Physio-
            therapy Association and then American Physical Therapy Association
            again)
1925   American Speech-Language-Hearing Association
1933   American Congress of Rehabilitation Medicine
1935   American Academy of Orthopaedic Surgery
1938   American Academy of Physical Medicine and Rehabilitation
1947   American Board of Physical Medicine (accrediting board)
1954   Residency Review Committee for Physical Medicine and Rehabilitation
1967   Association of Academic Physiatrists
1969   International Rehabilitation Medicine Association
1970   American Academy of Orthotists and Prosthetics
1975   American Spinal Cord Injury Association
1976   Rehabilitation Nursing Foundation
1981   Rehabilitation and Engineering and Assistive Technology Society of
            North America

Foundation. Pope also had an engineer with his company, Carl Hubbard, design the first "Hubbard tank" in 1928. A Hubbard tank is a keyhole-shaped tank for full-body immersion, used for hydrotherapy (Eisenberg, 1995). Pope and Bernard Baruch, the son of a physician/hydrotherapist at Columbia University, provided funds for Hubbard tanks to be installed in the therapy facilities at Warm Springs, Georgia. Plastridge later became director of physical therapy at Warm Springs and made important advances in physical therapy. Baruch would became an important supporter of rehabilitation in New York City.

World War II accelerated demands in military hospitals for rehabilitation professionals. During this period the focus of physical medicine began to broaden from the recovery of ambulation and low-energy activities in individuals with disabling conditions to the comprehensive restoration of an individual's physical, mental, emotional, vocational, and social capacities (Kottke and Knapp, 1988). Innovators such as Howard Rusk serving in military hospitals made great strides in rehabilitation, establishing the effectiveness of active rehabilitative processes that addressed the physical and emotional needs of the soldiers over the passive, nonphysical convalescence that had been standard. World War II furthermore made U.S. society as a whole become aware of efforts in rehabilitation and the necessity for more advanced treatments.

The rise of the rehabilitation movement can be traced to efforts in many areas, and orthopedic surgeons also played a significant role. Paul B. Magnuson, a powerful Chicago orthopedic surgeon who once served injured workers at the Chicago Stockyards hired John Stanley Coulter to be the medical director of physical therapy at the Northwestern University Medical School. Besides starting the VA hospital system, Magnuson also founded the Rehabilitation Institute of Chicago and believed devoutly in vocational rehabilitation.

Following World War II orthopedic surgeons influenced rehabilitation programs all across the United States, being particularly known for their work with children, human ambulation, amputation, and prosthetics and orthotics. In physiatry, Frank Krusen was one of the earliest disciples of physical medicine and he along with Henry Kessler, Howard Rusk, and George Deaver are regarded by many as pioneers of physical medicine and rehabilitation. Rusk served in the Army Air Corps as director of reconditioning and recreation. From his experiences with injured airmen, he established many of the principles of rehabilitation that were later incorporated into the programs of the Institute of Rehabilitation at New York University, an institution that had a large impact nationally and internationally on the field of rehabilitation. Rusk and Deaver, as with Sauerbruch and Biesalski before them, advocated the team approach, which has become an essential element of good rehabilitation.

This work in New York and all around the country was facilitated by private citizens like Bernard Baruch and Mary Lasker. In Washington, D.C., it was supported by the VA, by the Vocational Rehabilitation Act of 1954, which permitted research and training funding for rehabilitation through the U.S. Department of Health, Education, and Welfare (DHEW), and by the Children's Bureau of DHEW. Washington, D.C., administrators like Mary Switzer and James Garrett of DHEW, Robert Stewart of the VA Prosthetics and Sensory Aids Service, and General S. S. Strong, Jr. of the National Academy of Sciences/National Research Council, Committee on Prosthetics Research and Development are just a few of the many people who played instrumental roles in launching rehabilitation in the United States.

Research in rehabilitation science and engineering mushroomed after the war—stimulated partially by veteran amputees who were languishing in hospitals and who were disappointed by the state of limb prosthetics in 1945. Federal grants that funded those studies were the first such grants issued to advance science and engineering in rehabilitation. As a consequence of their lobbying, U.S. Army Surgeon General Norman Kirk called for a meeting to select which prostheses would be best for World War II veterans. That meeting, held in Chicago in January 1945, produced recommendations for scientific and engineering studies of limb prostheses. The federal grants that funded those studies were the first such grants issued to advance science and engineering in rehabilitation.

The early studies were dramatically successful, and the period from 1945 to 1975 was one of the most productive periods in U.S. prosthetics research. In 1945, Americans again looked to Europe for prosthetics ideas, but this time these ideas were combined with an active research and development program, coordinated by the Committee on Prosthetics Research and Development (CPRD) of the National Research Council. Since then, research and development efforts in the United States, particularly work sponsored by VA but also Army and Navy research laboratories and by the National Institute of Disability and Rehabilitation Research (NIDRR), have made the United States a world leader in the field of prosthetics and rehabilitation in general.

Among the noteworthy events and achievements during this developmental phase of rehabilitation science and engineering is the 1954 publication of the classic book *Human Limbs and Their Substitutes*, edited by Paul E. Klopsteg, an engineer/scientist, and Philip E. Wilson, an orthopedicist/rehabilitationist and published under the sponsorship of the National Research Council (Klopsteg and Wilson, 1954). The book is a milestone of the early results of federally funded research and development in limb prosthetics. It illustrates the union of engineering and science with medicine and rehabilitation. In the foreword to that book, Detlev W. Bronk, President of the National Academy of Sciences, said, in part:

> Science and technology have enabled man to increase the natural powers of his body. . . . This notable and significant book reveals how scientists have extended that function by augmenting the powers of those whose bodies have been crippled [*sic*] by injury or disease. . . . The great accomplishments set forth in [this book] are in large part due to cooperation of physicists and surgeons, of engineers and mathematicians. . . . The designers of the devices and methods for rehabilitation here described have made a lasting contribution of great benefit to mankind. They have done more. They have given amputees courage and have healed the psychological trauma, which is no less grievous than the bodily loss itself. I like to think that this furtherance of spiritual well-being is the greatest contribution . . . [and] deserves special comment at a time when human values could be obscured by too great emphasis on material objectives (p. vi of Foreword).

The initial research work described in that book, conducted largely through the military and VA, was so successful that it was soon copied by civilian agencies and may be viewed as the beginning of most federal support involving science, engineering, and technology in disability and rehabilitation-related research. NIDRR's predecessor agencies noted the success of the prosthetics program and began funding similar research for

civilian amputees. After all, the United States had more amputees resulting from war industry injuries (60,000) than from wartime combat (20,000).

This expansion of services from veterans to the general public spurred
an increase in research and training as the demand for new knowledge
and rehabilitation professionals still outweighed the growth of each. The
American Occupational Therapy Foundation, for example, was established in 1965 to advance the science of occupational therapy, supporting
the education and research of its practitioners. Likewise, the Association
of Academic Physiatrists was formed in 1967 explicitly to increase opportunities in research and education.

In 1970, prosthetists and orthotists formed the American Academy of
Orthotists and Prosthetists, and research began to expand beyond amputations to other disabling conditions such as spinal cord injury, stroke,
and cerebral palsy. At about that time a new field called *rehabilitation
engineering* began to emerge, and the field has flourished in the United
States for the last 25 years, enabling many Americans with disabling conditions to have access to the leading rehabilitation technologies in the
world. This did not happen by accident, but rather as a direct result of
federal research and development activities, including in particular those
sponsored by VA and NIDRR.

Rehabilitation Science and Engineering in the
U.S. Government

The year 1995 marked the 75th anniversary of the passage of the
Smith-Fess Act (Public Law 66-236), which originally authorized $750,000
for a program of federal grants-in-aid to state departments of education
for the vocational rehabilitation of civilians (nonveterans) with disabling
conditions (see Box 1-2). This "experimental" program, administered by
the Federal Board of Vocational Education, was reauthorized several times
and received permanent authority (and an annual budget of $2 million)
under the Social Security Act of 1935. Further amendments under the
Barden-LaFollette Act of 1943 (Public Law 789-113) expanded the program to include disabled veterans and placed it under the Office of Vocational Rehabilitation (OVR).

Much of the success of rehabilitation research within the OVR program in the 1950s resulted from the strong leadership of one of OVR's
early leaders, Mary Switzer. Committed to the improvement of the quality of life for people with disabling conditions, she was a strong advocate
for people with disabling conditions before the U.S. Congress, resulting in
greatly increased budgets not only to provide rehabilitation services but
also to support training programs, fellowships, and support for research
in medical rehabilitation. During her administration, the concept of re-

BOX 1-2
Time Line for Development of Federal
Rehabilitation-Related Programs

1920 Smith-Fess Act established the Vocation Rehabilitation Program under the Federal Board of Vocational Education

1943 Barden-LaFollette Act expanded the Vocation Rehabilitation Program's scope to include physical restoration services
Office of Vocational Rehabilitation established within the Federal Security Agency Administration

1945 The Committee on Prosthetics Research and Development formed at the National Research Council

1954 The Office of Vocational Rehabilitation (OVR), under the U.S. Department of Health, Education, and Welfare (HEW), expands to include private, community-based rehabilitation programs and established a research program within OVR)

1962 First rehabilitation research training centers (RRTCs) funded through the OVR research program (RRTCs at the University of Minnesota and New York University)

1963 Office of Vocational Rehabilitation is reorganized as the Vocational Rehabilitation Administration (this included a division of research with a specific appropriation for research and training grants) [Frank Corrigan, NIDRR, personal communication, 1996])

1965 The Vocation Rehabilitation Program expands to include individuals "disabled by a lack of education and social skills."

1967 Vocational Rehabilitation Administration reorganized as the Rehabilitation Services Administration

1972 Rehabilitation Engineering Research Centers

1973 Rehabilitation Act replaces Smith-Fess Act

1978 The Rehabilitation, Comprehensive Services, and Developmental Disabilities Act becomes law
Title VII (Independent Living) is added to Rehabilitation Act
National Institute of Handicapped Research (created from Rehabilitation Services Administration Division of Rehabilitation Research)

1979 Department of Education created out of HEW
Office of Special Education and Rehabilitative Services established within Department of Education
Rehabilitation Services Administration and National Institute for Handicapped Research moved from the U.S. Department of Health, Education, and Welfare to Office of Special Education and Rehabilitation Services, Department of Education

1986 Amendments to the Rehabilitation Act
National Institute for Handicapped Research renamed National Institute for Disability and Rehabilitation Research

1988 Technology-Related Assistance for Individuals with Disabilities Act

1990 Americans with Disabilities Act

1991 National Center for Medical Rehabilitation Research formed within the National Institutes of Health

gional rehabilitation research and training centers was adopted and funded by Congress and became a major resource for rehabilitation research and research training.

An early need in the growing constellation of federal programs was simple coordination. U.S. Army Surgeon General Norman Kirk saw the need for better coordination of the emerging Army programs with those in the Office of Scientific Research and Development and VA. As mentioned previously, he asked the National Research Council to form the Committee on Prosthetic Devices—a joint effort by the Division of Medicine and Surgery and the Division of Engineering—which advised the agencies on how best to join the physicians and rehabilitation professionals with physical scientists and engineers to plan, undertake, and disseminate research. The committee lasted almost 20 years, although its name changed to the Advisory Committee on Artificial Limbs and then to the Committee on Prosthetic Research and Development, and it witnessed many changes in federal administration and organization.

One of the largest changes came about as a result of the Vocational Rehabilitation Amendments of 1954 (Public Law 83-565), which instituted a multiple-program approach that included a separate system of grants for rehabilitation-related research. OVR became part of the U.S. Department of Health, Education, and Welfare and formed the National Advisory Council on Vocational Rehabilitation to review its research and training programs in rehabilitation science and engineering. In 1978, to provide a focus for these activities, the U.S. Congress created the National Institute of Handicapped Research (NIHR), which was initially staffed by researchers from OVR, the predecessor of the Rehabilitation Services Administration (RSA).

Thus, by congressional action, NIHR became the lead agency for coordinating disability research, development, demonstration, dissemination, training, and related activities. Renamed NIDRR in 1986, it also has responsibility for coordinating rehabilitation research activities among other federal agencies, including the National Institutes of Health, National Science Foundation, National Aeronautics and Space Administration, and the U.S. Departments of Veterans Affairs, Education, and Labor.

The Rehabilitation Act of 1973, as amended, with its authorizations for the research and other programs of RSA, expires in 1997. A thorough review and possible change can be expected under the 105th Congress in preparation for reauthorization.

ORIGIN, SCOPE, AND ORGANIZATION OF THE REPORT

In light of the many and varied programs in rehabilitation research and the growing number of people with disabling conditions, Senator

Robert Dole introduced the following into Senate Report 103-318, from the Committee on Appropriations:

> Advances in rehabilitation science are essential to realizing the Nation's commitment to equal opportunity, economic self-sufficiency, and full participation of Americans with disabilities. There are important questions of the adequacy of Federal efforts in both meeting the needs of the rapidly growing number of Americans with disabilities, and in realizing the new opportunities of science and technology on behalf of people with disabilities. The committee believes an independent assessment of the current Federal efforts in rehabilitation science and engineering is warranted and requests that the Secretary [of Health and Human Services] make appropriate arrangements with the Institute of Medicine or a similar independent entity to undertake such a review. The study should include an assessment of funding and manpower development, and make recommendations for the improvement of Federal rehabilitation science efforts (Senate Report 103-318).

In response to this congressional request and subsequent negotiations with the Office of the Assistant Secretary for Health in the U.S. Department of Health and Human Services, the Institute of Medicine appointed a committee to review and consider (1) the current status of research in rehabilitation science and engineering, (2) the unmet needs of rehabilitation that require new approaches from science and engineering and that take into account the social and behavioral contexts of the individual, and (3) the best strategies for achieving the necessary level of research and medical expertise to address those needs.

More specifically, the Institute of Medicine assembled a committee with expertise in rehabilitation science and engineering, health policy, basic biomedical rehabilitation and clinical research, assistive technology, social science, program evaluation, economics, and public administration and policy to address the following tasks:

• *Assess and evaluate the current content, quality, and adequacy of the knowledge base in rehabilitation science and engineering.* Therefore, in this report the committee evaluates the status of professional disciplines involved in rehabilitation science; the related needs for education, training, and research; and the potential need for a new discipline in rehabilitation science and engineering.

• *Evaluate the utility of current rehabilitation models as they reflect the interdisciplinary and multidisciplinary nature of rehabilitation and the interaction of the person with the environment.* To do this, the committee examines the integration of the various professions in rehabilitation science and considers the potential benefits of improved rehabilitation science and engineering in terms of clinical practice, individual function, quality of life, independence, and work productivity and reduced costs in health care and long-term care.

• *Describe and recommend mechanisms for effective transfer and clinical translation of scientific findings, advances, and information that will promote health and health care for people with disabilities and disabling conditions.* The committee does this by identifying obstacles and barriers to the effective translation of progress in science and clinical practice.

• *Review and critically evaluate current federal programmatic efforts in rehabilitation science and engineering as to their productivity, relevance, and coordination.* The committee thus describes potential organizational and administrative options for implementing an enhanced national program, establishes priority research categories within the context of resource limitations, and makes recommendations for enhanced coordination among federal researchers and research programs.

The remainder of this report is organized into Chapters 2 to 11 and Appendixes A to D. Chapter 2 describes the magnitude, costs, and potential savings associated with disability and rehabilitation; Chapter 3 discusses a new model of the enabling–disabling process as a framework for the discussion and analyses that occur in the subsequent chapters. Chapters 4, 5, and 6 present the status and needs for research in the areas of pathology and impairment, functional limitation, and disability, respectively. Chapter 7 describes health services research in rehabilitation science and engineering. Chapter 8 discusses issues related to technology transfer, and Chapter 9 discusses education. Chapter 10 discusses the organization and administration of rehabilitation-related research in the federal government and makes recommendations for improvement. The final chapter of the report (Chapter 11) provides overarching recommendations, identifies general priorities for future research, and presents a table that shows the relationship of the overarching recommendations and general priorities to the recommendations in the preceding chapters.

The appendixes present a description of the committee's data collection and analysis methods (Appendix A), summary descriptions of federal research programs in disability and rehabilitation-related research (Appendix B), a preliminary draft taxonomy (Appendix C), and brief biographies of the committee members and staff who prepared the report (Appendix D).

Table 1-2 lists each of the individual tasks that the committee addresses in this report and the chapter(s) that contains the majority of the committee's response to them.

TABLE 1-2 Addressing the Charge

Task	Committee Action
Assess and evaluate the current content, quality, and adequacy of the knowledge base in rehabilitation science and engineering.	• Chapters 4–6 address research and the knowledge base in each state of the enabling–disabling process (i.e., pathology, impairment, functional limitation, and disability). • Chapter 7 discusses health services research. • Chapter 9 discusses rehabilitation science and engineering as a scientific and academic field of study.
Evaluate the utility of current rehabilitation models as they reflect the interdisciplinary and multidisciplinary nature of rehabilitation and the interaction of the person with the environment.	• Chapter 3 describes current models of disability and presents the committee's enhancements for a model of the enabling–disabling process.
Describe and recommend mechanisms for effective transfer and clinical translation of scientific findings, advances, and information that will promote health and health care for people with disabilities and disabling conditions.	• Chapter 8 identifies both barriers and current mechanisms for technology transfer.
Review and critically evaluate current federal programmatic efforts in rehabilitation science and engineering as to their productivity, relevance, and coordination.	• Chapter 10 describes the federal effort in funding research in rehabilitation science and engineering, and the strengths and weaknesses of the individual programs as well as the combined, overall effort. • Chapter 11 describes overarching recommendations and general priorities and shows their relationship to recommendations in the individual chapters.

2

Magnitude and Cost of Disability in America

Understanding the importance of rehabilitation science and engineering and the potential impact that it might have on improving the health of the nation first requires an understanding of the current status of the incidence, prevalence, costs, and potential savings associated with rehabilitation. This chapter describes the various types of disabling conditions and their frequencies of occurrence in the United States as measured by various surveys and other means. It also attempts to characterize the associated costs and savings that can be realized through effective rehabilitation.

The most recent estimates of the number of people with disabilities is 49 million noninstitutionalized Americans (McNeil, 1993). Almost 4 percent of the U.S. population have disabling conditions so severe that they are unable to carry out the major activities of their age group (playing, attending school, working, or attending to self-care) (Institute of Medicine, 1991). An additional 6 percent are restricted in their major activities, and another 4 percent are limited in other types of activities.

In addition to and partly as a result of the loss of human function, enormous economic costs are associated with disabling conditions. Estimates vary but seem to hover around an aggregate annual cost of approximately $300 billion, including the cost of the medical resources used for care, treatment, and rehabilitation; reduced or lost productivity; and premature death.

As described in several reports, including *Disability in America* (IOM, 1991), numerous federal programs exist for people with disabling conditions. Most recently, a report by the National Academy for State Health Policy identified 129 separate programs administered by 14 different federal agencies, with annual funding of $175 billion. Approximately 95 percent of this money is allocated for income support and medical coverage. The remainder is divided among research and a variety of service-related activities, especially in the areas of education, housing, and transportation.

The federal government's largest program in rehabilitation research is located in the National Institute on Disability and Rehabilitation Research (NIDRR) in the U.S. Department of Education. As mandated by the U.S. Congress, NIDRR also has primary responsibility for coordinating rehabilitation research among federal agencies. The NIDRR director is the chair of the Interagency Committee on Disability Research (ICDR), which is charged with promoting communication and joint research activities among the committee's member agencies.

Other agencies involved in conducting rehabilitation research include the National Institutes of Health (NIH) and the U.S. Department of Veterans Affairs (VA). In 1984, NIH described 688 rehabilitation-related research projects in addition to other basic studies that help to elucidate the biological underpinnings of impairment and disability. In 1990, a new center, the National Center for Medical Rehabilitation Research (NCMRR), was established at NIH to help coordinate and focus specifically on medical rehabilitation research. VA supports a rehabilitation-related research program that allocates approximately $22 million to fund more than 175 separate projects at 60 VA medical centers.

MAJOR NATIONAL SURVEYS

The main source of statistics on people with disabling conditions are the federal surveys based on nationally representative samples of the noninstitutionalized U.S. population.

National Health Interview Survey

The National Health Interview Survey (NHIS) is a household survey sponsored by the National Center for Health Statistics (NCHS) and is designed to assess the health status of Americans. In 1994, the survey consisted of interviews with 116,179 people in 45,705 households. It includes questions related to disability such as degree of activity limitation and provides information by demographic variables such as age, race, and gender.

Activity Limitations

In NHIS terminology, disability is defined as activity limitation. Activity limitation is defined at three levels: (1) inability to carry out a major activity, (2) limitation in the amount or kind of major activity that can be carried out, and (3) limitation in carrying out a nonmajor activity. Major activities considered usual for one's age group are defined as ordinary play for children under 5 years of age, attending school for children ages 5 to 17, working or keeping house for people ages 18 to 69, and capacity for independent living (ability to bathe, shop, eat, and care for oneself without the assistance of another person) for people ages 70 and older. Nonmajor activities include social, civic, or recreational pursuits. The 1994 NHIS estimate of the number of people limited in activity because of chronic conditions was 39 million, or 15 percent of the civilian noninstitutionalized population. Of these 39 million people, 18.2 million were male and 20.8 million were female; 32.4 million were white and 5.4 million were African American. Residents of the South (16.3 percent) and rural areas (17.6 percent) had a slightly higher prevalence of disability than did residents of other locations.

Table 2-1 presents disability rates by demographic characteristic for the 1992 NHIS. Table 2-2 indicates the prevalence of activity limitations, limitations in the self-reported ability to work among people 18 to 69 years, and limitation in activities of daily living (ADL) and instrumental activities of daily living (IADL) among people over age 5 years by the impairments and diseases or disorders causing the limitation. The data summarize information from LaPlante and Carlson (1996) and are derived from analyses of the 1992 National Health Interview Survey (NHIS) conducted by the Bureau of the Census for the National Center for Health Statistics. NHIS surveyed a stratified random sample of the noninstitutionalized population of the continental United States and had approximately 110,000 respondents. Sampling weights associated with each respondent allowed for the estimation of the total number of people in the continental United States with limitations associated with impairments and conditions.

Total Prevalence Table 2-2 presents data on the prevalence of activity limitations associated with major classifications of impairments and diseases or disorders, including the number of people with the particular classification and limitation and the proportion of all activity limitations attributed to the classification. Overall, in excess of 61 million impairments or diseases and disorders contributed to activity limitations in 1992; of these, 16.3 million were impairments (26.7 percent of the total) and the remaining 44.7 million were diseases or disorders (73.3 percent). Among

TABLE 2-1 Crude and Age-Adjusted Rates of Limitation in Activity, by Selected Sociodemographic Characteristics, 1992

Characteristic	Crude Rate (percent)	Age-Adjusted Rate (percent)
Gender		
Male	14.6	15.2
Female	15.4	14.8
Race or origin		
Native American	17.6	20.8
Asian or Pacific Islander	7.2	9.0
Black non-Hispanic	15.9	18.3
Black Hispanic	13.7	16.5
White non-Hispanic	15.8	14.9
White Hispanic	10.4	14.1
Other and unknown	10.3	13.1
Education		
≤ 8 years	38.4	28.5
9–11 years	25.6	24.6
12 years	17.1	17.6
13–15 years	13.9	16.6
16 years	11.5	13.0
Unknown	21.3	18.9
Geographic region		
Northeast	13.7	13.1
Midwest	14.7	14.7
South	16.3	16.3
West	14.5	15.2
Urban/rural		
Metropolitan area	14.4	14.6
Central city	15.4	15.9
Not central city	17.3	13.8
Nonmetropolitan area	17.3	16.4
Nonfarm	17.6	16.8
Farm	13.6	11.2

SOURCES: LaPlante and Carlson (1995), Table A; 1992 National Health Interview Survey.

impairments, orthopedic impairments were the most common classification contributing to limitations, with a total of 8.6 million conditions accounting for 14.1 percent of all conditions that contribute to limitations. In excess of 1 million cases each of visual or hearing impairment, learning disability or mental retardation, and paralysis contributed to limitations, although none of these classifications individually accounted for more than 2.6 percent of all conditions contributing to an impairment.

The most common major classifications of disease and disorder contributing to activity limitations included musculoskeletal and connective

TABLE 2-2 Prevalence of Activity Limitations, Work Limitation, and Need for Assistance in ADLs and IADL, by Impairments and Diseases and Diagnoses Causing the Limitation, Continental United States, 1992

Impairment and Disease or Disorder	All Causes		Main Cause		Work Limitation		ADL or IADL Limitations	
	No. (thousands)	Percent	No. (thousands)	Percentage of Main Cause	No. (thousands)	Percent	No. (thousands)	Percent
All impairments and diseases or disorders	61,047	100	37,733	61.8	31,323	100	9,243	100
Impairments								
All	16,327	26.7	10,992	67.3	8,551	27.3	2,320	25.1
Visual	1,294	2.1	558	43.1	580	1.9	254	2.8
Hearing	1,175	1.9	654	55.7	396	1.3	85	0.9
Speech	545	0.9	315	57.8	145	0.5	9	0.1
Impairment of sensation	141	0.2	94	66.7	94	0.3	20	0.2
Learning disability-mental retardation	1,575	2.6	1,389	88.2	546	1.7	399	4.3
Absence of body part	788	1.2	477	60.5	437	1.4	140	1.5
Paralysis	1,071	1.8	546	51.0	552	1.8	278	3.0
Deformities	900	1.5	628	69.8	429	1.4	117	1.3
Orthopedic impairments	8,608	14.1	6,111	71.0	5,273	16.8	988	10.7
Other	230	0.4	150	65.2	99	0.3	30	0.3

Diseases or disorders								
All	4,716	73.3	26,813	58.9	22,703	72.5	6,923	74.9
Infectious diseases or disorders	378	0.6	250	66.1	206	0.7	600.6	
Neoplasms	1,628	2.7	1,087	66.8	899	2.9	348	3.8
Endocrine, nutritional, metabolic, and immunologic	3,409	5.6	1,525	44.7	1,875	6.0	331	3.6
Blood and blood-forming organs	217	0.4	103	47.5	82	0.3	210.2	
Mental disorders	2,035	3.3	1,494	73.4	1,296	4.1	367	4.0
Nervous system and sensory organs	4,373	7.2	2,585	59.1	2,114	6.8	8,849.6	
Circulatory system	10,170	16.7	5,396	53.1	5,143	16.4	1,624	17.6
Respiratory system	4,774	7.8	3,279	68.7	1,850	5.9	436	4.7
Digestive system	1,727	2.8	730	42.3	1,007	3.2	133	1.4
Genitourinary system	778	1.3	407	52.3	450	1.4	72	0.8
Skin and subcutaneous tissue	362	0.6	175	48.3	173	0.6	240.3	
Musculoskeletal and connective tissue	10,530	17.2	7,211	68.5	5,446	17.4	1,856	20.1
Congenital anomalies	287	0.5	210	73.2	137	0.4	27	0.3
Symptoms, signs, and ill-defined conditions	2,843	4.7	1,691	59.5	1,313	4.2	601	6.5
Injuries and poisonings	1,205	2.0	670	55.6	692	2.2	139	1.5

SOURCE: LaPlante and Carlson (1995).

tissue disorders (accounting for 17.2 percent of all conditions contributing to limitations), circulatory conditions (16.7 percent), respiratory conditions (7.8 percent), and nervous system and sensory organ conditions (7.2 percent).

Disability with a Primary Cause Table 2-2 also presents estimates of the major classifications of impairments and diseases or disorders reported by NHIS respondents as the main cause of their limitations; the number of people with each major classification as the main cause of their limitation and the proportion of all causes of limitation for which the particular classification is the main cause are presented. A total of 37.7 million people reported activity limitations in 1992. Of these, 10.9 million (roughly 2/3 of all 16.3 million individuals with an impairment) stated that any form of impairment was the main cause of their limitation. The probability that a condition will be reported as the main cause of limitation differs dramatically among impairments. Thus, only 43.1 percent of visual impairments were said to be the main cause of limitation, whereas 88.2 percent of the cases of learning disability or mental retardation were reported to be the main cause of limitation. In terms of prevalence, orthopedic impairments were the most common main cause of limitation.

More than 26.8 million people, or just under 60 percent of all 44.7 million people with diseases or disorders contributing to limitation, stated that a disease or disorder was the main cause of their limitation. Digestive, endocrine, nutritional, metabolic, immunologic, blood and blood-forming organ, and skin and subcutaneous conditions are least likely to be reported as the main cause of activity limitation, whereas respiratory, musculoskeletal, and connective tissue conditions, mental conditions, congenital anomalies, neoplasms, and infectious diseases are most likely to be reported as the main cause of activity limitation. In terms of prevalence, musculoskeletal and connective tissue and circulatory conditions are the most common diseases and disorders listed as the main cause of limitation.

Impairment and Work Limitation NHIS asked people 18 to 69 years of age questions about work limitations. Table 2-2 indicates the frequency of conditions contributing to work limitations and the proportion of all work limitations associated with each major classification of impairment or disease and disorder. In 1992, more than 31.3 million people reported having a condition that contributed to a work limitation. Of these, in excess of 8.5 million (27.3 percent of all people with conditions contributing to work limitations) had impairments that contributed to work limitations. Orthopedic impairments were again the most common form of impairment contributing to work limitations; more than 5.2 million cases of orthopedic impairment were cited, which represents 16.8 percent of all conditions affecting work capacity. Other impairments that were common causes of work limitation included visual impairments (mentioned 580,000 times), paralysis (552,000 times), and learning disabilities or mental retardation (546,000 times).

In excess of 22.7 million cases of disease or disorder were reported to contribute to work limitations, representing 72.5 percent of all conditions contributing to such limitations. The most common diseases and disorders contributing to work limitations include musculoskeletal and connective tissue disorders (5.4 million individuals), circulatory diseases (5.1 million individuals), and nervous system and sensory organ conditions (2.1 million individuals).

Impairment and Daily Life Finally, Table 2-2 indicates the number of conditions contributing to limitations in ADL or IADL and the proportion of all such limitations associated with each major classification of impairment or disease or disorder. The data concerning ADL or IADL limitations are limited to persons age 5 years or older. In 1992, in excess of 9.2 million individuals indicated that they had conditions that contributed to ADL or IADL limitations. Of these, 2.3 million (about 25 percent of all people with conditions contributing to ADL and IADL limitations) had impairments that contributed to ADL and IADL limitations. A total of 988,000 individuals had orthopedic impairments that contributed to ADL or IADL limitations; other impairments mentioned included learning disabilities or mental retardation (399,000 individuals), paralysis (278,000 individuals), and visual impairment (254,000 individuals). All forms of diseases or disorders contributed to ADL or IADL limitations in more than 22.7 million individuals, or roughly 3/4 of the total. The most common major disease classifications contributing to this form of limitation included musculoskeletal and connective tissue disorders (1.9 million individuals), circulatory conditions (1.6 million individuals), and nervous system and sensory organ conditions (884,000 individuals).

Prevalence of Activity Limitation in Children Among children under the age of 18 years, an estimated 4.0 million (6.1 percent of the U.S. population under the age of 18 years) have some type of disabling condition.* Disability in this age group is defined differently from disability in adults and includes any limitation in activity due to a chronic health

---

*The committee believes that, given the potential for effective interventions that can enable people with disabling conditions, most of these conditions should be strictly defined as *potentially* disabling conditions. For the sake of readability, however, we use the term disabling condition throughout this report with the intent that "potentially" is understood.

condition or impairment. Work limitations for adults are translated to limitations in play (under age 5 years) and school-related (ages 6 to 17 years) activities, because these are major activities for children. Play is one of the most important ways that children learn about the world. If play and activity are absent during early life, an important part of the foundation on which the child's life is based will be missing. Engineering and technology, in association with rehabilitation science, can provide substitute play and activities to compensate for the typical play and activities that may be missed. Like those for adults, the findings presented in this section were derived from analysis of data from the 1992 NHIS. Data were collected from households of the noninstitutionalized U.S. population by asking questions of parents and guardians. Children were not interviewed or observed.

Play and School Activities The prevalence of children with disabling conditions is greatest in those attending school and represents 7.4 to 7.6 percent of all children ages 5 to 17 years (Wenger et al., 1996) (Table 2-3). The majority of these children with disabling conditions are unable to perform a major activity or are limited in the amount or kind of major activity that they can perform. More males than females are represented among children ages 5 to 17 years with disabilities (Wenger et al., 1996) (Table 2-4).

Distinct Childhood Pattern The data on impairments and diseases associated with all children with disabling conditions reveals a pattern distinct from that for adults. The major impairment associated with disabilities is mental retardation or Down's syndrome, occurring in 15.8 percent of all children with disabilities (Wenger et al., 1996) (Table 2-5). This is followed by speech impairments (6.7 percent), hearing impairments (3.8 percent), and learning disabilities (2.8 percent), whereas orthopedic impairments (2.9 percent) and deformities (e.g., spina bifida) (2.7 percent) are not as prevalent in children as they are in adults.

Similarly, the major disease or disorder (i.e., pathology) associated with children with disabling conditions differs from that for adults because diseases of the respiratory system (23.6 percent) supplant cardiovascular disease in adults. Asthma is the leading respiratory disease associated with disability in children (19.8 percent); mental disorders (8.8 percent) and diseases of the nervous system and sense organs (7.5 percent) are the second and third most prevalent causes, respectively, of disabling conditions in children. Diseases of the musculoskeletal system and connective tissue are not as dominant in children with disabilities as in adults with activity or work limitations (Table 2-5).

In summary, the pathologies and impairments associated with child-

TABLE 2-3 Number and Percentage of Children Under Age 18 with Disabilities, by Degree of Limitation and Age, 1992

Group	Under Age 5 Number (thousands)	Percent	Ages 5 to 13 Number (thousands)	Percent	Ages 14 to 17 Number (thousands)	Percent
With disability (limited in activity)	547	2.8	2,479	7.4	1,021	7.6
No disability (not limited in activity)	19,110	97.2	30,899	92.6	12,429	92.4
Definitions of "major activity"	Play activities		Attending school		Attending school	
Degree of activity limitation:						
Unable to perform major activity	123	0.6	185	0.6	88	0.7
Limited in amount or kind of major activity	280	1.4	1,674	5.0	607	4.5
Limited, but not in major activity	145	0.7	620	1.9	326	2.4
Total	19,657	100.0	33,378	100.0	13,450	100.0

SOURCE: LaPlante and Carlson (1995).

TABLE 2-4 Number and Percentage of Children Aged 5 to 17 with School-Related Disabilities, by Degree of Limitation and Gender, 1992

Group	Total Number (thousands)	Percent	Males Number (thousands)	Percent	Females Number (thousands)	Percent
Has school-related disability	2,554	5.5	1,520	6.2	1,034	4.5
Has disability, but not school related	946	2.0	561	2.3	385	1.7
No disability	43,328	92.5	21,888	91.3	21,440	93.8
Degree of school-related disability:						
Unable to attend school	273	0.6	154	0.6	119	0.5
Attends special school or classes	1,484	3.2	924	3.9	560	2.4
Needs special school/ classes but does not attend them	245	0.5	155	0.6	90	0.4
Otherwise limited in school attendance	552	1.2	287	1.2	265	1.2
Total	46,828	100.0	23,968	100.0	22,860	100.0

SOURCE: LaPlante and Carlson (1995).

TABLE 2-5 Health Conditions and Impairments Causing Disability in Children Under 18, by Broad Condition Category, 1992

Impairment, Disease, or Disorder	Prevalence (thousands)	Percent
Impairments	2,069	41.6
Visual impairments	83	1.7
Hearing impairments	190	3.8
Speech impairments	335	6.7
Learning disabilities	167	3.4
Mental retardation/Down's syndrome	786	15.8
Absence or loss	18	0.4
Paralysis	140	2.8
(cerebral palsy)	99	2.0
Deformities	134	2.7
(spina bifida)	17	0.3
Orthopedic impairments	144	2.9
Other and ill-defined impairments	69	1.4
All Diseases and Disorders	2,906	58.4
Infectious and parasitic diseases	47	0.9
Neoplasms	38	0.8
Endocrine, nutritional and metabolic diseases and immunity disorders	72	1.4
Diseases of the blood and blood-forming organs	32	0.6
Mental disorders (excluding mental retardation)	440	8.8
Psychoses	25	0.5
Neurotic, personality, and other nonpsychotic mental disorders	415	8.3
Diseases of the nervous system and sense organs	375	7.5
Diseases of the nervous system	214	4.3
(Epilepsy)	123	2.5
Diseases of the eye	72	1.4
Disorders of the ear	89	1.8
Diseases of the circulatory system	63	1.3
Diseases of the respiratory system	1,174	23.6
(Asthma)	987	19.8
Diseases of the digestive system	70	1.4
Diseases of the genitourinary system	33	0.7
Diseases of musculoskeletal system and connective tissue	48	1.0
Diseases of the skin and subcutaneous tissue	61	1.2
Congenital anomalies	108	2.2
Symptoms, signs, and ill-defined conditions	279	5.6
Injury and poisoning	66	1.3
All Conditions	4,974	100.0

SOURCE: LaPlante and Carlson (1995).

hood functional limitations and disabilities appear to be distinct from those for adults. This suggests that a research emphasis on pathology and impairment in rehabilitation science and engineering should reflect the fact that disabling conditions among children are distinct from those among adults. Also, the prevention or reversal of the most prevalent causes of activity limitations among adults might begin in childhood.

Functional Limitations

The questions in NHIS also address the need for personal assistance in activities of daily living, such as eating, bathing, dressing, and getting around the home, and instrumental activities of daily living, which are everyday household chores, necessary business, shopping, or getting around for other purposes.

Chronic Conditions Causing Disability

In the NHIS respondents identify chronic conditions that cause activity limitations. A condition is considered chronic if either (1) it was first noticed 3 months or more before the reference date of the interview or (2) it is a type of condition generally considered chronic by NCHS, regardless of the time of onset, such as diabetes. Most chronic conditions do not have high risks of disability. About 12 percent of conditions identified in NHIS cause activity limitations, the broadest measure of disability. Impairments have the highest risk of becoming a disabling condition. Of the conditions reported in NHIS to cause activity limitations, heart disease ranks first, followed by back disorders, arthritis, orthopedic impairments of the lower extremity, and asthma (LaPlante and Carlson, 1996) (Table 2-6).

Families and Disability

Prevalence estimates of disability have focused on the individual as the unit of analysis. A new study looks at disability prevalence with the family as the unit of analysis (LaPlante and Carlson, 1995). It examines the composition of families with members with disabling conditions in comparison with the composition of families without a member with a disabling condition, their demographic and socioeconomic characteristics, and their utilization of health services. The study found that an estimated 20.3 million families, or 29.2 percent of all 69.6 million U.S. families, have at least one member with a disabling condition. An estimated 2.3 million (4 percent) two-parent families contain one or more children with a disabling condition. The rate of disability is 29.1 percent for white families, 31.9 percent for African-American families, and 21.7 percent for other

TABLE 2-6 Conditions with Highest Prevalence, All Causes of Limitations, 1992

Condition Causing Limitation	All Causes	
	Number (thousands)	Percent
All causes	61,047	100.0
Heart disease	7,932	13.0
Deformities, orthopedic impairments, disorders of spine and back	7,672	12.6
Arthritis and allied disorders	5,721	9.5
Orthopedic impairment of lower extremity	2,817	4.6
Asthma	2,592	4.2
Diabetes	2,569	4.2
Mental disorders (excludes learning disability and mental retardation)	2,035	3.3
Disorders of the eye	1,577	2.6
Learning disability and mental retardation	1,575	2.6
Cancer	1,342	2.2
Visual impairments	1,294	2.1
Orthopedic impairment of shoulder and/or upper extremities	1,196	2.0
Other unknown or unspecified causes	1,188	1.9
Hearing impairments	1,175	1.9
Cerebrovascular disease	1,174	1.9

SOURCES: LaPlante and Carlson (1995), Table D; 1992 National Health Interview Survey.

ethnicities. Among Hispanic families, 23.4 percent have members with disabling conditions. In general, the median family income is substantially lower if a head of household has a disabling condition, whereas income is affected much less by the presence of other members of the family with disabling conditions. The highest poverty rates by disability status are among families with single heads of households with two or more children with disabling conditions. More than half of such families are headed by women living at or below the poverty level.

NHIS Disability Supplement

NCHS fielded a disability supplement to NHIS that began in January 1994 and that continued through 1996. This survey represents a consensus reached by researchers and policy makers and will provide comprehensive information for estimates of prevalence and for program and policy development. In the first phase of the survey, conducted during 1994 and 1995, basic information on disability was obtained by personal interviews for a national representative sample of 225,000 people, about 45,000 of whom had some indication of a disabling condition. In the second phase of the survey, which began in late 1994 and which continued through 1996, the 45,000 people with an indication of a disabling condition were reinterviewed to obtain additional information.

A separate questionnaire was administered to children, including a control group of children without special health needs. In the first phase, questions about developmental milestones for children under age 5 and about performance of activities of daily living for children ages 6 to 17 were asked. The second phase included questions on (1) utilization and barriers to utilization of medical and mental health services, assistive devices, case managers, home care services, child care services, and educational and recreational services; (2) functional status, including measures of emotional and behavioral development; and (3) impact of the child's health problem on the family. The data were collected over a 2-year period to ensure an adequate sample size. The following were among the topics covered:

- Physical health conditions
- Childhood development
- Mental health conditions
- Functional assessment
- Assistive technology devices
- Income sources and amounts
- Family impact of disability
- Personal assistance services
- Health insurance coverage
- Self-perception of disability
- Special education services
- Supplemental Security Income and Social Security Disability Insurance participation
- Transportation accommodations
- Work site accommodations
- Use of medical services
- Vocational rehabilitation

Data will be released on electronic files for statistical analysis. The first release was in mid-1996 and included data collected for Phase I in 1994. NCHS plans to publish several descriptive reports based on the disability data, but NCHS does not have staff or funds to support full-scale analysis of the data. Verbrugge (1994) has outlined the research potential of this new source of data. Efforts are under way to identify sources of funding for data analysis.

Survey of Income and Program Participation

The Survey of Income and Program Participation (SIPP) is a panel survey designed to provide detailed information about income distribution and federal and state income transfer and services programs. A supplemental survey containing extensive questions about disability status was performed as part of the sixth wave of the 1990 panel and the third wave of the 1991 panel. SIPP contains information on economic and social variables on people with disabling conditions that are not usually included in health surveys that ask about disability. McNeil (1993) has provided disability data from SIPP.

In SIPP, *functional limitation* is defined as the ability of people ages 15 years and older to perform a set of sensory and physical activities. Limitations are ranked as 1 (with difficulty) or 2 (not at all or only with aid).

SIPP also uses need for assistance in activities of daily living and instrumental activities of daily living as a measure of disability. Mobility limitations are reported separately, because assistive devices such as wheelchairs and canes, rather than another person, are often used to overcome such limitations.

On the basis of interviews conducted during the period from October 1991 through January 1992, SIPP found that the number of people with a disability was 48.9 million, or 19.4 percent of the total population at the time of 251.8 million. Disability was defined as a limitation in a functional activity or in a socially defined role or task.

SIPP identified the number of people with a severe disability to be 24.1 million, or 9.6 percent of the population. The 24.1 million people identified as having a severe disability were identified as people who were unable to perform one or more activities, people who had one or more specific impairments, or people who used a wheelchair or who were long-term users of crutches, a cane, or a walker.

Current Population Survey

The Current Population Survey (CPS), a monthly survey conducted by the Bureau of the Census for the Bureau of Labor Statistics, is designed to collect information on labor force participation and income. In March, supplementary questions are asked about income and work disability, defined as a limitation in the kind of work that a person is able to perform because of a chronic condition or impairment.

Work Disability

Data from the 1995 CPS indicate that among people ages 16 to 64, 16.9 million people (10 percent) had a work disability (LaPlante and Carlson, 1995).

In addition, 11.4 million people (67.9 percent) among those with a work disability were not working and were not actively seeking employment.

The percentage of the population with a work disability increased with age. The group ages 16 to 24 had the lowest proportion (4 percent). This increased to 22 percent for those ages 55 to 64. The percentage of the population with a work disability decreased with the level of educational attainment, measured in years of school completed. People with fewer than 8 years of schooling had a work disability rate of 30 percent, compared with a rate of 4 percent for those with at least 16 years of education. This education-based disparity increased for people with a severe work disability. Those who had completed less than 8 years of school had a severe work disability rate of 23 percent, whereas the rate was 1 percent for those with at least 16 years of formal education. This means that the severe work disability rate among those with little schooling is greater than the among college graduates.

African Americans have a much higher rate of work disability (14 percent) than either whites (8 percent) or people of Hispanic origin (8 percent) (U.S. Bureau of the Census, 1989).

Back disorders rank as the most frequent cause of work disability (16.4 percent), followed by heart disease (13.1 percent) and arthritis (8.1 percent) (LaPlante and Carlson, 1996).

Labor Force Participation

According to 1995 CPS data, of those with a disabling condition, 27.8 percent have jobs, whereas 76.3 percent of people without disabling conditions have jobs (LaPlante et al., 1995).

Income

SIPP data indicate a negative association between earnings and disability status. For example, among people ages 35 to 54, those with no disabling condition had mean monthly earnings of $2,446, those with a disabling condition that was not severe had monthly earnings of $2,006 and those with a severe disabling condition had monthly earnings of $1,562. However, there was a strong negative association between education and disability status. Therefore, one of the ways that a disabling condition may affect earnings is through its effect on levels of education and training (McNeil, 1993).

COSTS OF DISABILITY AND REHABILITATION

Cope and O'Lear (1993) reported that research firmly establishes the clinical benefit and economic savings associated with early, aggressive, and highly expert application of rehabilitation technology to both brain injury and spinal injury patients. Just as estimates of disability prevalence vary depending on the definition of disability, however, so do estimates of the costs of disability. Estimates of cost of disability are done by surveying populations of interest and by secondary analysis of large databases. Most of the cost estimates available are for traumatic brain injury or spinal cord injury. Direct costs include medical treatment and rehabilitation. Indirect costs include loss of earnings resulting from the disabling condition. Also included are studies of the cost savings resulting from rehabilitation. Hill (1991) presented a comprehensive study of direct costs (cash transfer programs, medical care expenditures, and costs of direct services) and indirect costs (reduced earnings) and found that direct costs for fiscal year 1986 were $86.5 billion in cash transfers, $79.3 billion in medical care payments, and $3.5 billion in direct services. Indirect costs can range from 10 to 37 percent of preillness income.

Traumatic Brain Injury

The Brain Injury Association estimates that each year more than 2 million people sustain a brain injury, and 373,000 of these are severe enough to require hospitalization. Brain injury ranks as the leading cause of death and disability among children and young adults. An individual with severe brain injury typically faces 5 to 10 years of intensive rehabilitation, with cumulative costs of $48 billion annually (Brain Injury Association, 1995). In addition to the costs of hospitalization and rehabilitation, head injuries result in 14 million person-days of restricted activity each year (Max et al., 1991).

Lehmkuhl et al. (1993) examined data for 301 patients in model traumatic brain injury systems and found that total charges for acute care and inpatient rehabilitation, exclusive of physicians' fees, ranged from an average of $73,000 for mild traumatic brain injury to $154,000 for very severe traumatic brain injury. A population-based study of persons surviving traumatic brain injury (Brooks et al., 1995) found that costs for acute care and rehabilitation ranged from $17,015 for mild injuries to $133,467 for severe injuries. The study also examined costs for people with traumatic brain injuries 4 years after the initial injury and found that follow-up charges ranged from a mean of $2,323 for mild injury to $54,701 for severe injury. Follow-up costs included rehospitalization, visits to physicians, outpatient services, medication, equipment, supplies, attendant care, and other services. At an incidence rate of 69 per 100,000, the investigators projected that the total cost for new patients with traumatic brain injury requiring hospitalization will exceed $8 billion over the course of the first 4 years following injury.

Spinal Cord Injury

Harvey et al. (1992) used data from a survey of the U.S. population with spinal cord injuries to estimate the direct costs of traumatic spinal cord injuries. Direct costs were defined as the value (in 1988 dollars) of resources used specifically to treat or to adapt to the spinal cord injury. Estimates are $95,000 for initial hospitalization, $8,000 for modifications to the person's dwelling, $8,000 per year for medical services, supplies, and adaptive equipment, and $6,000 for personal assistance and institutional care. These are average costs and will vary depending on the severity of the injury, age, and patient motivation.

The National Spinal Cord Statistical Center at the University of Alabama at Birmingham estimates that there are between 7,600 and 10,000 new patients with spinal cord injuries each year. The lifetime costs directly attributable to spinal cord injuries vary greatly according to the severity of the injury. Average yearly health care and living expenses in 1992 dollars varied from $417,000 for the first year and $75,000 for each subsequent year for individuals who sustained severe injuries to $123,000 for the first year and $9,000 for each subsequent year for individuals who sustained less severe injuries. The average costs for all groups was $198,000 for the first year and $24,154 for each subsequent year.

These figures do not include any indirect costs such as losses in wages and productivity, which could average almost $38,000 per year but vary substantially on the basis of education, severity of the injury, and preinjury employment history (National Spinal Cord Statistical Center, March 1996).

Cost-of-Illness Framework

The impact of illness on society is frequently estimated by calculating the amount of medical care expenditures on behalf of people with disabling conditions (called direct costs in the cost-of-illness nomenclature) and the amount of wage losses or its equivalent in services provided by homemakers (called indirect costs) (Rice and Cooper, 1967). In an alternative formulation, some economists seek to price losses in all domains of activity, including work and housework but also encompassing leisure, family, and voluntary activities, by asking individuals how much they would be willing to pay to forego an illness (Thompson et al., 1982). However, the methods used to assess willingness to pay are primitive, and results have not differed substantially from those obtained by the more traditional methods of assessing costs of illness (Thompson, 1984).

Using the cost-of-illness framework, it becomes possible to estimate the economic impact of disability. Trupin and colleagues (1996) used the National Medical Care Expenditures Survey for 1987 to estimate the medical care expenditures of people with and without disabling conditions. They reported that the approximately 17 percent of the population with an activity limitation accounted for 47 percent of total medical care expenditures. These individuals incurred medical care costs four times as great as those for people without disabling conditions, accounting for 38 percent of hospital admissions but 57 percent of total hospital costs and 19 percent of costs for visiting physicians but 42 percent of total physician service expenditures. (See Chapter 7 for an examination of the implications of these figures on health services research.) Overall, people with disabling conditions had $157 billion in medical care expenditures in 1987. Expressed in 1994 terms, medical care expenditures for people with disabling conditions would amount to $205.7 billion, or 3.1 percent of the gross domestic product (U.S. Bureau of the Census, 1995).

Chirikos (1989) estimated both direct and indirect costs of disability using 1980 data. He reported an aggregate economic cost of disability of $176.8 billion, 51 percent due to medical care expenditures and the remainder due to the lost productivity of people with disabling conditions or family members who had to stop working to care for them. Expressed in 1994 terms, medical care expenditures would amount to $163.1 billion and indirect costs would total $155.0 billion.

Using the cost-of-illness framework, the committee estimated the magnitude of the indirect costs of disability with more recent data. First, the committee used the 1994 NHIS to compare the labor force participation rates of people with and without disabling condition of working ages, ages 18 to 64. In that survey, people with disabling conditions are those who report that they are unable to do the major activities for people their age, who report being limited in the amount or kinds of these activities, or who report being limited in nonmajor activities. Of 158.6 million working people in the United States, 22.5 million (14.1 percent) reported that they had disabling conditions. Of these individuals, 51.8 percent were in the labor force, whereas 83.0 percent of people without disabling conditions are in the labor force, a difference of 31.2 percent.

Assuming that people both with and without disabling conditions earned median hourly wages, wage losses for the percentage of people with disabling conditions who could be working but were not amounted to $158.7 billion, or 2.4 percent of the gross domestic product for 1994. The foregoing figure assumes that both groups bring an equal mix of skills and experience to the labor market. However, people with disabling conditions typically have other potential liabilities that affect their position in the labor market and, thus, in recent years earned only about 70 percent as much as people without disabling conditions (Yelin and Katz, 1994). Assuming that the earnings gap reflects differences in skill and experience—that is, objective characteristics—rather than discrimination, the indirect costs due to lost wages would amount to $111.1 billion.

Second, the committee used the 1994 CPS to estimate lost wages among people with disabling conditions. CPS is the source of the monthly unemployment statistics for the United States. Once a year, respondents are asked about their disability status. In the CPS people with disabling conditions are those who self-report the presence of a limitation that prevents work or limits the amount or kind of work that they can do. According to CPS, 11.8 million people have such a disabling condition. CPS also collects data on hours of work among those with disabling conditions who are working, allowing one to estimate wage losses for those who have stopped working altogether and for those who are working fewer hours. Owing to the more stringent definition of work disability in CPS, only 21.1 percent of people with disabling conditions were working in the week before the interview, whereas the proportion was 68.6 percent among people without disabling conditions, a difference of 47.5 percent. In addition, the people with disabling conditions who were working averaged 36.4 hours per week on the job, compared with 41.3 hours among people without disabling conditions, a difference of 4.9 hours. Summing the wage losses of those who stopped working altogether and those with reduced hours of employment, indirect costs due to disability amounted to $133.0 billion, or 2.0 percent of the gross domestic product in 1994. After taking differences in skill and experience into account, wage losses would still amount to $93.1 billion.

The estimates of indirect costs due to wage losses in CPS are lower than the estimates in NHIS because of the lower overall prevalence of individuals with disabling conditions in the former survey. Nevertheless, both estimates are in the same range as those of Chirikos (1989), suggesting that the definition of disability aside, the indirect cost of disability is well in excess of $100 billion annually.

Studies of the cost of illness emphasize wage losses, because such costs are relatively easy to measure. This methodology underestimates the impact among women, however, both because women earn less than men for jobs requiring similar levels of skill and because homemaking activities are poorly remunerated in the labor market, even though families value them highly (Lubeck and Yelin, 1988). Women have higher rates of disability than men, accentuating the problem of estimating the costs of disabling conditions.

However, the impact of disability extends far beyond work. Indeed, people with disabling conditions are less likely to be involved in all domains of human activity than people without disabling conditions (Lubeck and Yelin, 1988). In addition, because they devote so much time to personal care activities and to the time required to secure medical care services, even when they do participate in the same activities as people without disabling conditions, they are able to devote less time to many of them. These "costs" of disability are not easily priced in the marketplace, but they are important to people with disabling conditions and to their families. Thus, the impact of disability is far larger than the costs accounted for by current economic methods.

Future Needs

The first National Disability Statistics and Policy Forum, organized by the Disability Statistics Rehabilitation Research and Training Center, was held in October 1994. The topic of the forum was the future of disability statistics. Participants at the forum identified the following needs for future data collection efforts: more emphasis on social participation of people with disabling conditions, designing data sets that respond to policy questions, more emphasis on mental illness data, the need for more state-level data, more sharing of data across agencies, and use of repeated cross-sectional data to identify trends.

The second National Disability Statistics and Policy Forum in June 1995 focused on employment statistics and policy. Participants emphasized the need for data on barriers to work; estimates of the number of people with disabling conditions who are working, looking for work, and out of the labor force; and earnings and benefits data by occupation, industry, impairment groups, and environmental barriers, all reported in a consistent time series. They agreed on the need to examine more closely the problems that make it difficult for people with disabilities to go to work. Surveys should be designed to collect data on health status separately from employment status and work limitations. Data on how the workplace accommodates impairment and on the costs of accommodations required under the Americans with Disabilities Act of 1990 need to be collected. These data are needed to respond to concerns that the American with Disabilities Act imposes costly burdens on employers.

The third National Disability Statistics and Policy Forum was held in May 1996 and was titled Housing and Disability: Data Needs, Statistics, and Policy. The conference examined ways in which the quantity and quality of statistical information on the housing situation of Americans with disabling conditions can be improved.

CONCLUSIONS AND RECOMMENDATIONS

Estimates of the prevalence and economic impact of disability are dependent on the definition of disability used. Differences in methods aside, the prevalence of disability may be as high as 14 percent of the population and in certain age-gender-race groups may be significantly higher. Direct costs of disability would appear to be as high as $200 billion dollars a year and indirect costs may be as high as $155 billion. Thus, regardless of the definition of disability used, disability affects a substantial portion of the population and exacts a tremendous economic toll on the nation. In addition to diminishing or reducing disabilities due to paralysis or to visual or orthopedic impairments, rehabilitation science and engineering can contribute handsomely to enabling people to work by modifying the work environment, providing special equipment at work sites, enabling people to work at off-site locations, or providing the personal aids needed to carry out work tasks.

The foregoing data on the prevalence of and costs associated with disability were collected without an explicit conceptual model of disability. Accordingly, disability is defined in different terms for each of the major statistical series. More importantly, the design of each of these series predates the development of a more contemporary understanding of the process by which pathologies, impairments, and functional limitations give rise to disability, suggesting that the emerging definitions of disability are yet to be reflected in data collected in current surveys. In the chapter to follow, the committee reviews how the prevailing wisdom about the cause of disability has changed in the last several decades and then shows how the emergent model of disability might structure the research agenda for the foreseeable future, including the collection of data on the prevalence and impact of disability.

Recommendation 2.1 The Disability Statistics Subcommittee of the Interagency Committee on Disability should foster research to design and evaluate survey items to be used to ascertain the prevalence and impact of disability that accord with the contemporary model in which disability is jointly determined by characteristics of individuals and of their environments.

Recommendation 2.2 These survey items should be incorporated in on-going surveys, including the National Health Interview Survey, Current Population Survey, and Survey of Income and Program Participation.

3

Models of Disability and Rehabilitation

Models assist understanding by allowing one to examine and think about something that is not the real thing, but that may be similar to the real thing. People use a variety of models to obtain a clearer understanding of a problem or the world around them. Such models include physical models, three-dimensional graphical models, animal models of biological systems, mathematical or ideal models, and computer models. When relationships are highly complex, however, as they are in rehabilitation processes and other areas of human endeavor, it is seldom possible to develop models that are quantitatively predictive. Nevertheless, it is often possible to establish rough relationships between various variables that are observable.

Models based on partial knowledge are often called *conceptual models*. Conceptual models may help people to think about behaviors of components in complex systems, even though they may not yield quantitative answers. They may allow one to understand general relationships without the necessity for an extensive verbal or written description. In this way they are like an out-of-focus picture that partially reveals relationships. It is common in science and engineering to use models to help develop hypotheses that can be examined experimentally, but even as models assist scientists in moving forward with new understanding, they are abandoned for new versions. Experimental results may suggest that the models must be altered or even abandoned in favor of new models.

The models discussed in this chapter are conceptual in nature.

Such models must constantly be changed as new knowledge is gained if they are to adequately represent processes or systems that are in flux. Rehabilitation science and engineering, at its current stage of development, does not have a comprehensive paradigm or a universally accepted theoretical model. It is an emerging field of study, and as such, is still evolving. This chapter presents a brief look at the history of models of disability, which is useful in understanding the current status and direction of disability and rehabilitation research, and then presents a model of disability that builds upon and elaborates previous models, as well as adding several new elements. It presents this model verbally, schemeatically, and mathematically. Finally, it introduces a matrix that defines rehabilitation research.

EVOLUTION OF MODELS OF DISABILITY

The prevailing wisdom about the causes of disability has changed in the last several decades. In the 1950s, impairment of a given severity was viewed as sufficient to result in disability in all circumstances; in contrast, the absence of impairment of that severity was thought to be sufficient grounds to deny disability benefits. Thus, the American Medical Association's Committee on Medical Rating of Physical Impairments stated that "competent evaluation of permanent impairment requires adequate and complete medical examination, accurate objective measure of function, and avoidance of subjective impressions and nonmedical factors such as the patient's age, sex and occupation" (American Medical Association, Committee on Medical Rating of Physical Impairment, 1958).

By the mid-1970s, Nagi (1976) outlined a process by which a pathology (e.g., arthritis) gave rise to an impairment (e.g., a limited range of motion in a joint), which may then result in a limitation in function (e.g., an inability to type), which, finally, may result in a disability (inability to work as a secretary). While outlining a process that would seem to move inexorably from pathology to loss of a job, Nagi noted that correlations among impairments, functional limitations, and work loss were poor, and he speculated that the extent to which the environment accommodated limitations largely determined whether disability would result from the onset of a medical condition. In the interim, at least three others have developed models or modifications: the WHO (International Classification of Impairments, Disabilities, and Handicaps, 1980), the IOM (*Disability in America*, 1991), and the NCMRR (1993). All of these models attempt to facilitate and improve understanding by describing the concepts and relationships among medical conditions, impairments, functional limitations, and the effects of the interaction of the person with the environment (i.e., handicap, disability, societal limitation) although each uses different nomenclatures for the components.

Nagi's model of disability explicitly brought the environment into the conceptualization. His model initiated a search for the factors in family, community, and society that affect disability as an outcome. With respect to disability in the work setting, for example, research has focused on the social and demographic characteristics of the individual and family, the individual's prior occupation and the industry in which the individual was previously employed, the flexibility of the workplace with respect to the physical tasks of work and hours of work, the nature of the local economy, customs and laws governing employment, and the extent of income transfer programs (Yelin, 1992).

Although the Nagi model included the environment, it was limited in how it conceived of the environment. In his model, the environment impinges on individuals only when activity limitation interacts with the demands placed on those individuals; the process that gives rise to disability is still inherently a function of the characteristics of medical conditions and attendant impairments.

The IOM model (IOM, 1991) was derived directly from Nagi, defining disability as "a function of the interaction of the person with the environment" and beginning to describe certain subsets of environmental factors that could potentially affect the development of and movement within a disabling process. In this model, physical and social environmental risk factors (as well as biological and lifestyle risk factors) were described as independent variables that exist at all stages of the process. These factors affect progression within the model, and their control therefore affects (prevents) disability.

The NCMRR model adds emphasis to the importance of environment by adding a category called *societal limitations* to account for restrictions that society places on individuals and that limit their ability to participate independently in tasks, activities, and roles. The unwillingness of employers to provide accommodations and the lack of ramps that deny access to public buildings to persons with disabilities are given as examples.

Building on these models, this committee describes a model where the environment interacts with the individual to determine whether disability will result. Nagi's nomenclature is used in describing the stages of the model and the relational nature of disability, as described in the IOM model, is now enhanced and clarified. In this new model, the environment plays a critical role in determining whether each stage occurs and if transitions between the stages occur.

A NEW MODEL FOR THE
ENABLING–DISABLING PROCESS

A common understanding of such terms as injury, impairment, handicap, functional limitation, disabling conditions, and disability is essential to building effective, coherent programs in rehabilitation science and engineering. As described above, several frameworks have been advanced to describe disability-related concepts, but none of these has been universally adopted. The lack of a uniformly accepted conceptual foundation is an obstacle to research and to other elements critical to rehabilitation science and engineering. Using the definitions laid out in Chapter 1, this committee presents a new set of models, based primarily on the previous IOM model (1991), designed to enhance the robustness of the previous models with respect to reversing the disabling process, i.e., rehabilitation. This section presents an overview of "the enabling–disabling process," explains its stages, and describes the nature of disability.

An Overview of the Enabling–disabling Process

An overview of how disabling conditions affect a person's access to the environment is shown in Figure 3-1. Access to the environment, depicted as a square, represents both physical space and social structures (family, community, society). The person's degree of physical access to and social integration into the generalized environment is shown as degree of overlap of the symbolic person and the environmental square. A person who does not manifest disability (a) is fully integrated into society and therefore has full access to both: 1) social opportunities (employment, education, parenthood, leadership roles, etc.) and 2) physical space (i.e. space access equivalent to persons without disabling conditions). A person with potentially disabling conditions[1] has increased needs (expressed by the size of the individual) and is dislocated from their prior integration into the environment (b).

The rehabilitative process attempts to rectify this displacement, either by restoring function in the individual (c) or by expanding access to the environment (d) (e.g., building ramps). This model does not mean to imply that the two methods (which may be generally characterized as cure and care) are mutually exclusive. Indeed, the most effective rehabilitation programs include both. The model separates the two only to illustrate that disability is the interaction between the potentially disabling

---

[1]It is important to note that a *potentially* disabling condition becomes an actual disabling condition once the person is dislocated from the environment as a result of that condition.

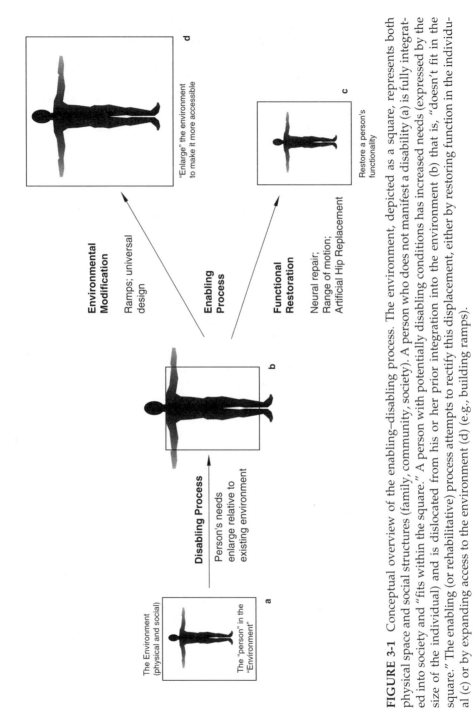

FIGURE 3-1 Conceptual overview of the enabling–disabling process. The environment, depicted as a square, represents both physical space and social structures (family, community, society). A person who does not manifest a disability (a) is fully integrated into society and "fits within the square." A person with potentially disabling conditions has increased needs (expressed by the size of the individual) and is dislocated from his or her prior integration into the environment (b) that is, "doesn't fit in the square." The enabling (or rehabilitative) process attempts to rectify this displacement, either by restoring function in the individual (c) or by expanding access to the environment (d) (e.g., building ramps).

conditions of an individual and the environment, and therefore strategies that affect the environment or the pertinent potentially disabling conditions both target disability. While this model provides an overview, more detail is provided below.

The New IOM Model

Looking at the enabling–disabling process with more scrutiny requires greater detail in the model. To this end, this report adopts the IOM model (1991) and makes some modifications designed to both improve the model and to tailor it more towards rehabilitation (see Figure 3-2). The original IOM model was conceived with prevention in mind, and the need for identifying risk factors whose control would facilitate the prevention of disability. The 1991 IOM model (IOM, 1991) established a new conceptual foundation in the field of disability in that it analyzed and described the components of the disabling process in such a way as to allow for the identification of potential points for preventive intervention. Identifying and describing the importance of the different types of risk factors that affect the disabling process as well as the interaction and integral nature of quality of life were fundamental contributions to the emerging field of disability prevention. Over time, however, some shortcomings in the 1991 IOM model have emerged, including the implication that the disabling process is unidirectional, progressing inexorably toward disability without the possibility of reversal. The unidirectionality was implied by the arrows in the model that pointed only to the right, that is, toward the condition of disability. Although this may have been a result of that committee's focus on developing interventions to prevent progression in the disabling process rather than reversal, that is, rehabilitation, it is a shortcoming in the original model that needs correction and clarification, especially in the context of rehabilitation.

A second apparent shortcoming in the 1991 IOM model is its limited characterization of the environment and the interaction of the individual with the environment. Although the importance of the environment is discussed in the text in some detail, it is not clearly represented in the model except as a category of risk factors involved in the transition between the various categories of the disabling process.

The third apparent shortcoming in the 1991 IOM model that the committee identified as needing improvement is the representation of societal limitation. Some enhancements to the original model address these shortcomings.

The new IOM model (Figures 3-2, 3-3, and 3-4) is designed to show disability more clearly as the interaction of the person with the environ-

The Enabling–Disabling Process

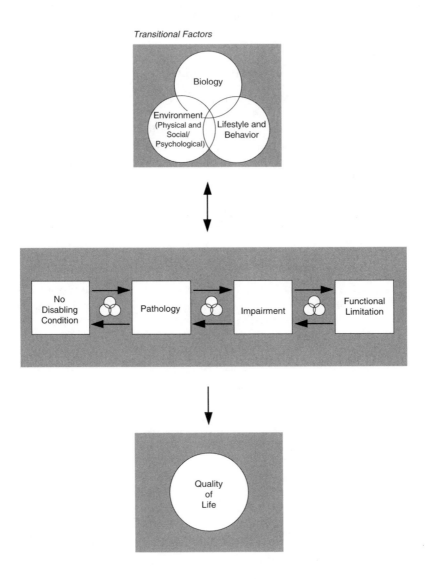

FIGURE 3-2 Modified IOM model. The *Disability in America* model (Institute of Medicine, 1991) is revised to include bidirectional arrows and a state of "no disabling condition," and to show transitional factors and quality of life interacting as part of the enabling–disabling process. The state of "disability" does not appear in this model since it is not inherent in the individual but, rather, a function of the interaction of the individual and the environment.

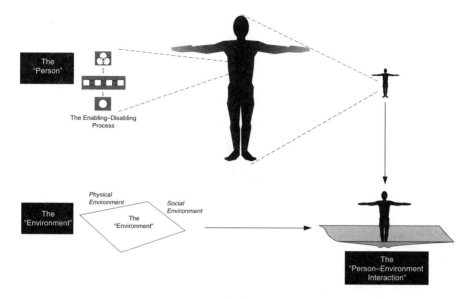

FIGURE 3-3 The person–environment interaction. The enabling–disabling process is depicted as being an active part of the individual person. The physical and social environments are depicted as a three-dimensional mat, with social factors on one side and physical factors on the other. The interaction of the person and the "environmental mat" is depicted as a deflection in the mat.

ment and also to show the possibility of movement in the direction of rehabilitation. To accomplish this diagrammatically, the new model is three-dimensional and has the following new features:

1. *The person*: Arrows pointing left were added to represent the potential effects of rehabilitation and the "enabling process" (risk factors and enabling factors are now combined into "transitional factors"). In addition, the new model includes the designation "no disabling conditions" to indicate that there is a beginning and an end to the disabling process when a pathology, impairment, functional limitation, or disability does not exist.

2. *The environment*: The shaded gray area from the 1991 model becomes "the environment," including the physical, social, and psychological components of the environment, and is represented as a three-dimensional mat that supports and interacts with the person and the disabling process, serving to highlight the importance of the person-environment interaction.

3. *Disability*: The box that was labeled "disability" in the 1991 model

**Disability is a function of the interaction between the
person and the environment**

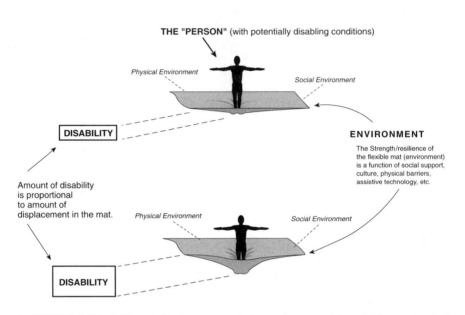

FIGURE 3-4 Disability as displacement of the environmental mat. The amount of disability that a person experiences is a function of the interaction between the person and the environment. The amount of displacement in the environmental mat is a function of the strength of the physical and social environments that support an individual and the magnitude of the potentially disabling condition. The amount of displacement represents the amount of disability that is experienced by the individual.

has been moved from being a part of the disabling process to being a product of the interaction of the person with the environment.

Each of these enhancements is described in greater detail below.

Assembling the Model

As shown in Figure 3-3, the new model can be shown as having three parts: the person, the environment, and the interaction of the person with the environment (disability).

The Person In the new model a new designation was added to indicate people with no disabling conditions. This feature of the model will allow for "complete" rehabilitation (designating also both the origin of the disabling process and the termination of the enabling process).

Transitional Factors In the new model, the committee defines the converse of risk factor as "enabling factor." Risk factors are phenomena that are associated with an increase in the likelihood that an individual will move from left to right in the new model, that is, from no disabling condition toward functional limitation. In contrast, enabling factors are phenomena that are associated with an increase in the likelihood that an individual will move from right to left in the new model, that is, toward less limitation.

The general types of enabling factors are the same as the general types of risk factors, that is, environmental (social, psychological, and physical) along with lifestyle and behavioral. So, for example, access to appropriate care and assistive technology would be an enabling factor (social environment), but lack of access would be a risk factor, or a disabling factor; curb cuts and universal design would be enabling factors (physical environment), but a lack of these would be disabling factors; the age of the person is a biological factor that can be either enabling or disabling; and compliance with pharmaceutical prescription regimens would be enabling, whereas drug abuse would be a disabling (behavioral and lifestyle) factor.

Thus, since both disabling and enabling factors affect transitions between the stages of the model, the committee groups them together as "transitional factors."

The Environment The environment is represented as a flexible three-dimensional mat in the new model. The strength and resilience of this mat are proportional to the quantity and quality of accessible support systems and the existence of various barriers. Stronger mats equate with more supportive environments, for example, access to appropriate health care, the availability of assistive technology and social support networks, and receptive cultures. Weaker mats equate with nonsupportive environments. For example, physical barriers, discrimination, lack of accessible and affordable assistive technology, and lack of appropriate health care result in greater displacement of the mat and, therefore, cause greater disability.

Thus, a person with a given level of impairment or functional limitation (i.e., potential disability) will experience greater disability (more displacement of the mat) in a less supportive environment than he or she would experience in a more supportive environment (indicated by a stronger mat and less resulting displacement). The amount of disability is proportional to the amount of displacement in the mat that represents the environment.

The environment is represented as having two general categories: the social-psychological and the physical. Examples of the types of things that might be included in each category include:

Psychological and Social Environments
- Discrimination
- Access to health and medical care
- Appropriate care
- Access to technology
- Culture
- Employment
- Family
- Economy
- Community organizations
- Access to social services
- Traits and personality factors
- Attitudes and emotional states
- Access to fitness and health-promoting activities
- Education
- Spirituality
- Independence

Physical Environments
- Architecture
- Transportation
- Climate
- Appropriate technology
- Geography
- Time

Each of the items listed in the social and physical environments could be thought of as layers in the mat; for example, access to assistive technology would be a layer in the environment mat, and so if an individual had good access to assistive technology, a strong layer for assistive technology would be added to the mat. If there were no access to assistive technology, then this layer would be missing from the mat, thus weakening the overall support and increasing the resultant disability.

In keeping with this model, it is important to note that the environment interacts at all points in the process (e.g., the environmental risk factors described in *Disability in America* [Institute of Medicine, 1991]).

Reflecting the increasing focus on the interaction of the individual and the environment, recent research on disability and rehabilitation has described the constituent parts of the environment in as much detail as Nagi's model gave to the individual pathway (Fawcett et al., 1994; Fougeyrollas and Gray, 1996; Fougeyrollas, 1997; Law et al., 1996). These researchers see the environment of the person with a disabling condition as including elements that are proximate, such as the immediate home and work environments (termed the *microsystem* of the individual), and distal, such as the community in which the individual lives (termed the *mesosystem*) and the society, economy, and, perhaps above all, the culture in which the local community is embedded (termed the *macrosystem*). However, these researchers do not include psychological or intrapersonal factors as part of the microsystem, an omission that the enhancements of the model described in this chapter are meant to rectify. In this chapter, psychological factors such as one's thoughts, beliefs, or expectancies are included in the intrapersonal environment.

Although the person with a disabling condition experiences the microsystem tangibly every day, the extent to which a particular condition is expressed as a disabling condition may be determined as much at the macro- or mesosystem level as by the nature of the local environment. For example, research on disability in the work setting indicates that the economic status of the overall labor market has a far greater impact on the employment status of people with disabling conditions than the willingness of individual employers to provide accommodations or the extent of the physical or mental impairment for that matter, even though both accommodations and extent of impairment do have some effect (Yelin, 1992). Similarly, the overall culture frequently determines whether a limitation will be considered disabling. In the broader U.S. culture, for example, a severe limitation in hearing is considered a disability. In a society in which the culture supports the use of sign language, a hearing loss may not be limiting (Groce, 1985).

The relative importance of the different elements of the environment may differ among kinds of activities. The extent of family help and the nature of the landscape and the built environment—microsystem and mesosystem characteristics, respectively—may affect an individual's ability to get around the community more than the overall culture (macrosystem characteristics). Even in that example, however, the importance of the overall culture becomes clear, because in some societies the provision of such services flows quite naturally from a communitarian ethos, whereas in others it is left to individuals and families to fend for themselves.

Disability The definition of disability has not changed, but its representation in the model has. In the new model, disability is a dependent variable whose value is determined by the relationship between two other variables: the person and the environment. Since disability is not a part of the person, but rather is a function of the interaction of the person with the environment, the box that represented disability in the 1991 IOM model has been removed from the person component in the new model (see Figure 3-4). Disability is now represented as the quantity of deflection in the mat that represents the environment.

Thus, in the new model disability is a relational outcome. Although many parts of the process are not well understood at present, the areas in which knowledge is strong and those in which it is weak can be specified in the new model.

Theoretical Quantification and Mathematical Model of Disability

As a relational concept, disability lends itself to mathematical modeling. At present this can be done only on a conceptual basis, since quantification of the variables is not yet reliable and reproducible. Nonetheless, a mathematical model is useful in further clarifying the relationship that exists between the person and the environment and how they interact to create disability.

Beginning with the variables of pathology (P), impairment (I), and functional limitation (FL), the first assumption is that the sum of these variables represents a quantity known as an individual's *potential disability*, or PD: $P + I + FL = PD$. Potential disability is referred to as "potential" because it is only the interaction of potential disability with the environment that creates true disability. In addition, some (or all) of these variables may be equal to zero. If all are equal to zero, then there is no potential disability.

Environment (E) is the denominator in the mathematical model, because it is the influence of the environment that creates disability from any given potential. The environment is the variable factor against which the other factors are measured and that determines the existence of disability. Without environmental factors there would be no disability. Thus, disability (D) can be represented mathematically as the relationship of potential disability $(PD$, or $P + I + FL)$ to environment (E): $(P + I + FL)/E = D$ or $PD/E = D$.

Take the following example. If the range of PD (i.e., the sum of $P + I + FL$) is 0 to 10 (where 10 is the maximum potential for experiencing disability) and the range of E is 0.1 to 10 (where 1.0 is a neutral environment, 10 is a very accessible and supportive environment, and 0.1 is a very inaccessible and nonsupportive environment), then the resultant quantity of D would range from 0 to 100 (where 100 is maximum disability).

So, for example, if PD were 5 and the environment were a very "good"

TABLE 3-1 Estimating the Effects of the Environment on Disability

Functional Capacity (qualitative)	Potential Disability (qualitative)	Potential Disability (range: 1–10)	Environmental Support (range: 0.1–10)	Disability Score (range: 0.1–100)
High	Low	1	10 (good)	0.1
		1	1 (neutral)	1
		1	0.5 (bad)	2
		1	0.1 (worst)	10
Moderate	Moderate	5	10 (good)	0.5
		5	1 (neutral)	5
		5	0.5 (bad)	10
		5	0.1 (worst)	50
Low	High	10	10 (good)	1
		10	1 (neutral)	10
		10	0.5 (bad)	20
		10	0.1 (worst)	100

one (e.g., $E = 10$), then the level of disability would be 0.5. However, with the same PD (i.e., $PD = 5$) but a less supportive environment (e.g., $E = 1$), then the level of disability would increase from 0.5 to 5. (When E is equal to 1, the effect of the environment is neutral and PD is equal to D.)

Mathematically, to allow the environment to exert a truly negative effect in the model, the range of quantities for the denominator (i.e., the environment) should be less than 1.0 but greater than zero; thus, the range would be from 0.1 to 10. Using the example above, if E is equal to 0.5 instead of 1, then the level of disability would increase from 5 to 10. If the environment was at its worst (i.e., $E = 0.1$), then the amount of disability would increase to 50 in this example.

In summary, maintaining the level of potential disability constant ($PD = 5$) and varying the quality of the environment (E is from 0.1 to 10) results in the moderate disability scores listed in Table 3-1 for the example cited above.

CONCEPTUAL MATRIX FOR REHABILITATION RESEARCH

The conceptual models presented here could form the basis for a new science—rehabilitation science and engineering—that embodies the underlying, rudimentary paradigm implicit in each. The committee believes that there is a legitimate and distinct field of study that justifies the term "rehabilitation science." Rehabilitation science emphasizes function, focusing on the processes by which disability develops and the factors influencing these processes. The vision of rehabilitation science is that better understanding of the causes and factors contributing to disability will lead to better treatments and technology for those with disabling conditions. To help define the parameters of rehabilitation science and engineering, the committee developed the conceptual matrix presented in Table 3-2. The matrix is useful as a tool for identifying the focus of rehabilitation science and engineering, defining which research activities address rehabilitation, and providing new possibilities for future research.

Table 3-2 demonstrates that rehabilitation science and engineering targets the enabling–disabling process, which runs across the stages of disability, and addresses the disabling conditions and the environment. The cells of this matrix (i.e., the different letters, A_1 through M_4) match disability-related variables in the rows to performance measures in the columns. A single cell (e.g., A_1 or C_3) in the matrix constitutes the minimum requirement for research classified as associated with the new academic field of rehabilitation science and engineering. If a row variable is studied across several performance states, the multi-cell begins to represent the enabling–disabling process. Every research study in rehabilitation science and engineering must have some measure of disability-related function (columns) and some measure of a disability-related variable, either of the person or of the environment (rows). It is not sufficient to study a classification of illness or disease without a measure of performance. This requirement defines the subset of pathology and pathophysiology research in medicine that overlaps with rehabilitation science and engineering. It also serves as a guide for defining the rehabilitation science and engineering relevant research in basic biological, physical, behavioral, and social sciences and in the health professional and engineering disciplines. The highest priority in rehabilitation science and engineering is for studies yielding causal explanations of disabling and rehabilitative processes.

The matrix also reveals the unique nature of rehabilitation science and engineering. First, rehabilitation science emphasizes function. Second, rehabilitation science focuses on factors that lead to transitions between pathology, impairments, functional limitation, and disability. Third, rehabilitation science examines physical, behavioral, environmental, and societal factors that influence these transitions. Although rehabilitation science is multidisciplinary and utilizes methods from many fields including medicine, biomedical engineering, material sciences, sociology, architecture, and even economics, it is distinct from other scientific disciplines due to its emphasis on function, factors, and interventions that disable or enable people. Rehabilitation science and engineering combines knowledge from these otherwise distinct disciplines to create a knowledge structure for the understanding of performance deficits un-

TABLE 3-2 Conceptual Parameters of Rehabilitation Science and Engineering

	Disability-Related Performance Measures (rehabilitation realms)			
	Pathology	Impairment	Functional Limitation	Disability
Personal and Environmental Variables	Enabling Processes <———————————— Disabling Processes ————————————————————————————————————>			
Personal (e.g., biology, behavior, resources)				
Natural processes (growth, maturation, development, aging, repair)	A_1	A_2	A_3	A_4
Disease (manifestations and progression)	B_1	B_2	B_3	B_4
Behavioral lifestyle	C_1	C_2	C_3	C_4
Experiential (e.g., perceptions, autonomy, well-being, quality of life)	D_1	D_2	D_3	D_4
Resources (e.g., physical, monetary, skills)	E_1	E_2	E_3	E_4
External environment				
Natural (e.g., climate, terrain)	F_1	F_2	F_3	F_4
Culture	G_1	G_2	G_3	G_4
Engineered (e.g., assistive technology, architecture, transportation)	H_1	H_2	H_3	H_4
Therapeutic modalities	I_1	I_2	I_3	I_4
Health care delivery systems	J_1	J_2	J_3	J_4
Social institutions (e.g., family, religion)	K_1	K_2	K_3	K_4
Macroeconomic indicators (e.g., gross national product, unemployment rates)	L_1	L_2	L_3	L_4
Policy and law	M_1	M_2	M_3	M_4
Resources and opportunities	N_1	N_2	N_3	N_4

derlying disability, the processes in which disabling conditions develop, progress, and reverse, and the factors that mediate the disabling and enabling processes.

Table 3-2 finally creates possibilities for new research. The matrix identifies combinations of variables which can be researched, but are not likely studied in the separate, existing basic science, health professional, and engineering disciplines. The variables in the rows (i.e., person and environmental variables) may be investigated as dependent or independent variables with the performance realms (columns) as the respective independent or dependent variable counterpart. Switching the independent variable from column to row will allow elucidation of the impact of disabling or rehabilitative processes on the person or society, on the one hand, or the impact of person or environmental variables (as positive or negative effectors) on enabling and disabling processes. The new knowledge of rehabilitation science and engineering will stimulate insights into rehabilitative processes and innovations into rehabilitation therapeutics.

The matrix in Table 3-2 can also be used to evaluate current data collection efforts with respect to the prevalence of and impact of disability. Currently, federal surveys routinely collect information on the extent of pathology, impairments, and on limitations in major classifications of activities. The National Health Interview Survey collects some information on behavioral factors and in the use of health care. In addition, some episodic surveys such as the Longitudinal Study on Aging and Health and Retirement Survey collect some information on accommodations provided by government, family, and employers. However, no ongoing surveys routinely collect information on the experiential and resource domains within personal factors and none collect information on such external environmental factors as the natural and engineered environment, access to rehabilitation specific therapies and health care, the availability of social supports, and the experience of the laws and regulations governing disability policy. In short, information on disability is almost exclusively within the personal domains and even so, tends to focus on definitions of disability that accord with much more primitive models of disability.

SUMMARY AND CONCLUSIONS

The prevailing wisdom about the causes of disability has shifted dramatically in the span of the last several decades. From the deterministic position of the American Medical Association Committee on Impairments of the 1950s, in which pathology was viewed as equivalent to disability, to the probabilistic one in more recent years of Nagi, IOM, and National Center for Medical and Rehabilitation Research (NCMRR) that, although still focusing on the characteristics of the individual, viewed the relationship among pathology, impairment, functional limitation, and disability as contingent, to the view espoused here, that the environment and characteristics of the individual conjointly determine disability, the underlying notion of why someone is unable to function in the major activities of life has been transformed.

The notion that disability arises from the interaction of a person's physical condition and the person's environment has several implications. These implications affect research, professional training, and policy. Although there is not space here to discuss these implications in depth, their outlines will be sketched briefly in the hopes that others will investigate them further.

One implication of the notion that environments can be enabling is that disability does not always have to be viewed through a "deficit" model. Rather, it should be recognized that in an environment that is strongly enabling, a person with a substantial physical impairment can live a life that is indistinguishable in important ways from that of a similar person without such an impairment. That is, the person with the impairment can hold a good job, be married and have a family, engage in non-work-related activities, enjoy social relationships, and be part of a community. Not much research has been done from this perspective. Some exceptions are the works of Gray (1996), and White et al. (1995). The committee strongly recommends that more research be done which emphasizes the effects of enabling environments on the lives of people with impairments and functional limitations. If disability is a function of the environment, it is not a stable attribute across situations. Rather, it will depend on the particular environment or the particular situation. For example, it is possible that a person with a certain type of impairment might be more disabled in his or her work environment than in the family environment. This would be true, for example, of a deaf person working with hearing coworkers who did not know how to sign, who worked for a company that provided interpreters only for large or important meetings, but whose spouse and children all signed fluently. Or an impairment might affect a person's ability to use public transportation, but not the ability to work once arriving in the workplace.

For research, this means that one measurement of impairment or functional limitation cannot be developed to indicate degree of disability in all situations. One measurement that attempts to indicate how disabled a person is would be misleading. If the measurement were limited to a specific, clearly defined situation, such as a workplace, it might be possible to include enough environmental indicators that a valid and reliable measurement might be developed; however, this measurement is unlikely to apply across all situations. This will, for the short run, make the tasks facing researchers much harder.

This conception of disability also carries with it implications for professional training. If the goal of professional training in rehabilitation is to impart the skills needed to reduce disability, training programs will need to teach many forms of environmental modification. Training may need to be broader than it has been, and it will need to include more professional fields and skills (see Chapter 9 for further discussion of this issue).

Finally, even though disability policy is not the focus of this report, it is worth noting that the policy implications arising from this definition of the concept are enormous. Disability determination will not be able to be a single event. Rather, a determination of disability status, for example, for the purpose of receiving Social Security Disability Income benefits, will have to be tied to a specific time, place, set of skills, and type of job. It cannot be permanent, for not only will changes in the person's own health or educational status change it, but so will changes in aspects of the work environment. Additionally, any single disability determination might not be acceptable across programs, since different programs apply to different environments.

RECOMMENDATIONS

Recommendation 3.1 Researchers and educators should adopt the model for rehabilitation and the enabling–disabling process presented here. Programs supporting rehabilitation-related research should adopt its terminology and use it as an organizing tool.

Recommendation 3.2 Based on the model of the enabling–disabling process described in this report, methods for quantifying disability should be developed that are sensitive to the characteristics of both the person and the environment. Such a metric would facilitate additional research into the factors that affect transitions between disability and other states of the enabling–disabling process, and the development of effective preventive and rehabilitative intervention strategies.

4

Pathology and Impairment Research

From a medical perspective, the most basic way of investigating potentially disabling conditions is to study them in the performance realms of pathology and impairment. As defined in the conceptual matrix for rehabilitation science and engineering in Chapter 3 (see Table 3-2), research in the pathology and impairment realms of rehabilitation science and engineering includes studies of isolated cells, tissues, and organs derived from human or animal subjects. The performance variables of interest are measures of molecular, cellular, and organ or organ system function. Although the performance of the cells and organs may be assessed in an intact human, humans are not absolutely required for pathology and impairment research; pathology and impairment research may be performed using isolated cells and organs from humans or animals. These preclinical studies are intended to (1) define significant parameters or valid markers of pathology and impairment, (2) illustrate relationships (causal and other) among significant parameters, and (3) identify the mechanisms and factors governing changes in significant parameters.

By examining the different sciences that contribute to rehabilitation science and engineering, the roles and uniqueness of rehabilitation science and engineering are defined. This chapter evaluates the multiple number of scientific disciplines that contribute to knowledge about pathology and impairment and the scientific research that generates it. To better understand the importance of research in these areas and to define their boundaries, the chapter also addresses the major categories of activity limitations experienced by adults and children and the impairments and pathologies associated with these limitations. These categories are presented not to suggest that these pathologies and impairments be studied exclusively but, rather, to prioritize the need for the development of knowledge related to significant functional limitations affecting human independence, autonomy, and productivity in society. The state of knowledge for selected pathologies and related impairments is reviewed to describe the gaps in knowledge that exist and promising areas in which knowledge can be developed through research from the perspective of rehabilitation science and engineering.

SCIENCES CONTRIBUTING KNOWLEDGE TO STUDYING PATHOLOGY AND IMPAIRMENT RESEARCH

Knowledge in the realms of pathology and impairment comes from a variety of disciplines that partially overlap. Biology, engineering, and the physical, social, and behavioral sciences all contribute to rehabilitation science and engineering, in that those disciplines provide knowledge related to the altered cell and organ functions that may lead to disabling conditions. Rehabilitation science and engineering is unique in that it melds the knowledge from these otherwise distinct disciplines and creates a multidisciplinary structure that allows one to understand the nature of disability, that is, how potentially disabling conditions develop, progress, or reverse and the factors that mediate disabling or enabling processes. So, although an array of biological sciences offers knowledge of the normal molecular-cellular and organ-organ system level of performance, as well as of the molecular, cellular, and organ defects that lead to various pathological states and impaired organ system function, many of the factors that determine enabling and disabling processes and movement between the realms of pathology and impairment are related to disciplinary knowledge beyond that from the biological sciences. For example, replacement of organ function may entail an artificial organ (e.g., kidney dialysis machine, mechanical heart, or artificial hip) that emanates from a combination of medical and engineering research. Developments in engineering offer the hope of providing environments to assist with human functioning in the face of disability and impairment. Social sciences provide knowledge of the influence of personal lifestyle and societal conventions on enabling and disabling processes, even disability-related changes in performance at the molecular and cellular (pathology) and the organ (impairment) levels. The health professional disciplines support and stimulate the basic science research relevant to rehabilitation science and engineering and, most importantly, see that new knowledge from the basic sciences and rehabilitation science and engineering is translated into therapeutics and clinical care.

Physiology, Cell Biology, Neuroscience, Developmental Biology, Gerontology, Vascular Biology, and Biochemistry

The knowledge generated in the biological sciences, including, physiology, cell biology, neuroscience, developmental biology, gerontology, and biochemistry, has a direct relationship to rehabilitation science and engineering to the extent that this knowledge explains the basis of pathological function of the human biological system. Scientists in these fields study the structures and functions of the molecular, cellular, organ, and organ systems known to be the cause of disabling conditions. Particularly useful to rehabilitation science and engineering are elements of pathophysiology that are specifically associated with disability, including injury processes and intrinsic mechanisms for recovery or compensation of function at the cellular and organ-organ system levels. Of particular interest are markers of disease and disease progression, including ones that vary by gender, race, and age or developmental stage. Because of their seminal contribution to knowledge of human cell and organ function, these sciences are also critical to the development of knowledge that allows investigators to identify and understand complications of disability that present as secondary conditions, such as decubiti, infections, pain, muscle spasticity, joint dysfunction, immunological deficiencies, disease atrophy of skeletal muscle, micturition dyssynergia, and sexual impotence.

The biological sciences are also critically important to rehabilitation science and engineering for the development of animal or surrogate (computer or tissue culture) models of disabling diseases and disorders. A major obstacle to effective rehabilitation research is the paucity of good nonhuman models of disabling conditions that can be used to accurately predict treatment efficacy in humans. For example, current animal models that are important to rehabilitation research include models of neuropathic pain, spasticity, decubiti, infection, contractures, arthritic disorders, abnormal ossification, skeletal muscle atrophy, locomotor deficits, scoliosis, bladder and sphincter dyssynergia, thrombophlebitis, peripheral ischemia, burns, visuomotor deficits, postural instability and vestibular ataxia, posture-related autonomic dysfunction, endocrinological deficits, and immunological deficits. Tissue cultures are used to model apoptosis or skin healing.

Genetics and Molecular Biology

Although many disabling conditions are not intrinsic but are acquired (e.g., because of trauma, aging, infection, or exposure to harmful environmental agents), a significant number have their origins in the genetic inheritance of the individual either as defects of a single gene or as multiple gene disorders or chromosomal abnormalities. Duchenne muscular dystrophy and cystic fibrosis, for example, are inherited genetic disorders that are associated with progressive pathology and impairment. These manifest primarily with aging and, perhaps, as a result of environmentally determined factors that influence the timing of expression of a defective gene, such as that linked to breast cancer (e.g., *BRCA-1*) (Hall et al., 1990; Easton, Bishop, Ford et al., 1993). Normal human processes of special interest to rehabilitation science and engineering are growth and healing, repair, and compensatory mechanisms; these processes are critically dependent on the up- and down-regulation of genes and gene products. Similarly, normal human development and maturation are the manifestations of genetics, and thus, genetic disorders and disability are intertwined. At present genetics and molecular biology offer unique perspectives and powerful investigative techniques for providing an understanding of the cause and nature of some diseases at their most fundamental biological levels. It is also hoped that genetics and molecular biology will provide markers of these diseases and that nonhuman animal models can be used to study the factors determining the resultant disabling and enabling processes. Although not yet realized, the promise of this realm of biological science is genetic and molecular biological therapies that will allow for the exogenous replacement of defective and missing genes or the stimulation of expression of existing genes, perhaps even to regrow cells, organs, and limbs.

Pharmacology

Many pharmacological agents are used in rehabilitation therapeutics. The specific cellular and organ actions of drugs and pharmaceutical agents are often not well understood. Basic pharmacological research focuses on the mechanisms of drug actions. Rehabilitation science and engineering critically needs knowledge of how pharmaceutical agents act on cells with existing pathology and on impaired organs so that agents useful in the management of potentially disabling conditions and the prevention of secondary conditions can be found. For example, the effects of 4-amino-pyridine on axonal conduction in an animal model of diabetic neuropathy or spinal cord injury shows promise for human study and application. Pharmacologic agents are also a means of regulating gene expression in the developing and mature organism.

Engineering and Physical Sciences

Engineering is traditionally viewed as the application of science to the needs of society. The application of engineering to problems of people with impairments and disabling conditions however, is still rather young. Continuity in the application of engineering in rehabilitation can be traced only to 1945, the end of World War II, as described in Chapter 1. Engineering in rehabilitation has given many people the opportunity to demonstrate what is possible when disabling conditions are transcended through technical assistance.

One of the contributions of engineering to rehabilitation science and engineering lies in creating altered, supportive environments (external or internal) for people with disabling conditions, because when engineering of the environment is maximized, the manifestations of pathologies and impairments as functional limitations and disabilities are minimized. In addition, virtual reality systems that are in development may allow for the remote control of function and communication through robots and other engineered devices, such as eye- or voice-controlled power wheelchairs. These engineered environments limit or reverse the functional manifestations of pathology and organ impairment by compensating for or replacing the altered or lost function with engineered structures and devices. The majority of current rehabilitation engineering research is in the fields of materials sciences, biomedical engineering, and engineering technology development. Prosthetics and orthotics, replacement of joints by endoprostheses, neuroprostheses, implantable lenses and pacemakers, and implantable drug delivery systems are examples of engineered exogenous devices that improve function by replacing diseased organs or compensating for their impaired function and that help investigators in rehabilitation science and engineering to build their knowledge of enabling processes. Similarly, pressure-distributed and regulated seat cushions and other devices for people who use wheelchairs exemplify how engineered environments can prevent secondary conditions.

Engineering and physical sciences are also critical to the development of tools that can be used to measure outcomes at the cellular, tissue, organ, and organ system levels of performance. These tools allow for the assessment of the development of pathology and impairment and the progression of disabling and enabling processes. The data are derived from biological science research, but the tools are from engineering and physical sciences. The usefulness of the data to rehabilitation however, depends on the validity, reliability, and sensitivity of the measurements of the relevant parameters. In particular, rehabilitation science and engineering research needs outcomes that can be obtained by noninvasive or minimally invasive means and measures that can be used to track pathology and impairment.

Social and Behavioral Sciences

The significance of social and behavioral sciences to knowledge of pathology and impairment stems from their importance to understanding the effects of the individual and the social environment. Knowledge from psychology, anthropology, sociology, political science, economics, epidemiology and communication science contributes to understanding of pathology and impairment. For example, smoking leads to progressive cellular and respiratory system disease and the resultant functional limitation. Social sciences help to pinpoint who is most at risk for this pathology as well as for other aspects of the enabling–disabling process. Social sciences help to isolate cultural or behavioral elements which contribute to the development of pathologies, including, for example, sexual behavior, dietary habits, and driving behavior. Studies in epidemiology indicate the role that behaviors play in contracting the spread of potentially disabling pathologies.

Health and Health Professional Sciences

The health professional disciplines are essential to understanding the dimensions of human health and assisting people with achieving health. These sciences, including medicine (physical medicine and rehabilitation), nursing (rehabilitation nursing), physical therapy, public health, exercise physiology and sports medicine, audiology, occupational therapy, speech-language pathology, audiology, and veterinary medicine, among others, are important to rehabilitation science and engineering in that they foster the development of basic and applied science relevant to rehabilitation science and engineering. Relevant and ongoing research is occurring in all these fields and in addition, biomedical engineering and rehabilitation engineering make contributions to solve problems in the area of rehabilitation. It is frequently the clinician-scientist who asks questions about pathology and impairment and the enabling and disabling processes. The non-clinician physiologist, in contrast, may be interested in a pathology only to explain a normal cellular process. The health professional disciplines are also important to rehabilitation science and engineering in that they translate theoretical knowledge in rehabilitation science and engineering into innovations in therapeutics and evaluate their effectiveness.

Veterinary science may also contribute to the knowledge of enabling processes in rehabilitation science and engineering. Animals offer companionship and, if properly trained, assistance with mobility, activities of daily living, and communication. There are many examples of animals creating a social and physical environment that limits the negative impacts of pathology and impairment on human function. Animals also offer a means of continuing exercise despite impairments or chronic disease, for example, horseback riding for people with leg paralysis or multiple sclerosis.

Uniqueness of Rehabilitation Science and Engineering

Although much knowledge of and research on pathology and impairment in rehabilitation science and engineering overlap those of basic biological, engineering, social and behavioral, and health and health professional sciences, rehabilitation science and engineering is unique in melding this research and knowledge into a conceptual matrix to address the problems of people with disabling conditions (see Table 3-2 in Chapter 3). Rehabilitation science and engineering also includes and combines variables in ways that would not occur in the separate existing sciences, for example, an epidemiological study of the association of a particular pathology (using a biological marker) with a disability (using a social role performance measurement) to evaluate the health of a population. Rehabilitation science and engineering has the potential to organize and coordinate research in the existing disciplines and to fill in gaps in research to ensure that there is an appropriate knowledge base to address disability and rehabilitation.

There is significant overlap between many existing sciences and the pathology and impairment realms of rehabilitation science and engineering, and these related sciences have the potential to meet the basic and applied research needs of rehabilitation science and engineering. The highest priorities for rehabilitation science and engineering should be to, from the rehabilitation perspective, focus, coordinate, and support currently fragmented research efforts. Researchers from many disciplines will address the questions of rehabilitation science and engineering if they are introduced to them as priorities and the work is supported.

STATE OF KNOWLEDGE FOR SELECTED MAJOR CAUSES OF PATHOLOGY IN ADULTS

Since orthopedic and musculoskeletal pathologies and impairments are those most frequently associated with the most prevalent adult activity limitations, the committee reviewed the state of knowledge in selected fields related to the control and function of the musculoskeletal system. The following sections address neural restoration and regeneration, synovial joints and soft tissue, the neuromuscular system, and skeletal muscle in terms of state of knowledge and potential for development as an area of pathology and impairment research in rehabilitation science and engineering. This material is not intended to be a comprehensive review, but rather a summary description.

Central Nervous System

The inability of the brain and spinal cord to repair and regenerate themselves is one of the most established dogmas in science. In the same way that infectious diseases were regarded as incurable a century ago, clinicians regarded with great pessimism the possibility of effective therapies for brain and spinal cord injuries. Rehabilitation research was dominated by the view not only that the brain and spinal cord are incapable of repair, growth, and reconnection, but that it was impossible to develop therapies to restore brain and spinal cord function. As a consequence, research on neurological impairments has been oriented toward assessing mechanisms of injury, epidemiology, improving outcome measures, and preventing secondary injuries and conditions.

This pessimism, however, is beginning to reverse. In the past decade, researchers have overturned the dogma that the brain and spinal cord cannot regenerate. A majority of scientists now believe that it is not a matter of if but when such therapies will become available. Neuroprotective therapies that can be given after injury are already available for spinal cord injury and are in development for traumatic brain injury and stroke. Remyelinative and other reparative treatments are being developed. Thus, the door has been open for new therapies that will have a large impact on preventing and reversing neurological impairments.

An exhaustive description of recent therapeutic advances is beyond the scope of this chapter. However, it should be noted that significant advances have been achieved for neural tissue with preventative and regenerative therapies. Preventative therapies stop the process developing from no pathology to pathology. Regenerative therapies reverse the process from pathology to impairment.

Prevention of secondary injury is one of the primary goals of rehabilitative therapy, since brain and spinal cord injuries are believed to be immediate and irreversible. Animal studies, however, have suggested for decades that some injuries can be reversed by treatments given shortly after an individual sustains an injury. In 1991, the National Acute Spinal Cord Injury Study showed that high-dose corticosteroids given to individuals within 8 hours after they sustain a spinal cord injury significantly improve their neurological recovery (Bracken et al., 1990, 1992). More than a dozen other therapies have been reported to be neuroprotective in people who have sustained acute spinal cord injuries (Nockels and Young, 1992). To identify the next generation of neuroprotective therapies, scientists are now collaborating in the first multicenter preclinical studies of promising therapies (Basso et al., in press).

Laboratory studies have revealed that several classes of therapies significantly reduce ischemic and traumatic brain injuries. One of these, the calcium (Ca^{2+}) channel blocker nimodipine, has been shown to improve neurological recovery after subarachnoid hemorrhage (Allen et al., 1983). Glutamate receptor blockers have shown substantial promise in animal studies and are beginning to be tested in clinical trials (Choi, 1992). Other treatments, including those with opiate receptor blockers and free radical scavengers, as well as hypothermia, reportedly have neuroprotective effects in individuals who have sustained ischemic and traumatic brain injuries (Dietrich, 1992; McIntosh, 1992).

The convincing evidence that the central nervous system can regenerate was reported 15 years ago when Aguayo and colleagues reported that central neurons send fibers (axons) into peripheral nerves that are inserted into the brain or spinal cord (Aguayo et al., 1981, 1983, 1990; David and Aguayo, 1981; Benfey and Aguayo, 1982). Although the axons grew long distances in the peripheral nerves, they failed to penetrate back into the central nervous system at the other end of the peripheral nerve inserted into the brain or spinal cord. Aguayo and colleagues suggested that factors in central nervous system tissues prevent growth.

In 1987, Schwab and colleagues identified two related proteins in the spinal cord (on the myelin) that appear to inhibit axonal growth (Caroni and Schwab, 1988 a,b; Caroni et al., 1988; Schwab and Caroni, 1988). Blockage of one of these proteins (neurite growth-inhibiting factor) with an antibody allowed regeneration to occur in injured rat spinal cords and improved locomotion (Bregman et al., 1995). This study established the concept that white matter-associated inhibitory proteins prevent regeneration.

Cheng, Cao, and Olsen (1996) recently used peripheral nerve bridges and a growth factor to produce functional regeneration in adult rats with fully transected spinal cords. They avoided the inhibitory factors in white matter by bridging spinal tracts from white matter (where the axon tracts are situated) to gray matter (where the neuronal cell bodies are situated). In addition, they used a growth factor called fibroblast growth factor.

Although this treatment strategy is not yet applicable to a majority of individuals who have sustained spinal cord injuries, these findings represent a strong refutation of the regeneration dogma. They further confirm the growing conviction of many scientists that regeneration is possible under some circumstances.

Several laboratories are working on alternative approaches. For example, several studies have suggested that fetal cells also provide a suitable bridging environment at the injury site. Other researchers have implanted genetically modified cells that express and secrete molecules known to support axonal growth.

Synovial Joints and Soft Tissue

The human body contains many synovial joints, which comprise capsules, ligaments, tendons, and articular cartilage. These joints vary in size and facilitate different motions to fulfill the activities of daily living. The hip, knee, ankle, shoulder, elbow, and various joints in the hand are synovial joints. Together, they act to guide articulating bones, smoothing the path of motion and reducing friction.

Much collaborative work has been done by biomedical engineers, biochemists, anatomists, and clinicians to gain a basic understanding of the function of articular cartilage, various ligaments and tendons, and the capsular structure around synovial joints. In addition, valuable gait analysis information has characterized the three-dimensional motion of joints, which act both individually and synergistically during ambulation.

Some soft tissues will heal spontaneously when they are injured, whereas others will not. Tissues that do not heal are often replaced by surgeons using autologous or allogeneic tissue grafts. Surgical treatment of soft tissue injury often requires a postoperative rehabilitation regimen of physical therapy and activity restrictions. These protocols are generally not based on scientific studies, and thus, considerable research is needed in the area of postoperative rehabilitation to define proper protocols. For example, not known are the acceptable mechanical loads for the tissues in the immediate postoperative period and how over time these loads can be adjusted as the tissue heals.

It is generally known that stress and motion are required to promote tissue healing. Without them, tissues will form contractures and joint motion will be limited. In some cases, the loss of function is permanent. Contractures are among the most difficult rehabilitation problems. Prevention of contractures requires placing a load on healing tissues, but the maximal safe load is still undefined. The type, intensity, and frequency of loading necessary to maintain the composition and properties of most nominal soft tissues can vary over a broad range. This is not the case, however, for injured or repaired tissues. It is therefore important to know how and what type of rehabilitation protocol can best maintain tissue composition properties and promote healing.

Rehabilitation of synovial joint injuries should focus on (1) regaining the range of motion and function of the joint and (2) restoring the tissue properties to those of normal tissue. To accomplish this, it is necessary to first understand normal tissue and joint function from the structural level all the way down to the molecular level. In this respect, knowledge can build on what has been learned from various biomechanical, biochemical, and molecular biology measurements of normal soft tissue. However, the knowledge base is much smaller when dealing with healing soft tissues.

For example, the anterior cruciate ligament of the knee, one of the most frequently injured ligaments, has no ability to heal once it is torn, especially if the injury falls in the midsubstance of the ligament. Clinical experience has shown that more positive results are obtained by replacement of the ligament than by repair. Popular techniques involve reconstruction with tissue grafts. However, there is a great deal of controversy regarding graft configuration, intra-articular graft positioning, initial graft tensioning, and postoperative rehabilitation protocols. Therefore, it is important that the stress and strain levels in the graft during the postoperative rehabilitation process be evaluated. With this information, the changes in graft tissue properties over time can be charted, yielding quantitative data on the maximal allowable forces and elongation in the anterior cruciate ligament graft and how they change with healing over time. This will allow for the development and optimization of rehabilitation regimens.

Articular cartilage repair is another area that has received much attention, because articular cartilage lacks the ability to repair itself. Recently, chondrocyte transplantation and various other surgical techniques have been developed to promote cartilage regeneration. The surgical procedures are controversial, and little attention has been paid to the design of postoperative rehabilitation. Yet, rehabilitation may be the key to the successful outcome of cartilage repair. Additionally, noninvasive probes need to be developed so that the pathological conditions and overall properties of the articular cartilage during the rehabilitation period can be determined.

The field of molecular biology has also contributed the idea of using various growth factors to improve the quality of healing tissues. In the proper setting, growth factors could be used as an adjunct to improve healing during the rehabilitation period. This area has a great deal of potential, and the techniques to be developed and studied include the vehicle that should have been used for growth factor delivery, types of growth factors to be used, and how the use of growth factors can be optimized to accelerate tissue repair.

It is also well documented that proprioceptive responses in the soft tissues around the synovial joints are important to injury prevention and rehabilitation. Scientific studies in this area have gained momentum in recent years, and this concept must be extended to the postoperative or postinjury rehabilitation of the soft tissues of synovial joints. Proper retraining of proprioceptive responses in injured soft tissues is critical to facilitating healing, restoring nominal kinematics and function, and preventing further injury.

Neuromuscular System

In peak performance, as exemplified in ballet, basketball, or simple ambulation, the ability of the human neuromusculoskeletal system to produce graceful, meaningful movements is one of the wonders of nature. Neuroscientists are interested in how the central nervous system controls the muscles that produce such graceful human movements. Such knowledge of the control of movement is likely to be important to understanding pathologies of the neuromuscular system. Impressive progress is being made in the motor control field by a large cadre of neuroscientists, and this progress bodes well for the future rehabilitation of people with neuromuscular disorders.

It is not enough, however, to understand the neurological control of the human motor system; the biomechanical system of the body must also be understood if there is to be a thorough understanding of the neuromuscular system. Biomechanicists have been investigating this system of muscles, tendons, ligaments, tissues, and bones almost from the time of Leonardo da Vinci and Galileo Galilei. Today the field of human biomechanics is burgeoning as never before. Throughout the world, thousands of investigators connected with fields such as biomechanical engineering, robotics, physical therapy, orthopedics, physical medicine and science, sports medicine, exercise science, limb prosthetics, orthotics, psychology, and behavioral science are working in the field of biomechanics. Some are beginning to pull together neuroscience and biomechanics, a union that is important to understanding the complete system. This multidisciplinary array of scientists, engineers, and clinicians is gaining knowledge that promises to provide not only an understanding of the complex human motor system, but also the scientific and technical knowledge required to assist impaired or nonfunctional neuromuscular systems.

Present research in neuroscience and biomechanics will enable clinicians, rehabilitation engineers, and others to provide effective assistance to people with neuromuscular impairments. This assistance may be provided through suggestions for structural modifications through surgery. On the other hand, it may be provided through suggestions for therapeutic modifications (i.e., exercise) or the use of implanted assistive technical systems such as muscle stimulators or external devices such as mechanical bracing or limb replacement. Effective replacement or artificial assistance for parts of the human neuromuscular system are some of the most challenging problems of biomedical science and engineering. Nonetheless, the possibilities have already been shown by the advances that have been made in the areas of limb prostheses, total joint replacements, and functional electrical stimulation of paralyzed muscles. The extensive and remarkable advancements in cardiac pacing provide an excellent example of what can be accomplished through human muscle stimulation. It should be remembered, however, that the advancement of cardiac pacemakers came about over a long period of time and as the result of extensive funding of a large number of investigators.

Engineers and scientists in the field of robotics research and design also have interest in the human neuromuscular system. Study of this system may assist with the design of new robotic arms or robotic walking systems. Such robotic designs might assist with obtaining an understanding of the human neuromuscular system itself, because often an understanding of simpler technical systems aids in providing an understanding of more complex biological systems.

Subtle aspects of the performance of the neuromuscular system may be observable by motion analysis equipment. Gait analysis has been helpful in providing an understanding of human and animal movement since the scientific work of Marey in France during the latter part of the 19th century and the photographic work of Muybridge in the United States at about the same time. Gait and movement analysis systems are ubiquitous today, and their use for neuromuscular investigations should be encouraged. Sensitive analysis of integrated activities such as standing, walking, and pointing may prove to be effective in the early diagnosis of movement disorders of the neuromuscular system. Measurements of this kind may also be useful in assessing the propensity for falling among people who are aging. Multidisciplinary efforts are necessary for rapid progress in these areas.

Engineering measurement equipment, coupled with knowledge of the neuromuscular systems, has the potential to quantify muscle spasticity. Quantification equipment of this kind, along with other kinds of instrumentation, will likely be important in measuring neuromuscular treatment outcomes and in monitoring patient compliance with the use of therapeutic and assistive devices supplied to assist them with their neuromuscular impairments.

Mathematical and computer modeling of the neuromuscular system can also have important impacts on understanding neuromuscular systems. Musculoskeletal models of the human arm and leg systems are already showing promise in understanding the "crouch gait" of people with spastic diplegia. Models of this nature can also be used to predict the results of surgical procedures involving muscle transfers. Likewise, biomechanical measurement equipment can assist surgeons with obtaining the precise "tone" desired in muscle transfers. Computer-aided surgery and computer-assisted surgical decision making are already prevalent in orthopedics, and their use will continue to expand.

Skeletal Muscle

Skeletal muscle is the largest tissue mass in the human body and as such, it plays a dominant role in metabolism, thermal regulation, and fluid and electrolyte balance in the human body, in addition to being the contractile tissue responsible for all voluntary movement. Skeletal muscle is also requisite for exercise and the beneficial physical and psychological effects of exercise conditioning. A considerable body of knowledge in the scientific disciplines of physiology, biophysics, anatomy, and biochemistry covers the normal physiology of muscle, including the molecular basis

of force production, muscle shortening, the intracellular cycling of calcium (transduction of chemical energy into mechanical energy), and the
steps in the excitation–contraction coupling process that transforms the
electrical signal on the muscle cell membrane into a chemical signal (Ca^{2+})
that activates the contractile proteins.

The field of skeletal muscle physiology has a long history, and much
of the definitive work has been through studies of nonmammalian, such
as amphibian, crustacean, and striated muscle. This information obtained
from studies of nonmammalian muscle is highly relevant, however, in
that the most basic structure–function relationships in skeletal muscle
hold true for species ranging from frogs to humans; even the diameters of
the cells of a skeletal muscle are in the same range in a variety of species.
What varies is the complexity of cell organization, their activation by
nerves, and the number of cell phenotypes expressed.

Interestingly, exercise physiologists have been a major force in advancing the study of mammalian tissue, and their work has been bol-
stered by the biochemists and anatomists interested in the more complex
mechanisms of mammalian tissue and seeking answers to the basis for
the different phenotypes of skeletal muscle cells in mammals, despite a
singular genotype. The normal physiology of human skeletal muscle appears to be the same as that of skeletal muscle from other mammals.

Paralysis

Any disruption of motor neuron function, in the neuromuscular junction, or in the spread of the action potential of the muscle fiber will cause
paralysis of that muscle fiber. This accounts for the skeletal muscle paralysis in individuals who have sustained spinal cord injury, in individuals with direct motor neuron or muscle trauma, or in individuals with the
disease myasthenia gravis, in whom the receptors for the chemical that
carries the signal from nerve to muscle in the neuromuscular junction
(acetylcholine receptors) are diminished by an abnormal autoimmune
process. Paralysis of skeletal muscle can have consequences beyond the
loss of voluntary limb movement. It can alter respiration, because the
diaphragm and intercostal muscles of the respiratory system are also skeletal muscles. The pelvic floor musculature is also made up of skeletal
muscle, and weakness is known to contribute to stress urinary incontinence (see Miller, Kasper, and Sampselle, 1994).

Normally, one motor neuron branches to supply a variable number of
muscle fibers within a given muscle. This organization of the motor neuron with multiple fibers is termed the *motor unit*. All of the fibers in a
motor unit are thus stimulated simultaneously and equally, and they all
respond by becoming the same phenotype. Each time the motor neuron

sends a signal to contract, each fiber in the motor unit contracts maximally in a twitch that lasts 100 to 200 milliseconds. In normal human skeletal muscles, the fiber type composition is cross-sectionally mixed, and the same type of fibers of each motor unit are distributed throughout the muscle rather than located in physical proximity to each other. Gradations in muscle force generation are achieved by activating motor units of various sizes over time (Henneman, Somjjn, and Carpenter, 1965a,b). This allows for delicate or forceful movement and for short-duration or sustained force generation. The normal compensatory mechanisms for the loss of the motor neuron in a motor unit include branching of a motor neuron from an adjacent motor unit to the denervated fiber this mechanism is operative in recovery from polio (Wiechers, 1985).

This knowledge of normal motor unit organization and function is significant to rehabilitation science and engineering, in that methods of exogenously stimulating skeletal muscle will best mimic normal movement if motor neurons are stimulated. The motor neurons in turn will activate skeletal muscle fibers in their physically distributed motor unit. This is in contrast to direct electrical stimulation of skeletal muscle by an exogenous electrode, which activates the clumps of fibers closest to the electrode and which, as a nonphysiological stimulus, can cause hypercontracture damage and pain.

Barring direct trauma, relatively few diseases are intrinsic to skeletal muscle per se. Most often these are genetic defects. If the genetic defect is severe, the animal dies at birth because it cannot sustain movement or respiration. However, because of the remarkable plasticity and compensatory processes of skeletal muscle, not all genetic defects are fatal. Duchenne muscular dystrophy is a notable example in which the gene for the structural protein dystrophin is defective or missing from a fiber and contraction causes abnormal damage to the skeletal muscle fibers. The damage increases as the developing child uses skeletal muscles to stand and walk. Attempts are being made to use genetic and molecular biological therapies to treat this disease, but they are hampered by the very large size of the gene to be transferred into the fibers and the structures of the fibers themselves.

Skeletal muscle fibers are multinucleated as a result of the fusion of mononuclear myocytes early in development. As a result, any gene replacement must occur in the many nuclei that are distributed along the length of each hairlike fiber. Some promising research on nuclei (Eppley, Kim, and Russell, 1993; Kasper and Xun, 1996) and their control in skeletal muscle fibers is in progress and will likely have relevance for gene therapies as well as growth, repair, and phenotypic determination of skeletal muscle fibers. At present the rehabilitation of individuals with pathologies and impairments such as muscular dystrophy is primarily supportive, engineered physical environments in which the individual uses assistive devices (braces, wheelchairs, etc.).

Atrophy

Atrophy of skeletal muscle is a term used to determine a complex process associated with a reduction in the size (diameter) of muscle fibers or cells. Among the changes associated with atrophy is the decline of metabolic enzyme content. Skeletal muscle may undergo atrophy from disuse secondary to many conditions. Atrophy from disuse is associated with reversible changes in the muscle fiber; however, athrophy caused by dennervation may or may not be reversible. The recovery of skeletal muscle from atrophy is an important aspect of recovery from spinal cord injury and other causes of paralysis or from bed rest with no inherent paralysis (i.e., individuals in a non-weight-bearing state). Similarly, decreased movement due to arthritic pain can lead to the secondary condition of skeletal muscle atrophy. Loss of weight-bearing activity for a period as short as days or weeks can cause significant skeletal muscle fiber atrophy and weakness, making it difficult for the person to resume standing or walking activities. Similarly, use of mechanical respirators can cause diaphragm and intercostal muscle atrophy, and may cause difficulty for people during weaning from these devices.

Some relevant and promising research related to the recovery of skeletal muscle from disuse atrophy is being conducted. Overuse, even in the form of normal weight bearing, can cause fiber damage (Kasper, White, and Maxwell, 1990); however, researchers are developing protocols that can be used to test for the degree of even initial postural use (i.e., intervals of standing before walking) of skeletal muscle while tracking recovery versus damage at the cellular and molecular levels. Skeletal muscle exercise and strengthening programs designed for people with postpolio muscular atrophy are a specific example of the use of findings from basic and applied research to understanding and monitoring use versus overuse of skeletal muscle fibers. The promising findings from this line of research is that muscle tissue remains highly plastic and adaptable well into old age (see Thompson, 1984). In addition, exercise for people with rheumatoid arthritis can result in recovery from skeletal muscle atrophy without exacerbating the joint disease (see Rall and Roubenhoff, 1996).

Future Needs

In terms of the conceptual model of rehabilitation science and engineering, basic and applied research studies of skeletal muscle need to continue and new studies should be initiated. Person-specific and social-

environmental influences that promote or discourage optimum maintenance of muscle function are significant, because optimum maintenance
will ultimately determine recovery from skeletal muscle disuse and paralysis and these influences need to be studied. Similarly, the impact of
the physical environment on skeletal muscle performance is very important and needs to be studied as well.

In summary, because of the importance of skeletal muscle tissue
and function to human performance and well-being, research on the
adaptability and usage requirements for maintaining adequate skeletal muscle strength and function is important to rehabilitation science and engineering. Research specifically related to maintenance or
recovery of skeletal muscle function for individuals with activity limitations is important as the scientific basis of rehabilitation and the
prevention of secondary conditions.

CONCLUSIONS

Based upon evaluation of the current state and relevance of knowledge in the pathology and impairment realms of rehabilitation science,
the committee determined that basic and applied research from many
sciences and engineering is essential to innovations in rehabilitation. Basic and applied research in the pathology and impairment realms is critical for the development of interventions that restore organ and cellular
function in the person and, thus, minimize the biological basis of functional limitations and disability. Basic and applied research relevant to
restoration of biological function might address repair or regeneration of
cell/organ/limb structure in the organism or might address replacement
of biological structure and function employing engineered devices. The
rehabilitation-related research in the pathology and impairment realms is
likely to employ animals and animal tissue culture models as well as
human subjects, organs, and cells.

Another significant real and potential impact of basic and applied
research in rehabilitation science is that of knowledge related to development of secondary conditions in the face of primary disabling conditions.
This knowledge is essential to the development of health strategies and
interventions as well as determining essential environmental factors that
are related and modifiable by engineering other approaches. Great
achievements in meeting the challenges of disability have emanated from
the melding of basic and applied research in the biological and engineering sciences. The committee determined that strength in basic and applied research in the pathology and impairment realms of rehabilitation
science has contributed significantly to the successful approaches in existing enabling processes and offers the promise of dramatic innovations of

the future. The new rehabilitation science offers the added benefit of integrating behavioral and social science perspectives into the pathology and impairment realms.

Given the past impact of basic and applied research in science and engineering on the advances in physical medicine and rehabilitation and on outcomes for persons with disabling conditions, the committee was surprised that the review of abstracts from the major federal funding agencies of research did not reflect an inclusion of this type of research in the portfolio identified as rehabilitation related. Only the VA portfolio reflected research utilizing animals and tissue culture subjects/cells and a balance of research activity across the research realms (pathology, impairment, functional limitations, disability) of rehabilitation science. The NIH and NIDRR portfolios of agency-identified rehabilitation-related research, reviewed as abstracts (see Appendix A), were less balanced in that pathology and impairment types of research were less prevalent and the subjects in these studies were primarily human. The committee was unable to ascertain the reason for noninclusion of basic science studies of animals, especially in the NIH portfolio.

However, the committee did feel a need to emphasize the significance of animal and basic science and engineering research and development to rehabilitation science. It also concluded that each of the research funding agencies might benefit from establishing specific research priority areas in basic science and engineering from the rehabilitation science perspective. At the very least this would help basic scientists in general to identify additional relevance of their work. It also might give impetus to basic research areas that are most likely to lead to applied advances in rehabilitation. It might also be useful to have the research review committees seeded with basic researchers who are also rehabilitation scientists, especially since part of the merit of a proposal is judged on the basis of its perceived relevance to science in general. The following recommendations of the committee reflect these suggestions to enhance the basic research activity in pathology and impairment realms of rehabilitation science.

RECOMMENDATIONS

Recommendation 4.1 Multidisciplinary research teams, including basic biological, behavioral, social, health and health professional, and engineering scientists are needed, to broaden the scope of molecular-cellular and organ-organ system research and increase its relevance to rehabilitation science and engineering. Additional funding would be needed to support these activities.

Recommendation 4.2 Based on the National Institutes of Health model, consensus panels should be used to identify areas of pathology and impairment research in rehabilitation science and engineering that are of high priority on the basis of the readiness of the knowledge of the basic science in these areas to be translated to clinical care and potential impact on quality of life and cost to society.

Recommendation 4.3 National Institutes of Health should increase the number of peer reviewers who are rehabilitation scientists on all research review committees that consider grants in the pathology and impairment realms of rehabilitation science and engineering.

5

Functional Limitations Research in Rehabilitation Science and Engineering

Although rehabilitation interventions can effectively target impairments that can be remediated, little is known about the relationship between impairment and functional limitations (Jette, 1995). This chapter reviews knowledge and research in the area of functional limitation in the context of the enabling–disabling model (see Chapter 3). In this conceptual framework, the functional limitations result from impairment, and functional limitation may result in a disability. Reduction of functional limitation from arthritis alone by only 0.5 percent per year over 50 years could reduce disability by 4 million person-years, a savings of nearly $100 billion in 1993 dollars (Boult et al., 1996). Proper measurement of functional limitations is difficult and expensive, and many clinicians are not aware of the extraordinary deficiencies that exist in the functional limitations literature. For example, the functional benefits of strengthening exercises for older people with one or more weakness-producing impairments are essentially unknown, despite the obvious appeal of such a commonsensical notion. Although intervention strategies may be offered by the clinician, valid treatment outcomes have not been reported. Strength may have a nonlinear relationship to functional locomotion, because strength changes beyond some threshold may not engender further gait improvement (Buchner and deLateur, 1991).

At the opposite extreme, however, is the obvious and well-documented relationship between impairment from a lower limb amputation and the functional restoration provided by a leg prosthesis. Just as clearly, however, impairment does not always lead to functional limitation; indeed, disfiguring dermatological impairments may cause societal disability but engender no functional limitations.

BACKGROUND

The term *impairment*, for example, describes abnormalities in specific organs or organ systems (see Chapter 4). Pain* and decrements in strength, range of motion, balance, and endurance are examples of impairments. *Functional limitations* are restrictions or lack of abilities in performance of the whole organism or individual, assessed in a manner to eliminate external environmental barriers to performance. An individual's gait and other locomotor activities as assessed in a gait laboratory are examples of functional limitations measures. As such, functional limitations reflect an attribute of the capacity of an individual. In this report *functional limitation* is used as defined and discussed by Nagi (1965) and further developed in *Disability in America* (Institute of Medicine, 1991).

Disability, in contrast to functional limitation, is a relational concept that describes any restriction or lack of ability to perform an activity in the manner or within the range considered normal for a human being. As a relational concept, disability reflects the individual's capacity to perform a task or activity necessary to achieve a role such as homemaker, worker, parent, or spouse, as well as the environmental conditions in which they are to be performed. These activities can be organized and assessed across different spheres of life. Thus, a subject's report of self-care performance (as reflected in the Sickness Impact Profile, Functional Independence Measure [FIM], Barthel, and other traditional activities of daily living [ADL] measures) is an activity, and measures of such are indicators of disability.

The link between changes in impairment and changes in functional limitation has long been assumed, but it has rarely been documented scientifically. New impairments have been shown to engender locomotor compensatory mechanisms; to date, however, no data are available to link impairments to such compensatory mechanisms in individuals with specific functional limitations or disabilities. Until this link is established, it will be impossible to discern compensatory mechanisms such as Trendelenburg gait resulting from primary disabling and functionally limiting mechanisms such as hip abductor muscle weakness or range of motion limitation.

---

*Most often, pain is considered an impairment, a result of a pathology or impairment, and a cause for functional limitation. Chronic pain, pain that persists for 3 months or longer, has implications across the enabling–disabling process, with most significant impact at the level of disability and quality of life. Thus, pain may be identified at multiple areas of the model and may be modified through a variety of interventions.

It is therefore not known at present whether rehabilitation interventions should focus on the impairment, the primary functional limitation, or the compensatory functional limitations level. Rehabilitation demands that all levels of disability be addressed. Until more functional limitations research is done, however, it will be impossible to know how much activity limitation is imposed by the environment and how much is imposed by the whole person's functional capacity.

Virtually all rehabilitation texts suggest that strength, restriction of movement, and other impairments be measured during assessments of people with disabling conditions, but the current emphasis of health maintenance organizations and preferred provider organizations on rapidly returning patients to premorbid functional status is beginning to cause this paradigm to shift. Assessments of the level of home care support available and barriers to returning to work are causing disability and functional limitations to be measured first. Once established, the clinician can work to obviate the functional limitation by addressing it directly or, in the traditional way by fixing the impairment. Little research, however, supports either approach, and many more data are needed before such methods can be proven to be scientifically sound.

Cross-Cutting Issues

Two particular issues relative to functional limitations research must be addressed: (1) measurement of functional limitations and (2) time of onset or duration of impairment and functional limitation. Both of these issues affect the research and science in this area. Measurement in functional limitations research is essential, but it is poorly developed and often costly to complete. Measurement must be standardized for the age of the person with a disabling condition. It must also be recognized that people with disabling conditions age with their disabling conditions, and aging and secondary conditions affect the functional limitation and disability of those people.

Measurement

Measuring the effects of interventions has traditionally been at the impairment level. For example, clinicians frequently measure the levels of certain substances in blood, range of motion, and change in range of motion or strength in the laboratory. As well, burden of care or disability measures of performance are often confused as representing functional capacity measures. Typical examples of these measures are the FIM, Barthel, and other traditional measures. More recently, the FIM has been more consistently utilized to determine aggregate outcomes of a program rather than individual measurement. Measuring functional capacity outcomes requires determination of the performance of the whole person. Standardized measures of functional outcomes for use in evaluation or diagnosis are being developed, but they are not routinely used to obtain outcomes measurements for specific interventions. Contextual and environmental factors, however, must be noted and controlled: frequently, there is a difference between capability (the ability to complete a task in an ideal situation) and real-life performance (the ability to complete a task in a typical situation). Such standardized measures would be important for monitoring individuals and for determination of the costs–benefits of rehabilitation programs and interventions to society. Care must be taken in using existing outcomes measures accurately, because measurement at the functional limitation level is expensive and difficult.

Functional limitations measures—obtained, for example, through gait studies and gait analysis—are few and incompletely validated. Although computerized locomotion analysis laboratories have been widely available for many years, few data support the need for gait analysis in clinical decision making, with the possible exception of presurgical decisions for children with cerebral palsy (Krebs, 1995). More studies of locomotor activities of daily living (ADL) are needed to assess functional performance pre- and postintervention and to provide descriptions of the nature of functional limitations. For example, it is known that people with balance disorders may have ataxic gait, but there is no quantitative clinical, bedside, or laboratory measure of ataxia. As a result, treatment for ataxia resulting from cerebellar lesions is entirely empiric. Measurement at the level of functional limitation requires at least whole-body, person-level measurements of performance of ADL. Such measures should include not only the gait on smooth, level surfaces but also sit-to-stand, stair ascent and descent, turning, reaching, and other locomotor ADL.

Basic ADL include locomotor ADL and bowel, bladder, and sexual functions; that is, those ADL that are usually performed without aids or instrumentation. Instrumented ADL (IADL), by contrast, include some device such as a telephone or toothbrush in the performance of a task. Thus, the adaptation (or lack thereof) of the device will affect performance capacity. For example, a child may write or brush her teeth much better with a large-diameter pencil or toothbrush than with regular devices designed for use by adults. Elderly people with impaired vision will perform as well as subjects without impaired vision if the numbers on an instrument are large and have high contrast. Functional limitations research usually attempts to obviate such IADL differences, but in practice, some standardization is required even in basic ADL. For example, stair or chair height contributes substantially to performance variation (Krebs et al., 1992). Burden-of-care measures such as the Functional Independence

Measurement usually attempt to estimate the impact of functional limitations on care providers, but they often ignore differences among IADL. As noted, these measures are disability-level measures.

Aging and Secondary Conditions

The age of onset of an impairment and the duration of impairment are recognized as important aspects of functional limitations knowledge and research. Aging must be considered in evaluating the functional status of a person with a disabling condition over time and in evaluating the appropriate interventions. Aging is a conception-to-death series of events that includes attaining, maintaining, and losing skills. Therefore, functional capacity changes with age. Growth and development affect the functional outcomes of interventions for infants and children with disabling conditions. No validated methods of discriminating between development and interventions in children with developmental disabling conditions exist.

The process of aging discriminates against no person. Everyone is a participant in the process of growing older—including people with disabilities. "Nondisabled Americans are getting older; they're living longer, there are vastly more of them, and they're getting old nonfatally. In short, they're becoming more disabled. . . . All at once, it seems, there are a lot of formerly nondisabled people around." (Corbet, 1990) In the last two decades increasing attention has been directed toward disability and aging.

In people with disabling conditions, depending on the compensatory strategies used, secondary conditions and comorbidities, can affect functional status throughout a person's life. Secondary conditions are impairments, functional limitations, disabilities, diseases, injuries or other conditions that occur during the life of a person with a disability, where the primary disabling condition is a risk factor for that secondary condition, or may alter the management of health and medical conditions. This of course is based on the new paradigm that people with disabilities are healthy, that is a disabling condition does not imply illness and disease. Each factor in the interaction of disability and aging has the capability to become a "negative feedback loop" (Guralnick, 1994) which may lead to further disability or a new medical condition.

In recent years, a body of literature regarding the effects of aging and secondary conditions has been developing. Spinal cord injury and aging is the best developed, with information available in the areas of quality of life (Evans et al., 1994), functional changes over time (Gerhart et al., 1993; Pentland and Twomey, 1994), premature and interactive effects of disability and aging (Ohry et al., 1983; Lammertse and Yarkony, 1991; Bauman and Spungen, 1994), aging and secondary conditions (Charlifue,

1993), and psychological adjustment (Krause and Crewe, 1991), among other issues. Cerebral palsy (Turk et al., 1996), spina bifida (Lollar, 1994), and polio (Maynard et al., 1991), among other disabling conditions, have also been studied.

Identification of age-related changes and secondary conditions and their risk factors has been better developed (Whiteneck et al., 1992; Charlifue, 1993; Turk et al., 1995, 1996; White, Seekins, and Gutierrez, 1996) than prevention or intervention strategies. To illustrate, Table 5-1 provides some examples in various body systems of age-related changes, potential secondary conditions, and prevention strategies for people with mobility limitations such as spinal cord injury. This provides a heuristic and practical guide for examining the interactive effects among disabling conditions, aging, and secondary conditions.

The issue of disability and aging is one more dimension that should be considered with the enabling–disabling model. As a person with a disability ages, a series of new pathologies, impairments, and functional limitations become placed over the previous pathologies, impairments, and functional limitations. Thus, the model is a snapshot in time of an individual's status in the disabling process.

Relationship Between Functional Limitations and Impairments

The committee searched Medline files to determine the quantity of peer-reviewed publications from 1966 to November 1996 addressing functional limitations. Of the 31,612 publications that used the term *rehabilitation* anywhere in the Medline file, only 34 used the term *functional limitations*.

There were 4,980 publications that included the term "function," which might better represent "functional limitations" in rehabilitation research. Yet most of these articles focused on cell or organ function rather than whole-person function. Of the 34 publications that used the term "functional limitations," only a few examined changes in functional limitation. Therefore, it can be said that there is a paucity of published reports that truly represents research in functional limitations. This is in contrast to the relatively good support for functional limitations research by federal agencies as noted in Appendix A. This apparent mismatch of publications and funded research is likely related to confusion in terminology, difficulty in tracking systems, and unknowingly mixed impairment-functional limitations identifications, interventions, and measures. Funding agencies are increasingly supporting research intending to measure functional limitations, but few reports have emanated in part because functional limitations research is expensive and difficult to conduct.

TABLE 5-1 Lifelong Motor Disabilities, Aging, and Secondary Conditions

Body System	Pathology, Impairment, or Other Conditions Leading to Potential Secondary Conditions	Potential Prevention Strategies
Skin and Subcutaneous Tissues	Insensate skin; increased areas of pressure due to poor positioning, obesity, or limited weight shifts because of cognitive, behavioral, or personal care issues; decreased elasticity or turgor in aging with top layer thinning resulting in increased susceptibility to shearing and tearing; urinary or bowel incontinence.	Regular weight shift routine; appropriate seating systems and surfaces; good nutrition and hygiene habits; social or cognitive support to follow through with prevention.
Musculoskeletal System	Decreased strength and endurance; decreased range of motion; pain; osteoporosis (must recognize hereditary and all acquired forms); asymmetric motor performance; overuse or repetitive activities on unprepared system; aging issues of decreased flexibility, strength, endurance, and balance; risk of falls; obesity.	Maintenance of exercise programs (endurance, strength, flexibility); falls avoidance practices; osteoporosis prevention or management—must determine type of osteoporosis and state of clinical/scientific information; use of proper body mechanics and posture; appropriate assistive devices utilization; environmental accessibility; consideration of ergonomically correct work and activity surroundings; use of energy conservation and joint protection techniques.
Cardiovascular System	Hypertension; atherosclerosis (similar risk factors as in nondisabled individuals); limited activity and exercise; deep venous thrombosis and resulting pulmonary emboli—more often an early complication; obesity; age-related changes of slower responsiveness to position or heart rate change.	Health practices to identify risk factors for atherosclerosis (hypertension, smoking, hypercholesterolemia or hyperlipidemia, diabetes, menopause, etc.) and initiation of prevention or management strategies; good nutrition; maintenance of exercise or activity programs.

Genitourinary System	Urinary retention or incontinence; change in urinary function from existing underlying condition (expected or unexpected progressive changes); progressive and chronic kidney filtration changes from poor or unchanged bladder management techniques; chronic urinary tract infections; kidney stones; prostate enlargement; urinary continence changes with menstrual cycle; changing urinary function from aging (e.g., reduced bladder capacity, decreased tissue compliance, reduced flow rate).	Monitoring of fluid intake and output; maintaining regular voiding schedule (e.g., intermittent cath program, use of medication, timed voiding program); achieving acceptable hygiene program; participation in regular evaluation of urinary management (e.g., urodynamics, renal scans, postvoid residual checks); reporting of urinary habit changes; consideration of surgical options when appropriate; education in the consequences of urinary management, pros and cons of suggested interventions.
Respiratory System	Compromised breathing or cough due to underlying weakness; aspiration; existing obstructive or restrictive pulmonary disease or progression; breathing changes associated with aging (e.g., loss of reserve capacity, decreased tissue compliance); obesity; progressive weakness due to underlying condition; recurrent pneumonia.	Monitoring pulmonary function as appropriate and reporting changes; cessation of smoking or contact with secondary smoke; use of assistive coughing; maintaining exercise or activity program and health diet; education of management strategies in progressive conditions; use of vaccinations when appropriate.
Gastrointestinal System	Decreased bowel motility with increased transit time; esophageal reflux; peptic ulcer disease; constipation or obstipation; megacolon; abnormal swallow function; hemorrhoids or risk for hemorrhoids with bowel program; malabsorption.	Good nutrition with diet modification (e.g., consistencies, textures, tastes); maintaining and monitoring routine bowel evacuation with consideration of fiber, fluid, and medication; review of routine medications which could contribute to decreased bowel motility; avoiding overuse of bowel medications; monitoring diet history and weights; reporting changes in bowel evacuation.

NOTE: This is not an inclusive table and serves as a practical guide only.
SOURCE: Adapted from S. W. Charlifue (1993)

FUNCTIONAL CAPACITY INDEX AND
THE 10 DIMENSIONS OF FUNCTION

As mentioned above, one of the current issues within functional limitations research is measurement and quantification of functional limitation in an individual. One proposed method of classification is embodied in the recently developed Functional Capacity Index (FCI). As a way to map out anatomic descriptions of the nature and extent of functional limitations, the FCI first defines 10 dimensions of function in which scientists can describe physical capacity (MacKenzie et al., 1996). Using the FCI as a guide to describing the different areas of research in functional limitation, this chapter reviews 10 dimensions of function: (1) locomotion, (2) hand and arm manipulation, (3) bending and lifting, (4) eating, (5) elimination, (6) sexual function, (7) visual function, (8) auditory function, (9) speech, and (10) cognitive function. The category of pain is excluded because it does not describe function but rather determines function. Thus, only to the extent that pain affects function in each of the dimensions will it be reflected in this schema. Pain can be considered an impairment, and intervention for pain is often at the organ system level. Cardiopulmonary function is not identified individually, but is felt to be included for performance of most of the functions. It should however be noted that rehabilitation science and engineering has had direct involvement in research and intervention in this area (e.g. cardiac rehabilitation, pulmonary rehabilitation, mechanical ventilation [noninvasive and invasive]). Psychosocial function is also excluded, consistent with the entire committee report.

It should be noted that much of what is reported in this section is a combination of impairment and functional limitations research, and at times consideration or recognition of disability and quality of life measures. This points out the difficulty in identification of this research realm, but as in rehabilitation science and practice, recognizes the often blurred and necessary distinctions.

Locomotion Functional Limitations

Strength Impairment Relationships to Locomotor Functional Limitations

Scant data exist on strength training among people with impairments, still fewer studies include people with functional limitations, and to date no reports relate strength changes to disability measures and locomotor activities among people with disabling conditions. "Although high-intensity training increases force-generating capacity, little is known about its effects on functional performance. Unless investigations are conducted in which different measures of functional performance are made prior to and following resistance training, the validity of this approach to improving the quality of life of older persons cannot be established" (Hopp, 1993, p. 371).

Studying only outcomes and not the mechanisms by which strength contributes to function has produced limited and contradictory results. For example, Fiatarone et al. (1990) found that frail institutionalized subjects with a mean age of 90 ± 1 years experienced highly significant strength gains (mean strength gain, 174 ± 31 percent) following an 8-week high-resistance exercise training program, but they did not measure functional locomotor benefits or the real-life role changes, if any, that resulted.

Using cardiopulmonary and musculoskeletal outcomes measures, Morey et al. (1989) reported significant improvements in endurance, strength, and flexibility following regular exercise for 49 elderly people with chronic diseases including arthritis, heart or lung disease, and diabetes. By contrast, Thompson et al. (1988) reported that 16 weeks of exercise among 22 elderly people with hypertension, chronic obstructive pulmonary disease, or osteoarthritis resulted in no changes in cardiopulmonary performance, timed tasks, balance tests, and extremity muscle performance. One of the few extant studies showing a clear relationship between isokinetic strength and objectively tested gait and locomotion variables was limited primarily to young subjects following knee arthrotomy (Krebs, 1989).

Lord and colleagues (1993) used retrospective data to suggest that strength exercises engender better balance and gait in women ages 57 and older. Gehlsen and Whaley (1990), however, reported a low correlation between balance and strength outcomes in elderly subjects divided into fallers and nonfallers. Judge et al. (1993b) reported that gait measures improved insignificantly among 31 exercising elderly subjects (mean age, 82.1 years); self-selected gait velocity improved 8 percent, but maximal gait speed increased only 4 percent. Judge and colleagues (1993a) did find that combined exercise training (resistance exercise, brisk walking, postural control, and flexibility exercises) produced improved balance outcomes compared with those from flexibility exercise training among 21 women with a mean age of 67.8 years.

No study has examined the extent to which potentially destabilizing postural compensations for weakness, such as excess abductor lurch or forward trunk rotations, are ameliorated following strength gains.

Balance Impairment Relationships to Locomotor Functional Limitations

Rehabilitation scientists have begun to study whether exercise improves impairments and performance of ADL; the important missing component that should be addressed includes the relationship of impairments and disabling conditions to compensatory mechanisms and functional limitations. Whole-body locomotor studies provide insight into postures substituted for or compensatory mechanisms for lower-limb weakness or other impairments.

One third to one half of all people over age 65 experience a fall, many of which are injurious, and most occur during locomotion (Overstall et al., 1977; Baker and Harvey, 1985; Pentland et al., 1986; Tinetti and Ginter, 1988). To date, most investigations of "balance" have investigated standing-still activities alone. Although compensating for an internal or external perturbation while trying to stand is still important, most exercise treatments have been developed in part because standing still is easily measured by timed tests or with force plates (Heitmann et al., 1989). Few facilities are capable of measuring whole-body posture and momentum during locomotor studies.

No studies have described objective changes in gait, balance, or locomotor function from exercise interventions among patients with cerebellar disorders (CbD). Rehabilitation of individuals with acute CbD has included the use of Frenkel's exercises, rhythmic stabilization (Littell, 1989), and walking aids and weights (Urbscheit, 1990; Morgan, 1975). Frenkel's exercises were the earliest exercises used to reduce lower-limb dysmetria. Frenkel's exercises can be performed in the supine, sitting, or standing position and can involve performance of slow active movements by the subject while the subject is carefully watching the extremity. Kabat described proprioceptive neuromuscular facilitation in 1955, including resistive exercises that were used to develop strength, endurance, balance, and gait (Littell, 1989). However, no systematic research studies of the efficacy of proprioceptive neuromuscular facilitation for patients with CbD have been reported. There is sparse evidence of successful treatment of chronic CbD, and it has been regarded as a condition refractive to treatment (Sage, 1984). Generally, rehabilitation intervention in individuals with chronic CbD has been restricted to substitution strategies and conservative management, such as recommending that affected individuals increase their base of support or use assistive devices (such as canes and wheelchairs) to improve stability and maintain their range of motion.

Most treatment-related publications lack adequate intervention descriptions. Balliet et al. (1987) were among the first investigators to propose neuromuscular retraining methods. They described five patients with chronic CbD and gait disorders who reacquired "proper motor control and associated balance through slow, successive adaptation to increasingly demanding conditions" (Balliet et al., 1987). All 5 individuals improved on all variables measured; however, the overall treatment duration varied from 3 months to 2 years. Brandt and colleagues (1981)

proposed similar ataxia treatment by progressively increasing body instability to activate "sensorimotor rearrangement."

To make rehabilitation science a secure and reliable science, descriptions of rehabilitative treatments are needed, as are more investigations of the benefits of such treatments to whole-body, functional
locomotor performance.

Mobility and Ambulation

Many disabling impairments involve the lower limbs. The IOM report *Disability in America* indicates that mobility limitations make up the
largest area of disability in the American population (38 percent). Because
mobility is so important to general health (physiological and psychological), it is of much significance to rehabilitation. The ability to walk can be
restored or assisted through the use of ambulation aids such as leg prostheses, leg orthoses, special shoes and shoe inserts, canes, crutches, functional electrical stimulation, and walkers. Engineering and technology,
when combined with appropriate surgical management, with appropriate prosthetics and orthotics assistance, and with proper therapy and
training will be able to advance the area of aided-ambulation at a rapid
pace. Upright mobility can be significantly improved for persons with
spinal cord injury, cerebral palsy, spina bifida, stroke, and other conditions through better engineering understanding of the biomechanics of
walking and of aided walking.

Ambulation Restoration of Mobility has been one of the big successes
of engineering in association with professionals in the fields of prosthetics
and orthotics. Today leg amputees and persons with leg impairments
ambulate with a speed and grace that was unthinkable at the end of
World War II. In the 1996 Paralympics a bilateral leg amputee ran the 100-
meter dash in 11.32 seconds. In limb prosthetics (artificial legs) and orthotics (limb and spinal bracing), biomechanics, biomaterials, materials engineering, bioelectronics, and other engineering areas are having increasing
impact on the ability of persons to ambulate efficiently. Even more impressive perhaps have been the engineering advancements made with
human joint replacements, particularly at the knee and hip. Bioengineering in combination with physicians and surgeons have had extraordinary
success in the improvement of ambulation and the relief of debilitating
pain in persons with severe arthritic joint conditions.

Future Needs and Best Strategies

Much of the locomotion literature concerning clinical evaluation has
focused on time–distance gait measures or, at best, has emphasized only

lower-extremity kinematics during gait. A number of studies have reported on differences between the gaits of young and old people that can be summarized follows: older people walk more slowly (Sudarsky, 1990). The most obvious conclusion to be drawn is that tests of exercise interventions among people with balance problems must include (although not necessarily be limited to) whole-body locomotor tests. A more subtle problem with current gait assessment is that studying lower-limb movements (kinematics) and forces (kinetics) can reveal only details of human locomotion. Hence, because most studies of the human gait have focused on these details, the few extant treatments that even address locomotor stability focus on the role of the lower extremities. The upper body's mass accounts for roughly two thirds of the total body mass, and its center of gravity (CG) is located nearly two thirds of the person's height above the ground (Winter et al., 1990). Ignoring upper-body dynamics provides at best an incomplete picture of locomotor functional limitations.

During dynamic activities such as locomotion, the body's mass must be displaced outside its support base, requiring either good muscle strength or compensatory postures. The key difference between static balance and dynamic stability is that static balance assumes the center of gravity control within the base of support, whereas dynamic stability encompasses CG control outside the base of support as well, such as in gait and stair climbing. Even standing still is not truly static; CG is in constant motion. Although the static standing impairment of excessive postural sway may contribute to a better understanding of standing balance, more research is needed to determine if static standing is related to dynamic locomotor stability. If so, then a continued focus on improving static standing may be beneficial for people with balance disorders; if static standing sway (impairment) improvements are not related to dynamic functional locomotor performance, then current impairment-level interventions should be abandoned.

More studies of whole-body locomotion during naturalistic gait, rising from a chair, climbing stairs, and other locomotor ADL should be investigated following the implementation of interventions to determine the relevance of such impairment rehabilitation to whole-person functional limitations (Krebs and Lockert, 1995).

The engineering design of technologies for aided ambulation is inhibited by lack of an effective theoretical and scientific foundation for human gait. The deep understanding of walking necessary to guide the design of ambulation technology for people who have walking impairments is still not available. The work needed to assist people with mobility limitations, whether through engineering, surgery, physical therapy, drug therapy, functional electrical stimulation, or some other approach, is handicapped by this lack of a theoretical foundation on which to base new designs.

Similarly, gait analysis studies cannot be really effective until there is a scientific paradigm that scientists and engineers can agree upon and work under. Less complex and lower-cost gait analysis instruments cannot be created until it is known what key variables should be measured. Although orthopedic surgeons have used gait analysis measurements to guide some decisions associated with the surgical management of children with cerebral palsy, the decisions could likely be much improved if a strong theoretical and scientific basis for human walking existed. It should be possible for future gait analysis data to be used in ambulation studies the way that electrocardiographic analysis is used in cardiology.

The field of orthotics has much unmet potential for ambulation assistance. There does not seem to be any technical reason why people who require orthoses cannot ambulate more rapidly, with more assurance, and with less expenditure of energy than is typical today. Improved understanding of human ambulation will enable functional electrical stimulation to be used more effectively. The orthotic field in general can be complemented with new engineering ideas and with advanced materials and fabrication techniques. Engineering and technology can improve upright ambulation of elderly people, reduce morbidity due to falls, provide better artificial limbs, walkers, and canes, and prevent foot ulcerations by creating improved footwear. In addition to restoring mobility, engineering and technology can be used to accurately measure human performance and to provide objective measurement systems for the evaluation of functional outcomes and for the evaluation of risk factors (e.g., risk of falling). In other cases, engineering contributes to mobility in another way: wheeled locomotion (see Box 5-1).

Manipulation and Physical Control

The hand is more than an unusual instrument of grasp and manipulation; it is also an important sensory organ (e.g., for touch and sensing temperature), as well as an important organ of communication (e.g., for touching, gesticulation, and making signs). The importance and the varied roles that hands play in people's lives make restoration, repair, care, or replacement of a damaged or dysfunctional hand an extremely important area of rehabilitation, that often involves psychological assistance as well as skilled surgical and rehabilitative care to maximize functional abilities.

The human hand is a complicated mechanism, and hand surgery has been one of the most successful approaches to caring for an injured or disfigured hand. Hand surgery is an advanced specialty within orthopedic surgery and involves not only hand repairs but also reconstruction of the hand to create new functional holding and grasping patterns. Recon-

BOX 5-1
Wheeled Locomotion

Body-powered, wheeled locomotion is an engineering success story of this generation. The performance of modern wheelchairs has advanced dramatically, and this advance has resulted from work by wheelchair users, research engineers, and designers in commercial companies. Wheelchair racers can now beat the best world-class runners in all races 800 meters and longer and the margin of victory increases as the length of the race gets longer. People such as these top athletes with limb paralysis, some with engineering degrees, have shown by using mobile, reliable, lightweight wheelchairs how technology can be used creatively in the lives of people with disabling conditions.

Many improvements can still be made, however. Weight can still be reduced without reducing reliability or other features. As people who use wheelchairs age, they may need lighter chairs to maintain the same level of mobility. Hybrid wheelchairs that use some body power and some electric power also have considerable potential, especially in work situations.

Comfort and prevention of secondary conditions are continuing issues with wheelchairs. Appropriate seating and positioning technologies have emerged over the last few decades for wheelchair users. These systems have improved function for the user and have helped to prevent secondary conditions due to improper positioning of the body or inappropriate tissue loading during sitting. The technology for customized seating is now highly automated, and new use of the materials and mechanisms has resulted in greatly improved seat cushions and the creation of proper seating support systems. Nevertheless, the creation of proper seating and positioning is still largely an empirical art that can be significantly enhanced through science and engineering.

Powered wheelchairs have advanced rapidly since federally funded research programs demonstrated new design possibilities and highlighted the deficiencies and limitations of the few systems that were available in the early 1970s. Nevertheless, current powered wheelchairs are often heavy and bulky and are difficult to control easily, for example, by people with high-level spinal cord injury who do not have the use of their arms, hands, or feet for control of the chair. Since powered wheelchairs are so heavy and large, they frequently require large vans for easy accommodation and are sometimes too large for small dwellings. Smaller powered wheelchairs are needed.

struction may involve transfer of toes to the hand. When coupled with good therapeutic follow-up—often by occupational therapists—remarkable rehabilitation of hand injuries can be achieved.

Amputation may be preferable when a hand is severely damaged because in the end surgery may not be successful, particularly from a functional point of view, and because over long periods of time surgical repairs can be debilitating and can keep patients from moving along with their lives. Decisions concerning amputation are almost always difficult to make and should be based on common sense, experience, consultations, and careful deliberations.

Hand surgery and hand rehabilitation are largely based on empiricism. Rehabilitation science and engineering will be able to enhance understanding of hand biomechanics, hand surgery, replacement parts, hand orthotics, and hand therapies and thereby enhance the hand and arm rehabilitation process.

Impairment Relationships to Functional Limitations

Arthritis is a common disabling pathology of the hand. Joint replacements for the fingers are still not as successful as they should be. The benefits of different kinds of physical medicine therapies for arthritis need further study.

Disabling conditions of the hand or arm system due to stroke, spinal cord injury, and brachial plexus injuries may be mediated through therapeutic techniques such as exercises, range-of-motion equipment, electrical stimulation, functional training, compensatory skill development, and splinting. Therapies should be used to keep the hand and arm supple and flexible, to avoid secondary conditions due to contractures and joint adhesions. Functional electrical stimulation is showing promise for controlling hand function in paralyzed hands following high-level spinal cord injury. Hand orthoses and orthoses for the arm can be helpful but are mostly successful only from a therapeutic (e.g., protection of joint tissues) rather than a functional viewpoint. The functional gains resulting from arm orthoses are often not great enough to compensate for the disadvantages of current arm orthoses, particularly those for the nonsensate flail limb. Arm orthoses are currently mostly of external design. It may be that internal designs based on surgical revisions, muscle transplants, electrical stimulation, and the implantation of artificial tendons (spring-like devices) could be successful, but time costs and benefits of such procedures would need to be considered closely. The disadvantages resulting from possible long periods of recuperation from surgery and rehabilitation also must be taken into account.

Environmental modifications based on good ergonomic practices and the use of protective devices can help avoid hand injuries or conditions such as carpal tunnel syndrome, arthritis, and trauma due to repetitive actions of the hand and arm during work or recreational activities. Similarly, the environment can be modified to enable dysfunctional hand to be functional through the use of lever handles on doors and on kitchen and bathroom faucets. Special tools such as devices for helping with the removal of jar lids, reachers for picking up light objects at a distance, and sliding boards in the kitchen that enable heavy objects to be safely moved from a countertop to a serving cart without heavy lifting are examples of environmental modifications. Modifications of living environments so that working surfaces are easily accessible, so that one does not have to reach for items above the shoulder level, or so that electrical outlets are available at convenient heights are ways to solve problems associated with poor hand or arm function.

Eating is important in social relationships, and being able to eat independently is a matter of dignity for many people. Consequently, the ability to eat with some degree of gracefulness and with a high degree of independence is an important ability for many people with impairments. Engineering and rehabilitation science has made a few inroads in the section of this field that is concerned with bringing food from the plate to the mouth, but much needs to be accomplished. One approach is the use of personal robots to pick up food and make it conveniently available. Another approach, when the lower limbs can be controlled, is to couple use of a leg or a foot through a linking mechanism to guide food to the area of the mouth. Both of these approaches have had limited success so far. A hybrid approach that uses some robotic features and some direct body-control features may perhaps be more practical. In any case, eating aids will likely have to be customized to the user in most cases.

Future Needs

Artificial hands, artificial arms, upper-limb orthoses, and robots that assist with rehabilitation provide the capacity for people with disabling conditions to physically manipulate unstructured environments (the kind most of people find on their desks). Artificial hands have made big strides since the 1960s. Control of paralyzed or prosthetic arms is more problematic, as is the control of robotic assistants, but progress is being made in these difficult areas of human–machine interaction. Prosthetic substitution of a hand or arm can be achieved in many ways through current prosthetics technology. Actually, replacement in the physiological sense is not possible, but it is possible to replace the missing hand–arm system with devices that are useful assistive tools for the wearers. Electrically powered prosthetic hands provide arm amputees with strong grip force and fairly rapid motion, and their external appearance has good resemblance to a natural hand. Nevertheless, they would be much more useful if their weight could be reduced by half or more, without the loss of function. Durability and high reliability need to be emphasized. Lighter-weight artificial arms should be a priority, along with lightweight orthoses. Body-powered components are still used by a majority of artificial arm users in the United States, and body-actuated systems should continually be improved. Body control through Bowden cable systems, not unlike the brake cables on bicycles, provide the user with good proprioceptive and sensory control of prosthesis usage. This kind of approach to control can also be advantageous for electrically powered prosthetic systems. The human–prosthesis interface needs to be ergonomically configured so that the user can achieve effective multifunctional control without much mental loading. Bilateral, high-level arm amputees have the most disabling upper-limb losses. Although they are few in number, their needs are great and special consideration (as with orphan drugs) and attention need to be given to the research and development of hand–arm prostheses on their behalf.

Rehabilitation of people with dysfunctional or missing upper arms is a difficult task because of the daunting engineering problems associated with arm and hand replacement or assistance, but also because of the psychological issues that greatly compound the problem. Much more research and development work is needed in the field of hand and arm rehabilitation, work that brings engineers, surgeons, physicians, and therapists together with the injured person so that problems that are priorities can be articulated and so that important problems that appear to have feasible solutions, that would be achievable within a reasonable time frame can be worked upon in a creative fashion.

Expertise needs to be increased in this area of rehabilitation engineering and occupational therapy. This expertise will lead, if not to theories, at least to general principles that can guide people with information and ideas on how to best provide eating assistance to the people who need it. Experimental technical equipment for this purpose needs to be developed and tested in close conjunction with the users, caregivers, and occupational therapists skilled in this area. The problem is somewhat similar to the provision of effective artificial arms for high-level bilateral arm amputees so that they can eat and do other thing independently. Occupational therapists have many tools and utensils with modifications that can assist people with managing foodstuffs, but these devices can be expanded and combined, where needed, with more technical devices of many sorts. Developing devices that work effectively, that are simple to use and not too expensive, that are generally small in size and aesthetically pleasing, and that can be customized for individual needs is a challenge, but one that is not impossible for science and engineering.

Bending and Lifting

Spinal dysfunction in general and back pain in particular, because they limit lifting capacity, are the leading causes of disability and result in lost workdays and restricted functioning related to the societal role. Pain as a cause of lifting functional limitations must be further delineated; most rehabilitation interventions address spinal mobility, trunk strength, and fatigue and deconditioning of peripheral muscle, as well as the cardiovascular system. For example, transporting loads and manual lifting capacity are key to manual laborers' productivity, but their supervisors also lose workdays because of back pain and an inability to transport paper file folders or to perform other light office tasks involving lifting.

Relationship of Impairment to Lifting Functional Limitations

Although few data comparing impairments and gait locomotor function are available, to date no studies have systematically reported on the relationship of specific impairments to lifting functional limitations. A definitional problem may be blamed in part: lifting capacity is an impairment-level measure of strength. Athletes in Olympic weight-lifting trials, for example, are judged solely by the total mass lifted. In people desiring rehabilitation, functional lifting capacity may be impaired by a lack of coordination, a lack of limb or spinal flexibility, a lack of movement speed, hypertension and other diseases and impairments that contraindicate Valsalva maneuvers, and pain, in addition to primary strength impairment such as that which occurs following neuropathy or muscular dystrophy. Therefore, in rehabilitation lifting impediments are considered in the context of daily activity limitations, including their restrictions on vocational and other social role functions.

Measurement of the disability caused by lifting limitations is relatively straightforward. Once the cause is defined as a lifting limitation, economic analyses of lost workdays and cost to society are quite direct (Troup, 1965). One of the major problems in determining lifting functional limitations, however, is the lack of standard, objective measures that can be applied by employers, insurers, and governments. Indeed, most employment disability eligibility determinations are performed by physicians with little or no data other than the patient's subjective complaints. Although one can take the position that reliance on the patient's assertions should be sufficient to determine eligibility for benefits, including paid time off, the experience of Scandinavian and, more recently, Polynesian social democratic societies is that such practices can prevent an equitable distribution of resources to other people with physical limitations (Moore, 1996). Hence, a "job test" that could objectively determine if the same or some less demanding job can be performed would benefit rehabilitation and society substantially. Indeed, any test that could be used to relate strength, range of motion, and other impairments to lifting functional limitations would provide an important improvement to rehabilitation strategies.

Future Needs and Best Strategies

Most prior and current research on lifting in general and back pain in particular focus on impairment and capacity measures, typically focusing on leg and back strength. Lifting style and coordination have received scant attention, probably because they require a whole-body, functional limitations level of analysis. For example, Hagen et al. (1994) reported that workers often prefer the more back-straining technique of lifting with the back because they are less metabolically costly than the correct techniques of lifting with the legs. As the lifted load increases, subjects tend to change from lifting with the legs to lifting with the back, further thwarting the advice of rehabilitation professionals (Schipplein et al., 1990). Hence, more research is needed to determine the most mechanically efficient and cost-effective means of lifting, with costs being determined for limb and spine wear and tear as well as metabolism (Luepongsak et al., in press).

Many resources have been devoted to research on the psychological factors that prevent a return to work following acute low back pain studies (Fordyce, 1995): it is now widely accepted that workers return to work if they get along well with their supervisor (Bigos et al., 1992). These psychological studies, however, typically ignore the impairment and functional limitations levels of analysis. For example, a double-blind study of chiropractic versus conventional medical care (Carey et al., 1995) reported the effects of various pathologies and impairment-level interventions on return to work and the Survey of Income and Program Participation (SIPP), but functional limitations were assessed only by asking patients "whether they had returned to their previous functional status." Hence, Carey et al. (1995) may have wrongly concluded that chiropractic care is just as effective as conventional medical care because the appropriate functional measurements were not obtained. An inability to validly quantify lifting functional limitations is an important shortcoming of the rehabilitation research arena (Vasudevan, 1992; Fordyce, 1995).

An important problem in lifting research is measuring impairments such as strength and mobility, but reporting these as if they are functional limitations measures. Functional limitations reports must include the context and environment in which the person was asked to perform the lifting. Clearly, isometrically pulling a floor-mounted cable tensiometer in a quiet laboratory is very different from lifting materials in an unpredictably busy construction site.

In summary, substantial research resources should be devoted to determining the relationship between the easily studied pathology and impairment measures of lifting capacity and the functional limitations induced under more natural, usual conditions in the workplace where lifting is performed. Objective measures that are not effort dependent and, especially, that are not dependent on the person's psychological state must be developed.

Eating

Difficulty eating is characterized by problems with chewing, swallowing, and digesting food. In traditional rehabilitation research, issues of dysphagia and drooling are notable, and these two topics are covered here. It should be noted that by this definition, the ability to eat is independent of the ability to hold and use utensils. Problems with the use of eating utensils is covered above in the section "Manipulation and Physical Control."

Impairment Relationships to Functional Limitations

Dysphagia is difficulty in eating as a result of disruption in the chewing and swallowing process. The inability to swallow without coughing or choking, and the inability to control drooling with or without eating can be caused by a variety of impairments and diagnoses. An estimated 6 million to 10 million Americans have been found to have some degree of dysphagia. It has been reported that more than 40 percent of patients in acute-care rehabilitation settings have dysphagia (Logemann, 1995).

The coordinated swallowing process is divided into three stages, and impairments can be noted at any and all three stages (Noll, Bender, and Nelson, 1996). The first phase, the oral stage, is chewing and preparation of a food bolus for transport. It requires proper oral motor structure activity for lip closure, tongue mobility, mastication muscle function, and saliva production. The pharyngeal stage is the second stage and involves food bolus transport without aspiration. More coordinated oral motor pharyngeal structures must be intact to prevent oral and nasal regurgitation, to prevent tracheal aspiration, and to allow bolus transport through the pharynx. The pharynx is a used for both deglutition and respiration. Hence, prevention of regurgitation and aspiration is of significance. The third and final stage is the esophageal phase, which completes the bolus transport to the stomach with limited gastroesophageal reflux. This stage inquires coordinated peristalsis of the esophagus and control of the esophageal sphincter.

The organization of deglutition is generally highly complex. The process requires an intact central and peripheral sensory input, a functioning coordinating center, and a subsequent motor response. Impairments at any stage from mechanical or neuromusculoskeletal disorders, and with consideration of age and state of development, can result in an eating functional limitation. Dysphagia can result from congenital or acquired central neurological disorders (e.g., stroke, cerebral palsy, traumatic brain injury, or polio), treatment for head and neck cancer, progressive neurologic diseases (e.g., Parkinson's disease, myasthenia gravis, motor neuron disease, multiple sclerosis), or systemic diseases (e.g., scleroderma or dermatomyositis).

Drooling is an inability to manage secretions. This problem involves impairment at the oral stage and as in dysphagia, requires a certain level of cognitive function. Drooling can often be seen in individuals with cerebral palsy, traumatic brain injury, stroke, and mental retardation. Often, an association between drooling and dysphagia is found.

Current Status of Science and Research

The majority of research has been in documentation of the impairment, visualization of treatment strategies, and case reports or case series identifying the problem or evaluating interventions. Logemann has contributed significantly to this body of literature (Logemann, 1983).

Technical assessment of dysphagia has progressed considerably with this research. Visualization techniques have allowed investigators to have a better appreciation of the phases of swallowing and has allowed knowledge related to pathology and impairment to progress. Videofluoroscopy of swallowing (modified barium swallow study) has become the diagnostic tool of choice (Splaingard et al., 1988). The procedure has been standardized and individualized (DePippo et al., 1992; Gray et al., 1989), and seating issues for the study have also been addressed (Cameron and Guy, 1990). Other imaging techniques have been explored (Holt et al., 1990; Langmore et al., 1991; Silver et al., 1991; Schima et al., 1992). Positional or textural intervention strategies are also viewed by videofluoroscopy to determine success (Johnson et al., 1992; Rasley et al., 1993).

Dysphagia in people with specific disorders has been better described. Dysphagia in individuals with cerebral palsy, stroke, and brain injury have been studied the most. Dysphagia in people who have had a stroke has been reported to be as high at 30 to 45 percent (Horner et al., 1990; Teasell et al., 1993). The occurrence of dysphagia in individuals who experienced a brain injury is reported to be about 27 percent, and cognitive impairment is often the most significant factor (Winstein, 1983). Children with cerebral palsy often require treatment programs that address tonal abnormalities, postural control, adverse behavior, and primitive reflexes, along with the specific oral motor dysfunctions (Morris, 1989; Morton, 1993). Aspiration pneumonia and malnutrition are common secondary conditions associated with dysphagia (Sitzmann, 1990; Martin et al., 1994).

Review of interventions include compensatory strategies, direct treatment strategies, and surgery, which often result in reduced aspiration and pneumonia, improved nutrition, and improved quality of life and socialization (Logemann, 1995). Compensatory strategies such

as postural techniques of head turning or body positioning can eliminate aspiration of thin liquids in about 75 to 80 percent of people with
dysphagia (Logemann, 1983). Exercises designed to facilitate oral
motor strength and coordination, to facilitate a swallow reflex, and to
desensitize oral structures have been described, but with limited supporting research (Braddom, 1996). Surgical interventions are focused
and individualized; other than those have received tracheostomies,
few individuals who have received surgical interventions have been
studied and generalization is difficult (Baredes, 1988; Lindgren and
Ekberg, 1990).

Interventions for drooling include oral motor exercises, behavior
modification programs, medications, and surgery. Case series and controlled studies are at the base of the research. Behavior modification programs require reenforcement. Medications with anticholinergic properties have been helpful, but not universally.

Future Needs

More rigorous research is needed to determine the effectiveness of
interventions for dysphagia and drooling. In particular, exercise and direct feeding techniques need to be evaluated in a controlled manner and
over an extended period to determine their efficacy.

Videofluoroscopy is used diagnostically, and in some cases periodically, for ongoing evaluation but standardized interpretation is lacking.
The indications for its use initially and for periodic follow-up have not
been determined. In addition, individuals with acute and chronic conditions may have different requirements.

Issues of cost-effectiveness for diagnostic testing and interventions
have not been defined. Suggestions of cost-containment are based on pro-
jections and limited hospital costs. Standardized outcomes measures regarding functional limitations are needed for better comparison of different studies and different interventions. Finally, research is needed to
determine the impact of different interventions on disability and quality
of life, particularly over a lifetime.

Elimination

Bladder

A pathology of the central or peripheral nervous system's supply to
the bladder may result in a neuropathic bladder or, as it is more commonly termed, a neurogenic bladder. The neurogenic bladder has partial
or total loss of normal function (impairment), which may be caused by

different types of pathology such as spinal cord injury, stroke, multiple sclerosis, or a tumor.

Micturition or voiding requires fine coordination between the bladder and the urethral sphincter such that bladder contraction is associated with urethral sphincter relaxation. Any pathological process that causes a neurogenic bladder may result in the following problems or functional limitations: (1) the inability to void voluntarily, (2) the inability to empty the bladder completely with voiding, (3) the inability to remain continent of urine between voids, (4) the inability to sense bladder fullness, and (5) the inability to inhibit the urge to void.

Bladder Impairment Relationships to Functional Limitations Urinary incontinence (UI) affects approximately 13 million Americans and 30 percent of those over age 60. Estimates of the cost of managing this problem are $15 billion annually (Agency for Health Care Policy and Research, 1996). The etiologies of UI vary. Although much research on the best methods for treatment has been conducted, less is known about the relationships of UI to functional limitation or disability. In one of the few studies to address the impact of UI on function, McDowell et al. (1996) described the characteristics of UI in 90 homebound adults over 60 years of age with good cognitive skills. The subjects had a mean age of 75.8 years and reported a mean of 8.4 medical problems, and 80 percent had functional limitations in ambulation. Eighty were women and 10 were men. The majority (73.3 percent) had more than 10 episodes of UI per week. About half (54.4 percent) reported that UI further restricted their activities, and 52.2 percent reported that UI was extremely disturbing. However, 90.5 percent believed that UI could be treated.

Most studies of interventions for UI do not use a functional outcomes measure to determine success but often count the number of pads used, the number of leakage episodes, or the amount of leakage. Geriatric patients with urge incontinence lose different amounts of urine and respond differently to pharmacological treatments. Some of the factors that predict the severity of UI are underperfusion of the cerebral cortex, reduced bladder sensation, and impaired orientation (Griffiths et al., 1996). In a descriptive study, 251 consecutive geriatric patients admitted into a geriatric rehabilitation unit received medications and teaching about medication during each daytime administration of medication by nurses. The authors reported a decrease in the incidences of UI and urinary retention and an increase in the level of knowledge about medication regimens (Resnick et al., 1996).

Complicating matters is a trend to avoid seeking health care for such problems. Talbot and Cox (1995) examined 117 adults ages 58 to 93 who were mentally competent, not confined to bed, and residing in the community. The subjects were divided into three groups: those with dysfunctional continence (ineffective coping mechanisms; 28.2 percent), those with functional continence (effective coping; 32.5 percent), and those with UI (39.2 percent). Coping methods were determined with a four-point Likert-like scale. A total of 73 to 85 percent of the groups with dysfunctional continence and actual UI never talked to any health care provider about their UI-related concerns.

Many older adults with UI or other problems of bladder control are deterred from seeking treatment by factors such as social disapproval and a belief that bladder symptoms are normal or untreatable (Umlauf et al., 1996). Elderly people who experience loss of bladder or bowel control are frequently depressed, isolated, and fearful of being discovered. Left untreated, these individuals are prone to mental and social deterioration that may lead to social isolation or institutionalization (Gray et al., 1996).

Quality of Life and Urinary Incontinence A few studies have begun to examine the issue of quality of life and UI. In one study pelvic floor electrical stimulation therapy daily or every other day was effective in treating genuine stress incontinence. No differences in leakage episodes, pad count, leakage amount, subject subjective assessment, and quality of life were found comparing daily and every other day electrucak stimulation (Richardson et al., 1996).

A self-report quality-of-life measure specific to urinary incontinence (I-QOL) was developed and tested for its validity and reproducibility with a group of 62 people with UI (Wagner et al., 1996). The I-QOL, developed as an outcome measure for clinical trials and patient care, was compared with measures of psychological well-being and functional status (Short Form 36-Item Health Survey). The I-QOL was more sensitive at detecting levels of self-perceived UI severity than either the psychological general well-being or the Short Form 36-Item Health Survey).

Jackson et al. (1996) developed the Bristol Female Lower Urinary Tract Symptoms questionnaire that is sensitive to changes in the symptomatology of the female lower urinary tract, particularly UI, providing an instrument that can characterize symptom severity and effect on quality of life, and that can evaluate treatment outcome.

Functional Limitations and Disabilities The function of the bladder should be viewed from the total aspect of the person's ability to function in the society in which he or she lives (Cardenas, 1992). The expectations of society are that older children and adults can maintain continence and empty the bladder at acceptable intervals, usually not more than once in 3 to 4 hours. Certain working conditions are less conducive to frequent voiding, for example, truck driving and assembly line work. People with neurogenic bladders who must void frequently, even if they are ambulatory, might become disabled in such a job setting. In other job settings toilet facilities may not be wheelchair accessible. The most obvious examples are portable toilets at construction sites, but even some office buildings have minimal or no wheelchair-accessible bathrooms. The person with a neurogenic bladder who is unable to void and performs intermittent catheterization, one of the preferred methods of drainage from a health perspective, is often using a wheelchair for mobility and thus needs access to an adequately constructed wheelchair-accessible bathroom. If the job site or office building does not offer a wheelchair-accessible toilet, such people also become disabled because of a nonaccommodating environment.

Another alternative to bladder emptying used by some people with neurogenic bladders is an external or an internal indwelling catheter that is connected by a tube to a plastic receptacle (leg bag). Even with such a system, emptying the plastic bag is necessary after several hours of filling. Again, a wheelchair-accessible toilet is needed or the person will likely become disabled.

The following case report exemplifies the predicament of people with disabling conditions. A young man with a spinal cord injury that resulted in paralysis of most of the muscles of his arms and all of his trunk and leg muscles was hired at a bank in an urban community. The bank building did not have a wheelchair-accessible toilet, and the young man managed his neurogenic bladder by performing intermittent catheterization every 6 hours. He was forced to go to his wheelchair-accessible vehicle, a van, in the parking lot each midday to perform intermittent catheterization. As society complies with the legal mandates established under the Americans with Disabilities Act of 1990, increased physical access will allow people with disabling conditions to live and work in environments that allow their full participation.

Related Secondary Conditions More than 1 million nosocomial (hospital-acquired) urinary tract infections occur each year in the United States (Haley et al., 1985), and about half of these originate in the urinary tract in association with urinary catheters and other drainage devices (Kunin, 1994). Although no randomized comparative trials have been performed to determine the relative risks of indwelling catheterization, intermittent catheterization, and condom catheterization in predisposing patients to urinary tract infections, there is a general consensus that the greatest risk is with the use of indwelling catheterization (Cardenas and Hooton, 1995). Most studies on the urinary tract have not been conducted with patients with neurogenic bladders. Long-term complications of neurogenic bladders also have not received much attention. It is known, however, that the incidence of renal failure as the cause of death in individuals with spinal cord injuries has been reduced during the past two decades and that during this period intermittent catheterization replaced indwelling catheters as the major mode of bladder management. Other changes in the treatment of spinal cord injury have also occurred, however, including the introduction of newer antibiotics and formalized systems of rehabilitative care and follow-up. Physiological urinary tract changes over time have received minimal attention. A recent cross-sectional study showed that bladder pressures were lower in those who use intermittent catheterization with a longer duration of spinal cord injury, regardless of age (Cardenas and Mayo, 1995). Adequate longitudinal studies determining the effects of both aging and the duration of impairment of the bladder have not been performed. The roles of health beliefs, nutrition, and hygiene have received minimal attention in the research literature on the prevention of urinary tract infection in patients with neurogenic bladders.

Future Needs Research is needed not only to determine optimal strategies for bladder management but also to determine the educational needs of primary care providers in the appropriate management of urinary tract infections in those with neurogenic bladders. Research is also needed to determine the optimal duration of antimicrobial treatment of urinary tract infections in the person with a neurogenic bladder.

Longitudinal studies are needed to determine the long-term consequences of asymptomatic bacteriuria for the neurogenic bladder. Funded workshops are needed to train urologists in the state-of-the-art surgical options that may reduce the functional losses of the bladder, such as electrode implantation. New stimulation methods and approaches for the control of micturition and defecation are making bowel and bladder continence practical for persons with spinal cord injury and other pathologies. Dramatic advances are possible and should be pursued. Research is needed to determine the best prevention strategies for complications associated with a neurogenic bladder. Such secondary conditions include urinary tract infections; stones in the kidneys, ureters, or bladder; and renal insufficiency. Research on methods for changing the role expectations of employers and others toward the person with a neurogenic bladder, and on newer pharmacological agents or other treatments that can improve bladder functioning, including UI is also needed.

New electrical stimulation methods and approaches for the control of micturition and defecation are making bowel and bladder continence practical for people who have sustained spinal cord injuries and those with other pathologies. Investigators have devised technical stimulation methods that can stimulate small nerve fibers before they stimulate the large nerve fibers. This stimulation approach, along with other techniques, promises to provide dramatic advances in the voluntary control of micturition and defecation through the use of implants and small external technical apparatuses. Engineering and medicine appear to be on the brink of making significant practical advances with these technologies. These potentially major breakthroughs may dramatically alter the future care of people with bladder and bowel control problems.

Bowel

Functional Limitations The normal function of the bowel, like the bladder, may be altered by various types of pathologies, especially those that cause primary damage to the central nervous system and autonomic nervous system. This can result in the loss of the urge to defecate or an inability to inhibit a bowel movement. The impairment is the loss of normal bowel function, whereas the functional limitation relates to the possible loss of the normal ability to sit for prolonged periods of time without a potential "bowel accident," to loss of the ability to travel, and to a loss of potential cleanliness and personal hygiene.

An uncontrolled bowel movement with fecal incontinence may lead to loss of employment. The expectation of society is that older children and adults will not have fecal incontinence or soiling that can produce odor and lead to leaving the job task at hand to clean up and change clothing, tasks with which a person with a neurogenic bowel may require assistance. The person with a neurogenic bowel who has difficulty controlling "bowel accidents" may thus have a disability.

Historically, occupational therapists have worked with clients, their families, and caregivers to facilitate use of the bathroom and toilet for elimination of wastes and bathing, washing, brushing, shaving, etc. As with systems for assistance with eating, bathrooms must be customized for people with disabling conditions, their families, and their assistants. Again, as with eating assistance, there is a need to develop principles of bathroom treatments, if not theories, that will help guide families, architects, carpenters, and plumbers in creating customized facilities that make ergonomic sense, that can be altered as the level of disability increases or decreases, and that are compatible for use by other members of the family (universal design). Sensitivity needs to be given to issues of privacy. Independence of use needs to be maximized where possible. Engineers, architects, therapists, and others need to give more attention to the bathroom and toilet needs of persons with disabling conditions, particularly those people with significant disabling conditions.

Current Status of Science and Research No data are available on methods for changing the role expectations of employers or others toward people with functional limitations as a result of a neurogenic bowel. Minimal research regarding optimizing bowel management for avoiding fecal incontinence exists, although much clinical experience has provided good bowel care for many.

Future Needs Methods for reducing the time necessary for adequate bowel evacuation need further study. More research is needed on methods of triggering defecation, such as electrodefecation by sacral root stimulation. Additionally, research is needed to empirically examine the long-term effects of aging with a disability in noninstitutional settings, and how to maintain maximal bowel function over the lifespan. Research is also needed on methods for changing the role expectations of employers and others toward the person with a neurogenic bowel.

Sexual Functioning

Functional Limitations

Sexual functioning is an important aspect of human life and well-being. Impairment of sexual functioning may result from disease processes that alter neurological, vascular, or endocrine function such as spinal cord injury, multiple sclerosis, atherosclerosis, and diabetes mellitus, as well as from mental disorders and even common medications used to treat numerous conditions. Sexual functioning encompasses arousal, lubrication, erection, ejaculation, and orgasm. Sexual functioning involves reflex (neurogenic), hormonal, and psychogenic mechanisms that have not been completely described for humans with or without dysfunction. Loss of genital sensation or loss of motor input to the genitalia can result in severe loss of sexual function.

Functional limitations in sexual functioning involve (1) the inability to become aroused or lubricated, (2) the inability to develop adequate erections, (3) the inability to ejaculate, and (4) the inability to experience orgasm.

Loss of erectile function can be treated with various technologies, but not always successfully. Some men do not accept artificial methods for achieving an erection. Others are unable to afford treatment, which is not funded by many health plans. Owing to the role expectations of sexual functioning in marital or intimate relationships, the loss of erectile functioning may result in a disability. The same can be said for the loss of ejaculation, which affects not only sexual functioning but also the ability to procreate naturally. Again, technological advances such as electro-ejaculation are not always available or affordable.

Current Status of Science and Research

Research into sexual functioning related to neurogenic or vascular causes has focused primarily on men. For example, estimates of the incidence of erection after spinal cord injury have been determined for individuals with complete injuries according to the level of injury, but the incidence has not been determined for individuals with incomplete injuries. Testicular biopsies have revealed a high incidence of abnormalities of spermatogenesis in those with spinal cord injuries. Pregnancy and delivery may be associated with certain risks such as autonomic dysreflexia in women with spinal cord disorders, but with appropriate obstetrical care, minimal increased morbidity to the mother or baby her infant is achievable (Baker et al., 1992). Orgasm is less well studied than erection, lubrication, or ejaculation. The subjective experience of orgasm is paralleled by certain physiological changes, but measuring these changes has not received much attention in those with a loss of sensation such as may occur after spinal cord injury.

Future Needs

Psychological factors such as stress and anxiety as well as medications can affect all aspects of sexual functioning, but the disability that results is not well documented.

More research is needed on sexual functioning in women with impairments, such as loss of genital sensation, and research is needed to determine the educational needs of obstetricians and family practitioners caring for pregnant women with spinal cord dysfunction. More research is needed to determine the causes of abnormal spermatogenesis and methods for improving spermatogenesis.

Vision

Relationship of Impairment and Functional Limitation

Vision, the most developed sense in humans, provides people with most of their knowledge of the external world (Zeki, 1993). The visual system allows for the visualization of detail (acuity), color, form, movement, depth, and contrast (Livingstone and Hubel, 1987) and contributes to a capacity to attend to tasks of daily living. The visual system is complex and includes numerous structures, from those that receive stimuli from the environment (e.g., the cornea, lens, aqueous humor, and retina) to the areas of the brain where visual function becomes specialized at interpreting and combining stimuli (e.g., the retina, lateral geniculate nucleus, superior colliculus, and the various areas of the visual cortex). Maturation problems, diseases, and injury can cause functional limitations of low vision or blindness. Common impairments are cataracts, macular degeneration, which results in the gradual loss of central vision, and glaucoma, which results in loss of peripheral vision. These impairments often result in disability when they affect driving, reading, taking medications, and walking.

The higher areas of visual performance, the P pathway and the M pathway, can also be affected by disease (dementia of the Alzheimer's disease-associated type and Parkinson's disease), lesions (stroke or trauma), or aging. Insults to the visual pathways can cause the slowing of information processing. The functional impairments that result are impaired depth perception, contrast sensitivity, movement detection, and form recognition. The perception of depth is a complex process involving the unconscious interpretation of multiple visual cues and physiological responses. The primary visual cues are all binocular in nature, meaning that they require the use of both eyes to be effective. One of the most important binocular cues is known as stereopsis. In stereopsis, a phenomenon called binocular disparity occurs, which is a direct result of having two eyes separated horizontally on the head (DeAngelis et al., 1991). The loss of stereopsis can result in falls due to misjudging short distances between objects (e.g., steps) and vehicle accidents (e.g., errors in parking, merging, stopping, and turning across traffic). Loss of these visual processes may contribute to personal-injury accidents. When depth perception is adversely affected by poor lighting, lack of color or visual contrast, or deceptive visual patterns, depth cues send the brain erroneous information about one's immediate environment, and then a loss of function can occur.

Another functional limitation is contrast sensitivity, which is a function of the M pathway and which is the difference in light intensity between an object and its immediate surroundings. People with impaired contrast sensitivity cannot see objects in their environment, and it is believed to be a cause of vehicle accidents. Gunsburg et al. (1982) found that pilots who saw an obstacle from the greatest distances were those who had the highest contrast sensitivities. Pilots who had to get close to the obstacle before seeing it had the lowest contrast sensitivities. People with multiple sclerosis, a disease that attacks the insulation on nerve fibers, complain that the world appears "washed out." Presumably, this washed-out appearance of the world is related to the nervous system's diminished capacity to code contrast.

Movement detection helps with sight. For example, one may not notice an insect on the wall until it starts to move. Movement can also provide information about form. Motion serves several different perceptual purposes, including detection, segregation of an object from its background, and definition of an object's shape. The brain sees form before it sees detail. Research shows that types of dyslexia may result from the inability to see form before detail; also, some types of dyslexia result from an individual's inability to detect movement patterns (Frith and Frith, 1996). Parkinson's disease offers insight into how these impaired visual processes affect performance. Hunt et al. (1995) reviewed how Parkinson's disease impairs vision and, consequently, function in reading, balance, driving, and socializing.

Vision: Technical Aids and Advances

Computers and other technologies now enable machines to read printed text and to turn it into speech with considerable ease. Electronic text is easily converted into voice or braille output at reasonable speeds and at reasonable cost. Interfaces for graphical information such as that found on the Internet are being developed. Modern communications systems help facilitate safe travel by people without vision and future geographical positioning systems may be able to provide these people with highly accurate positioning and orientation information. Many technologies such as video magnification and other aids are benefiting persons with partial sight. Restoration of human vision through technical and biological means remains a long-range possibility.

Rehabilitation science and engineering has much potential to assist in the further development of technical aids for people with low vision or blindness. If the science and engineering can be carried out in close proximity to rehabilitation centers for blind people and in close proximity to blind and partially sighted people and their caregivers, the potential for major practical advances is enhanced.

Future Needs

The mechanisms of vision are beginning to be understood. How visual impairments relate to disability and the strategies used to support recovery in individuals with neurological damage provide challenges to rehabilitation scientists. Visual impairments can complicate assessment and rehabilitation. The process of learning required for recovery is best accomplished by a person with good visual and visual processing skills. Visual perception problems are prevalent in people with neurological damage. Vision scientists are not normally involved in the rehabilitation process, so that there is a gap between rehabilitation and vision scientists. This gap should be filled by multidisciplinary research that could lead to improvements in rehabilitation outcomes and in the quality of life for people with functional impairments that, in the absence of proven intervention strategies, have limitations that lead to disability.

Research needs to be done to gain an understanding of how damage to the visual pathways affects disability. This may help in the development of visual training programs, behavioral strategies, and environmental adaptations that can contribute to the optimal functioning of individuals with disabling conditions that otherwise may be ignored.

Hearing

Relationship of Impairment and Functional Limitation

The sense of hearing is used primarily for communication, for localizing sounds in the environment, and for aesthetic purposes such as the enjoyment of music. For most people, the communication function is by far the most important for carrying out the everyday activities of life. The ability to talk relies on auditory capability (Newby and Popelka, 1992) in concert with the capacity for language (Gleason, 1985) and the ability to produce speech sounds (Hegde, 1995). This ability develops naturally and functions effectively when the auditory system, a speech production system, and a central nervous system capable of language are in place at birth. Furthermore, the communication ability will be sustained if these separate systems remain functional throughout life. Thus, the auditory system plays a substantial role in the development and maintenance of the communication ability after oral language and speech abilities have developed.

An impairment of the auditory function affects the communication ability in ways that depend on the magnitude of the hearing loss, when the hearing impairment occurred in relation to the individual's stage of language and speech development, and the portion of the auditory system that is affected. A significant auditory impairment that is present at birth or that occurs before language and speech ability have begun to develop can interfere with the development of language and speech and may affect the ability to communicate. This type of hearing impairment has been termed *perilingual* and can result in a hearing disability that substantially affects oral communication ability. However, those with prelingual hearing impairments can learn to communicate effectively through the use of sign language. Neither their communication abilities nor their other academic abilities need be affected. In fact, "baby talk" in deaf children raised by signing parents will begin earlier than will baby talk in hearing babies. The key factor here is that early and consistent exposure to signing, lipreading, and speaking can be taught as successfully later as earlier, but linguistic ability will be lost if accessible language is not provided during critical developmental periods.

A significant hearing impairment sustained in later life, after language and speech abilities have developed fully, is termed a *postlingual hearing impairment*. This type of hearing impairment does not affect the development of language and speech but can affect the ability to communicate, resulting from an inability to perceive speech correctly. A significant hearing impairment that occurs at a point during speech and language development, termed perilingual, can result in a disability with some characteristics of both pre- and postlingual hearing impairments.

The peripheral auditory system consists of a right and a left side and includes the external ear and a variety of internal structures that process auditory information and send it to the brain. Some of these peripheral structures optimize sensitivity to sounds; that is, they increase the ability of the ear to hear the quietest sounds. Other peripheral auditory structures optimize sound discrimination, which is the ability of the ear to discriminate among different sounds. A peripheral auditory impairment often reduces hearing sensitivity so that sounds may not even be heard. A peripheral auditory impairment also can reduce the ability to discriminate sounds so that, for example, the "t" sound cannot be discriminated from the "d" sound in speech, even if the speech sounds are intense enough to be detected. Virtually all peripheral hearing impairments result in some degree of hearing loss, that is, a reduction in hearing sensitivity, and as a result, sounds must be made more intense for the individual to detect them. In many cases, the peripheral hearing impairment also results in a decrement in the ability to discriminate sounds, so that even if the sounds are made intense enough to be detected, they are still not perceived correctly.

Deficits of central nervous system function that do not involve the peripheral auditory system also may affect auditory capability, particularly regarding the ability to understand speech (Katz, 1994). A head injury or stroke usually does not cause a peripheral hearing loss, but may impair the communication ability related to deficits in the auditory processing capability in the central nervous system. Auditory processing associated with the auditory portions of the central nervous system generally does not include auditory sensitivity or simple sound discrimination, but it does involve more complex processing such as the ability to separate or integrate auditory input from both ears, interpret timing effects such as the temporal order or sequence of auditory sounds, separate speech sounds from background noise, and other kinds of processing that may interact with language functions and even learning and memory.

Hearing loss is defined in terms of hearing sensitivity for particular pitches in each ear and the average hearing sensitivity for speech categorized in increments ranging from mild to profound. Hearing loss is further defined in terms of the ability to understand speech including speech that is amplified enough to overcome the hearing loss and be detected. The disability resulting from the hearing loss involves a consideration of the magnitude of the hearing loss, the measured decrement in speech discrimination ability if any, and many other factors including when the hearing loss was sustained (pre-, peri-, or postlingual), whether or not both ears were affected, and the types of sounds most important to the individual (speech, music, etc.) (Newby and Popelka, 1992). A person with a profound, bilateral, perilingual hearing loss who relies on sign language may not have any disability related to the hearing loss because of his or her reliance on a communication system that does not require auditory function. A person with a severe, bilateral, postlingual hearing loss may be significantly disabled as a result of difficulties in perceiving speech at normal conversational levels. A professional musician with a very mild hearing loss in one ear that may not affect communication ability but that may still reduce the ability to play a musical instrument may be considered substantially disabled.

Some hearing impairments are the result of transient diseases or are able to be corrected with medical or surgical intervention. If the surgical or medical intervention is successful and is invoked as soon as possible after the hearing impairment has been identified, the hearing impairment usually will have no long-term effect on the auditory capability. If, however, the medical or surgical intervention is ineffective or such an intervention is impossible for various reasons, the hearing impairment can be considered permanent and can affect the auditory ability. For people with permanent hearing impairments, rehabilitative strategies other than medical or surgical intervention can help ameliorate the effect of the hearing impairment. If the hearing impairment is severe enough and if it is pre- or perilingual, the educational setting itself is a consideration. Schools for people who are deaf use teaching techniques that foster the development of oral language and speech (oralism), sign language (manualism), or a combination of both (total communication) (Northern and Downs, 1991). These schools teach language and communication ability simultaneously with traditional elementary school subjects; however, those that emphasize oral skills spend a disproportionate amount of time teaching those skills.

For children with auditory impairments who rely on oralism for the development of language and speech or for adults with postlingual hearing impairments whose language and speech skills have already been developed, a variety of technologies are available to assist the impaired auditory system. The first of these is a conventional hearing aid. A hearing aid is a small, portable, battery-operated device worn in the impaired ear. The device has the capability of amplifying sounds in the environment so that they are intense enough to be detected. Furthermore, the hearing aid may be adjusted so that some pitches are amplified more than others and so that the hearing aid is tailored to the specific hearing loss, resulting in some improvement in sound discrimination ability. The use of hearing aids can be a very effective rehabilitation strategy, especially for individuals with mild, moderate hearing impairments and combined with rehabilitation strategies that capitalize on the visual perception of speech (lipreading).

For some individuals with hearing impairments, a cochlear implant may be an effective option. A cochlear implant is a small, portable, battery-operated device much like a hearing aid, but instead of providing more intense sounds, it electrically activates the remaining auditory nerve fibers over wires surgically implanted in the inner ear. A cochlear implant may allow more severely hearing impaired individuals to detect sounds in the environment and, if multiple wires have been implanted, to achieve some degree of sound discrimination ability through the perception of multiple channels of sound information. A comprehensive rehabilitation program that incorporates a cochlear implant may be able to enhance speech development in people with perilingual impairments and to enhance oral communication ability for those with pre-, or postlingual impairments. However, the evidence about cochlear implants remains controversial. It must also be noted that some members of the deaf community feel very strongly that cochlear implants are not needed, especially among children, for whom signing can provide an optimal, comprehensive, and noninvasive communication technique, while others believe that speech production is enhanced by cochlear implants, even in the prelingual deaf.

Much of the available technology can enhance a person's communication ability by using modes that completely bypass the impaired auditory system. Alarm systems such as smoke detectors, fire alarms, door bells, and alarm clocks can be modified to emit signals that can be detected by other senses such as vision (flashing lights) or touch (vibrators). Other technologies permit the simultaneous display of speech as text in closed-captioned television, and telecommunications devices for the deaf display telephone voices as text.

Environments can be restrictive in their accessibility for people with hearing losses, and technology or policies can be invoked to improve accessibility. In larger venues (theaters, churches, stadia, lecture halls, classrooms, etc.) a microphone (lapel microphone worn by the lecturer, classroom teacher, or performer) can be positioned to pick up the acoustic signals of interest and transmit the signals wirelessly to special earphone devices or personal hearing aids worn by the people in the audience with hearing losses. Captioning can be provided in real time for situations in which closed captioning is unavailable or not able to be prepared ahead of time. Public telephones can have amplifiers, hearing aid compatibility, or companion telecommunication devices for people who are deaf. Interpreters for both oral and manual communication can be provided in other situations. Strategies for enhancing visual communication, including lighting and seating positions, may be used.

An auditory impairment can greatly complicate assessment and rehabilitation of other physical impairments. Assessments of cognitive or receptive language ability following a stroke may be based on hearing-based tasks that usually assume that the auditory system is healthy. This is a tenuous assumption because of possible preexisting peripheral auditory pathology. Incorrect responses to certain questions by an individual who has experienced a stroke may be interpreted as a cognitive deficit when in fact the responses may be the result of misperceptions due to a preexisting, mild peripheral hearing impairment, a common condition in people who are elderly.

Hearing: Engineering Advances

Hearing loss, after having normal hearing, is common, particularly among elderly people. Engineering advances have made hearing aids much smaller and more effective than earlier versions. Although hearing aids are useful they have many shortcomings that signal processing theory, technology (e.g., digital processors), and better understanding of the auditory system and its pathologies should be able to improve. The ability to place computers within hearing aids opens up a whole new world for hearing assistance. These new technical opportunities may produce changes in hearing aid performance that are as dramatic in nature as the changes that computers have brought about in society in general.

Future Needs

All of the technological devices mentioned above can be improved. Furthermore, as the technology is improved, behavior-based rehabilitation procedures need to be modified accordingly. Therefore, research projects need to center on both improvements to the devices themselves and improvements related to rehabilitation strategies, particularly as they interact with various technologies. Research projects can be at the cellular level (e.g., development of improved electrodes for cochlear implants), the signal processing level (e.g., development of improved digital processing software for enhancing speech perception with computer-based hearing aids), the assessment level (developing physiologically based techniques for detecting and quantifying hearing impairments in neonates), and the environmental level (developing strategies for supporting the communications abilities of all people).

Speech

Limitations of speech include difficulties in voice production and articulation, not in language, content, or structure of communication. The latter group are determined by cognition and are noted in the "Cognitive Function" section. Speech function is characterized by articulation and audibility and ability to produce and sustain a reasonably fast rate of speech.

Impairment Relationship to Functional Limitation

The normal process of human speech is accomplished through controlled and sequenced respiration, phonation, and articulation, with adequate resonance from the cavities of mouth, nose, and pharynx. Voice production through the vocal mechanism is accomplished through active inspiration (through activity of thoracic and neck muscles and intrathoracic pressure changes), and expiration through the larynx that is both passive (muscle relaxation and gravity) and supported (abdominal and intercostal muscle activity) for prolonged exhalation for speech.

Phonation and articulation require steady maintenance of air pressures, balanced vocal cords, and coordinated actions of tongue, lips, jaw, and soft palate. Resonance in the pharyngeal, oral, and nasal cavities are modified by changing the shape of the vocal tract, again requiring intact musculature and intra vocal tract pressure control. The coordination, sequencing, and programming of these activities is directed by the brain, most specifically, the left frontal cortex. An impairment at any organ level involved in the process will influence speech production, and lead to a functional limitation in speech.

Assessment of the impairment focuses on the speech production process. Impairments often occur at varying levels of severity and at numerous points in the process, all of which are interdependent. The speech functional limitation is focused most on intelligibility, and measures have been used to determine intelligibility in the clinic setting (functional limitation). It is recognized that intelligibility scores can be influenced by the speakers' task, the transmission system, and the judges' task (disability) (Yorkston et al., 1984; Yorkston and Beukelman, 1981)

Current Status of Science and Research

There are a variety of conditions that describe limitations in speech. Etiologies for speech limitations can be at a central or peripheral area, can involve motor control, and can be mechanically related. Dysarthrias are characterized by slow, weak, imprecise, or uncoordinated movements of the speech musculature, which results in reduced speech intelligibility. A number of diagnoses can be associated with dysarthria, and includes cerebral palsy, stroke, parkinsonism, multiple sclerosis, brain injury, muscle diseases, and amyotrophic lateral sclerosis. All or several speech subsystems may be involved in varying degrees (respiratory, phonatory, pharyngeal, and articulatory) (Miller et al., 1993). The dysarthrias can be described and diagnosed based on a cluster of features. (Darley, 1969a,b; Rosenbek and LaPoint, 1985). There are a variety of assessments that measure speech performance (Netsell, 1973; Netsell et al., 1989; Gerratt et al., 1991), since intelligibility is the hallmark of functional speech. Most tools are perceptual, and rely on a trained observer. However, at an impairment level, respiratory performance can be measured aerodynamically (Netsell, 1973); acoustic analysis can be performed (Keller et al., 1991); and measures of laryngeal resistance can be obtained (Smitheran and Hixon, 1981). Application of these technologies as a measure of intervention assessment could be helpful, but measures only a limited portion of speech function. Standard tools have been developed to measure sentence and single word intelligibility and speaking rate in a more structured fashion (Yorkston et al., 1984).

Those with severe limitations in speech may require augmentative or alternative communication devices. Treatment goals are to establish a functional means of communication. Systems range from communication boards and books to computer based speech synthesis systems (Brandenburg and Vanderheiden, 1987; Yorkston and Beukelman, 1991). Simple low tech strategies must also be considered and may be preferred. The selection of the most appropriate intervention requires careful consideration of the individual's capabilities (e.g., cognitive function, vision, hearing, hand and arm manipulation, positioning for function), proposed use in the selected environments, and financial issues. Lifelong use of these devices or staging of interventions need to be investigated more fully.

A moderate or mild limitation in intelligibility may require exercises to improve respiratory control (Netsell and Daniel, 1979; Bellaire et al., 1986), change speech rate to improve intelligibility (Yorkston et al., 1990), or focusing on phonation (Ramig, 1992). Effectiveness of speech interventions for individuals with spastic dysarthrias has been documented through case reports, single-subject design studies, and uncontrolled group treatments (Aten, 1988). Study outcomes measure changes in muscle strength and control, reduction in consonant imprecision, and improved intelligibility and speaking rate (Yorkston, 1995). A prosthetic lift at the nasopharyngeal area may improve dysarthria by controlling oral air pressures (Gonzalez and Aronson, 1970). Interventions for persons with progressive disorders require changing interventions, based on function (Hillel et al., 1989).

Articulation and phonologic disorders comprise a large portion of speech limitations. Disruptions in speech, or stuttering, vary greatly in frequency, duration, type, and severity. Stuttering is characterized by hesitations, prolongations, and repetitions of speech. Treatment effectiveness studies in school aged children show about a 61% reduction (Conture and Guitar, 1993). In adults, 60 to 80% improve with treatment (Bloodstein, 1987). Treatment approaches are determined by a variety of factors, and may be intensive or extensive (Conture, 1995). Articulation and phonologic disorders are among the most prevalent speech limitation in preschool and school aged children, affecting 10% of this population (Geirut, 1995). Interventions in this age group have been longstanding (Sommers, 1992). Hearing impairments must be considered in the pediatric group in particular when speech delays are noted.

Laryngeal-based voice disorders are characterized by abnormal pitch, loudness, or vocal quality and ranges from mild hoarseness to complete voice loss. Voice therapy can improve the characteristics of voice and reduce laryngeal pathology (Ramig, 1995). Voice treatment has been found to improve vocal nodules and to reduce recurrence if instituted after surgery (Lancer et al., 1988). Speech options after laryngectomies include external prosthetic devices (electrolarynxes and pneumatic reeds) (Miller et al., 1993), tracheal-esophageal puncture (one-way valved voice prosthesis) (Singer and Blom, 1980), and esophageal speech (Gates et al., 1982). Outcome studies have shown both difficulties (Schaefer and Johns, 1982; Miller et al., 1993) and success (Singer et al., 1981; Wetmore et al., 1985; Miller et al., 1993). Technology has assisted speech production for persons with chronic tracheostomies. In particular, the Passy-Muir tracheostomy speaking valve allows speech production through a one-way valve which opens with inspiration, and closes with expiration, redirecting air into the trachea and vocal cords creating sound through the oral and nasal cavities.

Speech: Engineering and Technical Advances

Communication aids for people who are unable to speak came into existence about 30 years ago, and the application of the sciences of information theory, computational linguistics, and coding theory, along with new computer technologies, have had a material influence on the ability of people to generate messages through standard alphabetic notation, speech input, or symbolic methods. Nevertheless, not all people who are unable to speak are able to communicate in these novel ways. Engineering and rehabilitation science can make big advances in this area, as well as in the recognition of speech that is difficult to understand through the translation of utterances into understandable artificial speech.

Cellular telephone links (voice and data), fax services, e-mail, and the Internet have opened up wide communication channels for everyone and it is incumbent upon rehabilitation technology to make these links accessible to people with disabling conditions, using universal design where possible. These communications systems can also provide much assistance to people with sensory losses (e.g., hearing or visual losses).

Future Needs

Currently, the majority of outcome measures in speech rehabilitation are perceptual or observational, and lack standardization. Research into the development of standardized instrumental and observational measures would move evaluation to the functional limitations level. Research regarding the effectiveness of interventions using rigorous descriptions of interventions and outcome measures would provide a basis for duration and frequency of treatments and indications for treatment options. Application of speech intelligibility measures into the disability realm would allow a realistic measure of intervention success.

In addition to the specific areas identified above, research along the lifecourse regarding interventions and devices is needed. Issues of patient and family choices should be considered.

Cognitive Function

Relationship of Impairment and Functional Limitation

The performance of everyday activities is supported by a number of physiological and psychological processes. Cognition represents one of these processes that guides individuals as they acquire and use information to support their actions. Cognition at the impairment level involves the mechanisms of language comprehension and production, pattern recognition, task organization, reasoning, attention, and memory (Duchek, 1991). When these mechanisms are intact, they support the person in learning, communicating, moving, and observing. When the mechanisms are deficient, they create functional limitations for individuals who require rehabilitation services to learn strategies to bypass the deficit or compensate for the loss, or both. They also create functional limitations for the families of such individuals.

Cognitive problems are common following stroke or head injury in people with Parkinson's and Alzheimer's disease and in some people with multiple sclerosis and other chronic conditions. It is the beginning of a new era in the study of cognition as "we understand how experiences generate changes in the nervous system that shape our language, our visual world, our coordinated movements, our cognition" (Merzenich et al., 1993, p. 17). It should be the goal of rehabilitation to minimize the consequences of brain injury in the lives of those who suddenly are impaired by difficulties in living, social interaction, family life, and vocational and educational pursuits. The major cognitive deficits that create functional limitations are described below.

Aphasia is the term attributed to difficulties with language comprehension and expression. It is the absence or impairment of the ability to communicate through speech, writing, or signing and may limit the person's ability to comprehend or express language making it very difficult for the person to communicate wants, needs, and ideas to others.

Agnosia refers to problems with pattern recognition. Agnosia can impair the recognition of objects, facial discrimination (Allender and Kaszniak, 1989), and the recognition of voice tone (Eslinger and Damasio, 1986), making it very difficult to recognize familiar people and voices and common objects such as a fork, toothbrush, or razor. Agnosia presents a difficult challenge, requiring rehabilitation and education for the affected individual and the family.

Apraxia describes the deficit that occurs when an individual has difficulty in organizing and executing purposeful movements. Functional limitations occur when the person cannot perform tasks such as putting an arm in a sleeve, reaching for a glass to take a drink, or even putting one leg in front of the other to take a step.

Deficits in reasoning and problem solving are frequently the result of frontal and temporal lobe damage (Mayer et al., 1986; Sullivan et al., 1989). Functional limitations occur because a person cannot put steps together in a sequence to accomplish a goal or may not be able to choose the items or tools necessary to perform even a simple task such as putting on a robe. Such a deficit makes tasks such as driving a car, paying bills, preparing food, and using the telephone problematic without training in compensatory strategies and environmental modifications.

Executive function comprises the mental capacities required to formulate goals, plan how to achieve them, and carry out the task effectively (Stuss, 1992). A person with *impaired executive function* has a functional limitation that results in difficulty beginning an activity, monitoring his or her performance during an activity, inhibiting irrelevant information, and maintaining attention. This configuration of cognitive problems makes independent living and productive work a challenge for a person who has sustained an injury and for the rehabilitation professional who needs to help the person and the family learn how to give the cognitive support that will make performance possible.

Memory plays a very important role in everyday functioning. Different types of memory can be impaired, depending on the location of the brain damage. Deficits in short-term memory, which holds information for further processing, can make new learning difficult. Individuals with memory loss often need rehabilitation to develop strategies to access long-term memory for personal events and general knowledge, to remember future events, and to support the procedures required to perform an activity. Cognitive deficits that impair memory have a profound impact on the performance of people as they recover from physical impairments and move on to try to reestablish independence following injury or illness.

Cognitive Issues: Engineering and Technical Advancements

Few investigators have examined if or how technical devices might be helpful in cases in which and individual is impaired because of the loss of cognitive ability. Nevertheless, it is known that developments in this area will not occur de novo. Positive action needs to be taken to investigate how assistive technical aids may be useful in this area. Action needs to come through the interaction of scientists, clinicians, and engineers. Memory aids and the use of step-by-step instructions are areas tailor-made for providing technical assistance, and engineering may be able to help make significant advances in this area. However, collaboration with families and caregivers, will be necessary for the problems to be understood and for design iterations to be based on realistic clinical experiences.

Future Needs

Cognition plays a critical role in the performance of the tasks of living. When any of these deficits occur (and many of these deficits occur simultaneously), the person is disabled until environmental and compensatory strategies are put in place to support him or her. During the past decade, the emphasis on biomedical science has generated new knowledge about brain plasticity and brain structure–function relationships. As this emphasis expands to include issues of functional limitation and disability, it should be possible to test the application of these findings in clinical interventions to determine how individuals with brain injuries can improve their performance of functional, real-world tasks (e.g., self-care, meal preparation, parenting, and employment).

Most cognitive research has been performed at the impairment level and has involved the administration of experimental and neuropsychological tests. As more clinical studies have been funded, investigators have learned that patterns of behavior in the real-life context differ from those that would have been predicted from neuropsychological tests (Prigatano and Altman, 1990). When a cognitive deficit occurs, the person also experiences changes in emotion, social interaction, and communication; these changes can range from subtle to severe changes and can create complex difficulties for the individual and his or her family, coworkers, and friends.

Rehabilitation strategies to overcome problems presented by aphasia, agnosia, and apraxia require further development and testing and will be understood more fully when scientists and engineers interact with clinicians and patients to understand the impact of these conditions on people's lives.

The research needed to understand the impact of cognition on the individual and society and the potential of environmental and learning strategies on recovery and functioning is yet to be done. It will require research of issues beyond the current biomedical mechanisms that exist today and involve interdisciplinary teams of professionals from fields that span education, philosophy, cognitive psychology, and neuroscience, including neurobiology and neuroradiology. The research must also include rehabilitation professionals such as occupational therapists, speech language pathologists, physicians, and neuropsychologists.

Such teams working together may begin to obtain an understanding of the mechanisms that underlie the recovery and preservation of cognitive functions after brain damage. It will be important to determine if there are aspects of affective disorders that can be distinguished from the cognitive sequelae of acquired brain injury and determine if the brain has different processing pathways for different types of information after brain injury (Buckner et al., 1996). For example, it would be possible to explore whether the cerebellum's contributions to motor learning generalize beyond the purely motor domain and whether the preserved function demonstrated by some people with disabling conditions is mediated by sparing of critical tissue or by compensatory neural pathways. It would be important to know how a deficit in inhibitory control affects everyday function; that is, can different aspects of attentional processing (e.g., divided attention, visual search, and vigilance) predict everyday functioning, including a complex task like driving or work.

Not all disability comes from within the individual. Each person needs a supportive environment to perform at his or her best. A study of cognition prompts investigators to ask new questions. How does cognitive activity relate to specific environmental contexts? What is the role of mediated action in the actual performance of cognitive and functional tasks in people with acquired brain injury and those with no cognitive loss? What role does the environment play in the internal representation and processing of visual information? Also, how is it possible to prepare spouses and families for the multitude of tasks required for life with a person who is severely disabled because of an acquired head injury?

Such questions can only be addressed when there is a level of analysis and method of measurement that allows for the description of cognitive deficits in real-life activities. Functional means of measuring intellect, motivation, mood, judgment, visual perception, auditory perception, motor control, visual attention, vigilance and arousal, working memory, procedural memory, declarative memory, and motion in context must be developed. The challenge of preventing disabilities in those with cognitive loss cannot be left at the level of functional limitation. New means of addressing the cognitive needs of individuals must come to the forefront in science to reduce the devastation of a cognitive impairment on the lives of the people and their families who must live with the consequences of the functional limitations brought on by injury and disease.

CONCLUSIONS

Although there is little published research on functional limitations' responsiveness to rehabilitation, this is only partially traceable to the limited funded research in this domain. Functional limitations research requires whole-person studies, which are costly and difficult to perform. Only clinical research that involves the whole person is, by definition, relevant to functional limitations research. Until functional limitations are properly studied, the role of the environment in preventing the physical expression of the person's capacity (i.e., disability) cannot be understood. The process of rehabilitation has heretofore focused on impairment-level interventions, but the economics of rehabilitation, especially in the managed health care sphere, is requiring that people be discharged home as soon as possible. In turn, functional limitations become paramount concerns because they alone prevent the person from returning to the premorbid environment after rehabilitation. Altering the environment to accommodate functional limitations, such as by adding a raised toilet seat following hip replacement or providing durable medical equipment following major amputation or spinal cord injury, are time-honored rehabilitation approaches. The historic reluctance of insurers to pay for such environmental modifications is understandable if one appreciates that society, not the insurer, benefits from improved functional capacity and thus decreased need for "external" support. If the functional capacity of a person, for example, a person with chronic back pain, increases as a result of rehabilitation and the person is able to return to work, society obtains an income tax-paying and less healthcare resource-consuming, member. The insurer benefits directly only inasmuch as the person consumes fewer health care resources. More functional limitations research is urgently needed to determine the optimal role of rehabilitation for individuals with disabling conditions compared with interventions at the societal or environmental level.

RECOMMENDATIONS

Recommendation 5.1 The National Institutes of Health (NIH) should ensure that rehabilitation scientists in general, and functional limitation researchers in particular, are well represented on study sections. NIH also should expand the research capacity of its Institutes to include functional limitations and rehabilitation research as important aspects of their missions.

Recommendation 5.2 A mechanism should be established, possibly through consensus panels, to frame the questions about functional limitations that would help to draw the link between impairments and functional limitations for the purpose of building the science of rehabilitation.

Recommendation 5.3 The Computer Retrieval of Information on Scientific Projects system and other databases used to track research funded by federal agencies should use a governmentwide code or coding mechanism to describe rehabilitation research that includes the concepts and definitions of pathology, impairment, functional limitation, and disability presented in this report. This would allow for the more appropriate classification of functional limitations and rehabilitation research.

Recommendation 5.4 A commonly used terminology and taxonomy* should be developed and used that would allow scientists and professionals to communicate more effectively with each other across disciplines. This would include terminology regarding methodologies, measures, the enabling–disabling process, and other descriptors of performance and functional limitations.

Recommendation 5.5 More research is needed to obtain an understanding of the factors that determine the changes in and causal relationships among impairments, functional limitations, and disabilities, and move-

---

*Appendix C contains a preliminary draft of an outline of a taxonomy.

ment among these states. Such research should be clearly focused on improving public health from a lifelong perspective.

Recommendation 5.6 More research is needed to improve the understanding of the impact of aging and other lifelong disabling conditions on functional limitations and secondary conditions.

Recommendation 5.7 The science supporting functional limitations depends on integrative studies of the whole person. Behavioral measurement and the development of valid functional limitation measures, should be high priorities in rehabilitation research.

6

Disability and the Environment

In the past four decades the prevailing wisdom about the cause of disability has undergone profound change. Previous models of absolute determinism that viewed pathology and disability interchangeably and that excluded consideration of the environment have been replaced by models in which disability is seen to result from the interaction between the characteristics of individuals with potentially disabling conditions and the characteristics of their environment.

The 1991 version of the Institute of Medicine (IOM) model of disability did not explicitly identify the environment as a factor in disability. Building upon the model presented in Chapter 3, this chapter considers in some depth the ways that the environment can be either enabling or disabling for a person with a pathological condition.

The chapter describes in greater detail how cultural norms affect the way that the physical and social environments of the individual are constituted and then focus on a few—but not all— of the elements of the environment to provide examples of how the environment affects the degree of disability. The overall message of this chapter is that the amount of disability is not determined by levels of pathologies, impairments, or functional limitations, but instead is a function of the kind of services provided to people with disabling conditions and the extent to which the physical, built environment is accommodating or not accommodating to the particular disabling condition. Because societies differ in their willingness to provide the available technology and, indeed, their willingness to provide the research funds to improve that technology, disability ultimately must been seen as a function of society, not of a physical or medical process.

As described in Chapter 3, disability is not inherent in an individual but is, rather, a relational concept—a function of the interaction of the person with the social and physical environments. The amount of disability that a person experiences depends on both the existence of a potentially disabling condition (or limitation) and the environment in which the person lives. For any given limitation (i.e., potential disability), the amount of actual disability experienced by a person will depend on the nature of the environment, that is, whether the environment is positive and enabling (and serves to compensate for the condition, ameliorate the limitation, or facilitate one's functional activities) or negative and disabling (and serves to worsen the condition, enhance the limitation, or restrict one's functional activities).

Human competencies interact with the environment in a dynamic reciprocal relationship that shapes performance. When functional limitations exist, social participation is possible only when environmental support is present. If there is no environmental support, the distance between what the person can do and what the environment affords creates a barrier that limits social participation.

The physical and social environments comprise factors external to the individual, including family, institutions, community, geography, and the political climate. Added to this conceptualization of environment is one's intrapersonal or psychological environment, which includes internal states, beliefs, cognition, expectancies and other mental states. Thus, environmental factors must be seen to include the natural environment, the built environment, culture, the economic system, the political system, and psychological factors. The categories and factors in these tables are not exhaustive and are provided as examples of the very broad and pervasive influence of a person's environment. This chapter illustrates how each of these environmental factors can have an impact on disability.

IMPACT OF THE PHYSICAL ENVIRONMENT
ON THE DISABLING PROCESS

As discussed in Chapter 3, the environmental mat may be conceived of as having two major parts: the physical environment and the social and psychological environments. The physical environment may be further subdivided conceptually into the natural environment and the built environment. Both affect the extent to which a disabling conditions will be experienced by the person as a disability.

Three types of attributes of the physical environment need to be in place to support human performance (Corcoran and Gitlin, 1997). The

TABLE 6-1 Some Enabling and Disabling Factors in the Physical Environment

Type of Factor	Type of Environment	
	Natural Environment	Built Environment
Enabling	Dry climate	Ramps
	Flat terrain	Adequate lighting
	Clear paths	Braille signage
Disabling	Snow	Steps
	Rocky terrain	Low-wattage lighting
	High humidity	Absence of flashing light alerting systems

first attribute is object availability. Objects must be in a location that is useful, at a level where they can be retrieved, and must be organized to support the performance of the activity. Neither a sink that is too high for a wheelchair user nor a telecommunications device for the deaf (TDD) that is kept at a hotel reception desk is available. The second attribute is accessibility. Accessibility is related to the ability of people to get to a place or to use a device. Accessibility permits a wheelchair user to ride a bus or a braille user to read a document. The third attribute is the availability of sensory stimulation regarding the environment. Sensory stimulation, which can include visual, tactile, or auditory cues, serves as a signal to promote responses. Examples of such cues could include beeping microwaves, which elicit responses from people without hearing impairments, or bumpy surfaces on subway platforms, which tell users with visual impairments to change their location.

Table 6-1 presents some examples of enabling and disabling factors in the natural environment.

The Natural Environment

The natural environment may have a major impact on whether a limitation is disabling. For example, a person who has severe allergies to ragweed or mold, which can trigger disabling asthma, can be free of that condition in climates where those substances do not grow. The physical conditions still exist, but in one environment they may become disabling and in another environment they might not. Another example might be that a person who has limited walking ability will be less disabled in a flat geographical location such as Chicago than he or she would be in a hilly location such as Pittsburgh, although the person would also be more disabled in both places during the winter than during the summer. Thus, the natural environment, including topography and climate, affect whether or to what degree a functional limitation will be disabling.

The Built Environment

The physical environment is a complex interaction of built-in objects (Corcoran and Gitlin, 1997). Built objects are created and constructed by humans and vary widely in terms of their complexity, size, and purpose. Built objects are created for utilitarian reasons and also for an outlet for creativity. For instance, built objects such as dishwashers and computers have the potential to enhance human performance or to create barriers.

Assistive Technology

Another aspect of the built environment is assistive technology. The Technology-Related Assistance for Individuals with Disabilities Act of 1988 (Public Law 100-407), also known as the Tech Act, defines assistive technology devices as "any item, piece of equipment, or product system, whether acquired commercially off-the-shelf, modified, or customized, that is used to increase, maintain, or improve the functional capabilities of an individual with a disability." Thus, assistive technology affects the level to which a functional limitation is disabling. As an illustration, a person whose visual impairment can be corrected by corrective lenses does not technically have a disability. There are numerous other examples of how the environment affects the amount of disability associated with any functional limitation through the use of assistive technology. A person with a hearing impairment who has a TDD can make phone calls to other people who also possess such devices. If there is a relay service, in which an operator translates from TDD to voice telephone, the person who owns a TDD can call anyone. In these situations the impairment does not cause a disability. This example, however, illustrates the fact that it is the intersection of technology and social factors that can be more enabling than just the technology itself. Other examples are that a person who has a speech impairment can "speak" using a computer voice synthesizer or that people with low vision or blindness can read office memoranda or correspondence if he or she has the right computer software. These technologies do not always need to be complex: a person who uses a wheelchair and who works in an office could work effectively if the simple technology of an adjustable desk allowed the desk to be raised to allow the wheelchair to fit under the desk.

Through the passage of Public Law 100-407, the federal government affirmed the importance and benefits of assistive technology for the millions of U.S. citizens with disabilities who need this technology to make their lives more functional and independent. The goals of this law have been operationalized through the National Institute on Disability and Rehabilitation Research (NIDRR) with an annual budget of $39,065,414 (fiscal year 95 allocations for state technology assistance) for the 50 states and U.S. territories that are participating in this program. However, despite the money spent implementing the Tech Act amendments of 1994, many key issues still remain, according to a 1995 report on Technology and People with Disabilities prepared for the U.S. Congress by the Office of Technology Assessment. The report states that, in spite of states' technology-related assistance programs carried out under the Tech Act, there remains "a need to support systems change and advocacy activities to assist States to develop and implement consumer-responsive, comprehensive state-wide programs of technology-related assistance for individuals with disabilities of all ages." Even with these limitations, more individuals than ever before are using assistive technology to compensate for their disabling conditions and enhance the environment in which they live and work.

Universal Design

It is frequently the case that the built environment can be modified permanently so that functional limitations become less disabling and personal or temporary assistive technologies are not needed. For example, the presence of ramps increases the ability of wheelchair users to get around and thus decreases the degree to which the condition that led to their use of a wheelchair is disabling. White and colleagues, (1995) found an increased frequency of trips out of the house and into the community for two-thirds of wheelchair users after ramps were installed in their houses. Wider doors, lower bathroom sinks, and grab bars are other examples of modifications to built environments that decrease the degree to which a building itself may be disabling. Lighting patterns and the materials used for walls and ceilings affect the visual ability of all people, even though the largest impact may be on improving the ability of the person who is hard of hearing to hear in a particular room or the ability of a person who is deaf to see an interpreter or other signers.

Universal design is based on the principle that the built environments and instruments used for everyday living can be ergonomically designed so that everyone can use them. Traditionally, architecture and everyday products have been designed for market appeal, with a greater focus on fashion rather than function. However, as the population of older adults and people with disabling conditions increases, there has been a greater trend toward universal design.

Today, with the influence of consumer demand and through thoughtful disability policy, greater emphasis is placed on the development of built materials that are ergonomically friendly to users, regardless of their abilities. Universal design is an enabling factor in the environment that allows the user with a functional limitation to become more independent, yet without an additional cost or stigma attached to the particular product. For example, people who were deaf previously had to purchase an expensive closed-captioning unit to attach to their television sets to view closed-captioned programs. Today, as a result of new federal legislation, all new television sets are manufactured with a closed-captioning microchip that allows any user access to broadcast closed captioning. Thus, it is useful not only for deaf users but also for immigrants wishing to learn English, older individuals who are starting to lose their audio acuity, or a person watching a late-night talk show in the bedroom who does not want to wake his or her partner.

In all of these ways, the environment affects the degree to which a functional limitation is disabling for a person. However, decisions about the use of technology or built environments are social decisions. The next major section considers the effects of the social and psychological environments on the extent to which a particular functional limitation will be disabling or not.

Modifying the Environment

External environmental modifications can take many forms. These can include assistive devices, alterations of a physical structure, object modification, and task modification (Corcoran and Gitlin, 1997). Table 6-2 gives some examples of these.

The role of environmental modification as a prevention strategy has not been systematically evaluated, and its role in preventing secondary conditions and disability that accompany a poor fit between human abilities and the environment should be studied. Environmental strategies may ease the burden of care experienced by a family member who has the responsibility of providing the day-to-day support for an individual who does not have the capacity for social participation and independent living in the community. These environmental modifications may well be an effort at primary prevention because the equipment may provide a safety net and prevent disabling conditions that can occur through lifting and transfer of individuals who may not be able to do it by themselves.

Rehabilitation must place emphasis on addressing the environmental needs of people with disabling conditions. Environmental strategies can be effective in helping people function independently and not be limited in their social participation, in work, leisure or social interactions as a spouse, parent, friend, or coworker.

TABLE 6-2 Examples of Environmental Modification

Environmental Modification Can Occur Through the Use of:	Such as:
Mobility aids	Hand orthosis Mouth stick Prosthetic limb Wheelchair (manual and/or motorized) Canes Crutches Braces
Communication aids	Telephone amplifier or TDD Voice-activated computer Closed or real-time captioning Computer-assisted notetaker Print enlarger Reading machines Books on tape Sign language or oral interpreters Braille writer Cochlear implant Communication boards FM, audio-induction loop, or infrared systems
Accessible structural elements	Ramps Elevators Wide doors Safety bars Nonskid floors Sound-reflective building materials Enhanced lighting Electrical sockets that meet appropriate reach ranges Hardwired flashing alerting systems Increased textural contrast
Accessible features	Built up handles Voice-activated computer Automobile hand controls
Job accommodations	Simplification of task Flexible work hours Rest breaks Splitting job into parts Relegate nonessential functions to others
Differential use of personnel	Personal care assistants Notetakers Secretaries Editors Sign language interpreters

IMPACT OF THE SOCIAL AND PSYCHOLOGICAL ENVIRONMENTS ON THE ENABLING–DISABLING PROCESS

The social environment is conceptualized to include cultural, political, and economic factors. The psychological environment is the intrapersonal environment. This section examines how both affect the disabling process. Table 6-3 provides an overview of some of the points to be made below.

Culture and the Disabling Process

Culture affects the enabling–disabling process at each stage; it also affects the transition from one stage to another. This section defines culture and then considers the ways in which it affects each stage of the process.

Definition of Culture

Definition of culture includes both material culture (things and the rules for producing them) and nonmaterial culture (norms or rules, values, symbols, language, ideational systems such as science or religion, and arts such as dance, crafts, and humor). Nonmaterial culture is so comprehensive that it includes everything from conceptions of how many days a week has or how one should react to pain (Zborowski, 1952) to when one should seek medical care (Zola, 1966) or whether a hermaphroditic person is an abomination, a saint, or a mistake (Geertz, 1983). Cultures also specify punishments for rule-breaking, exceptions to rules, and occasions when exceptions are permitted. The role of nonmaterial culture for humans has been compared to the role of instincts for animals or to the role of a road map for a traveler. It provides the knowledge that permits people to be able to function in both old and new situations (Geertz, 1973).

Both the material and nonmaterial aspects of cultures and subcultures are relevant to the enabling–disabling process. However, this section focuses primarily on the role of nonmaterial culture in that process.

Cultures have an impact on the types of pathologies that will occur as well as on their recognition as pathologies. The former case is the realm of epidemiological studies and so is not relevant here. (Albrecht [1992] has discussed the relationship between culture, social structure, and the types of disabilities that arise from the types of pathologies most likely to be present in those societies.) However, if a pathology is not recognized by the culture (in medical terms, diagnosed), the person does not begin to progress toward disability (or cure).

TABLE 6-3 Enabling and Disabling Factors in the Social and Psychological Environments

Type of Factor	Element of Social and Psychological Environment			
	Culture	Psychological	Political	Economic
Enabling	Expecting people with disabling conditions to be productive	Having an active coping strategy	Mandating relay systems in all states	Tax credits to hire people with disabling conditions
	Expecting everyone to know sign language	Cognitive restructuring	Banning discrimination against people who can perform the essential functions of the job	Targeted earned income tax credits (Yelin and Katz, 1994)
Disabling	Stigmatizing people with disabling conditions	Catastrophizing	Segregating children with mobility impairments in schools	Economic disincentives to get off SSDI[a] benefits
	Valuing physical beauty (Hahn, 1985)	Denial	Voting against paratransit system	No subsidies or tax credits for purchasing assistive technology

[a]SSDI, Social Security Disability Income.

Pathway from Pathology to Impairment to Functional Limitation

Culture can affect the likelihood of the transition from pathology to impairment. A subculture, such as that of well-educated Americans, in which health advice is valued, in which breast cancer screening time-tables are followed, and in which early detection is likely, is one in which breast tumors are less likely to move from pathology to impairments. In a subculture in which this is not true, one would likely see more impairments arising from the pathologies.

Cultures can also speed up or slow down the movement from pathology to impairment, either for the whole culture or for subgroups for whom the pathway is more or less likely to be used. For example, in Bangladesh, where Muslim rules of purdah apply, women are less likely to seek health care because it means a man must be available to escort them in public, which is unlikely if the males are breadwinners and must give up income to escort them, and women are also less likely to seek health care if the provider is male. Thus, their culture lessens the likelihood that their pathology will be cured and therefore increases the likelihood that the pathology will become an impairment.

Culture clearly has an impact on whether a particular impairment will become a functional limitation. Impairments do not become limiting automatically. Rather, cultures affect the perception that the impairment is in fact the cause of the limitation, and they affect the perception that the impairment is in fact limiting.

If a society believes that witchcraft is the reason that a woman cannot have children, medical facts about her body become irrelevant. She may in fact have fibroids, but if that culture sees limitation as coming from the actions of a person, there is no recognition of a linkage between the impairment and the functional limitation. Rather, any enabling–disabling process must go through culturally prescribed processes relating to witches; medically or technologically based enabling–disabling processes will not be acceptable.

If the culture does not recognize that an impairment is limiting, then it is not. For example, hearing losses were not equivalent to functional limitations in Martha's Vineyard, because "everyone there knew sign language" (Groce, 1985). Or, if everyone has a backache, it is not defined by the culture as limiting (Koos, 1954). There are many cross-cultural examples. In a culture in which nose piercing is considered necessary for beauty, possible breathing problems resulting from that pathology and impairment would be unlikely to be recognized as being limiting. Or, in a perhaps more extreme case, female circumcision is an impairment that could lead to functional limitation (inability to experience orgasm), but if the whole point is to prevent female sexual arousal and orgasm, then the functional limitation will not be recognized within that culture but will only be recognized by those who come from other cultures. In all these examples, if the culture does not recognize the impairment, the rehabilitation process is irrelevant—there is no need to rehabilitate a physical impairment if there is no recognized functional limitation associated with it.

Pathway from Functional Limitation to Disability

Perhaps the most important consideration for this chapter is the ways in which the transition from functional limitation to disability is affected by culture. A condition that is limiting must be defined as problematic—by the person and by the culture—for it to become a disability. Whether a functional limitation is seen as being disabling will depend on the culture. The culture defines the roles to be played and the actions and capacities necessary to satisfy that role. If certain actions are not necessary for a role, then the person who is limited in ability to perform those actions does not have a disability. For example, a professor who has arthritis in her hands but who primarily lectures in the classroom, dictates material for a secretary to type, and manages research assistants may not be disabled in her work role by the arthritis. In this case, the functional limitation would not become a disability. For a secretary who would be unable to type, on the other hand, the functional limitation would become a disability in the work sphere.

A disability can exist without functional limitation, as in the case of a person with a facial disfigurement (Institute of Medicine, 1991, p. 81) living in cultures such as that in the United States, whose standards of beauty cannot encompass such physical anomalies (Hahn, 1988). Culture is thus relevant to the existence of disabilities: it defines what is considered disabling. Additionally, culture determines in which roles a person might be disabled by a particular functional limitation. For example, a farmer in a small village may have no disability in work roles caused by a hearing loss; however, that person may experience disabilities in family or other personal relationships. On the other hand, a profoundly deaf, signing person married to another profoundly deaf, signing person may have no disability in family-related areas, although there may be a disability in work-related areas. Thus, culture affects not just *whether* there is a disability caused by the functional limitation but also *where* in the person's life the disability will occur.

Culture is therefore part of the mat; as such, it can protect a person from the disabling process and can slow it down or speed it up. Culture, however, has a second function in the disabling process.

As discussed above, there is a direct path from culture to disability; the following section presents the indirect paths. The indirect function acts by influencing other aspects of personal and social organization in a society. That is, the culture of a society or a subculture influences the types of personality or intrapsychic processes that are acceptable and influences the institutions that make up the social organization of a society. These institutions include the economic system, the family system, the educational system, the health care system, and the political system. In all these areas, culture sets the boundaries for what is debatable or negotiable and what is not. Each of these societal institutions also affects the degree to which functional limitations will be experienced by individuals as disabling.

All of the ways in which intrapsychic processes or societal institutions affect the enabling–disabling process cannot be considered here.

However, the remainder of this section presents some examples of how the enabling–disabling process can be affected by three factors: economic, political, and psychological (see also Table 6-3).

Economic Factors and Disability

Chapter 2 described the economic impact of disability and rehabilitation on society. This section summarizes how economic factors affect the disability-rehabilitation process and the expression of disability.

There is clear evidence that people with few economic assets are more likely to acquire pathologies that may be disabling. This is true even in advanced economies and in economies with greater levels of income equality. The impact of absolute or relative economic deprivation on the onset of pathology crosscuts conditions with radically different etiologies, encompassing infectious diseases and most common chronic conditions. Similarly, economic status affects whether a pathology will proceed to impairment. Examples include such phenomena as a complete lack of access to or a delay in presentation for medical care for treatable conditions (e.g., untreated breast cancer is more likely to require radical mastectomy) or inadequate access to state-of-the-art care (e.g., persons with rheumatoid arthritis may experience a worsened range of motion and joint function because disease-modifying drugs are not used by most primary care physicians). In turn, a lack of resources can adversely affect the ability of an individual to function with a disabling condition. For example, someone with an amputated leg who has little money or poor health insurance may not be able to obtain a proper prosthesis, in which case the absence of the limb may then force the individual to withdraw from jobs that require these capacities.

Similarly, economic resources can limit the options and abilities of someone who requires personal assistance services or certain physical accommodations. The individual also may not be able to access the appropriate rehabilitation services to reduce the degree of potential disability either because they cannot afford the services themselves or cannot afford the cost of specialized transportation services.

The economic status of the community may have a more profound impact than the status of the individual on the probability that disability will result from impairment or other disabling conditions. Research on employment among persons with disabilities indicates, for example, that such persons in communities undergoing rapid economic expansion will be much more likely to secure jobs than those in communities with depressed or contracting labor markets. Similarly, wealthy communities are more able to provide environmental supports such as accessible public transportation and public buildings or support payments for personal assistance benefits.

An earlier section of this chapter described how community can be defined in terms of the microsystem (the local area of the person with the disabling conditions), the mesosystem (the area beyond the immediate neighborhood, perhaps encompassing the town), and the macrosystem (a region or nation). Clearly, the economic status of the region or nation as a whole may play a more important role than the immediate microenvironment for certain kinds of disabling conditions. For example, access to employment among people with disabling conditions is determined by a combination of the national and regional labor markets, but the impact of differences across small neighborhoods is unlikely to be very great. In contrast, the economic status of a neighborhood will play a larger role in determining whether there are physical accommodations in the built environment that would facilitate mobility for people with impairments or functional limitations, or both.

Finally, economic factors also can affect disability by creating incentives to define oneself as disabled. For example, disability compensation programs often pay nearly as much as many of the jobs available to people with disabling conditions, especially given that such programs also provide health insurance and many lower-paying jobs do not. Moreover, disability compensation programs often make an attempt to return to work risky, since health insurance is withdrawn soon after earnings begin and procuring a job with good health insurance benefits is often difficult in the presence of disabling conditions. Thus, disability compensation programs are said to significantly reduce the number of people with impairments who work by creating incentives to leave the labor force and also creating disincentives to return to work.

Political Factors and Disability

The political system, through its role in designing public policy, can and does have a profound impact on the extent to which impairments and other potentially disabling conditions will result in disability, as a few examples from recent legislation may indicate. Until the passage of the Americans with Disabilities Act of 1990 (ADA), the civil rights legislation for people with disabilities, employers were free to suppose that people with disabling conditions did not have the capacity to take on certain, specific jobs. With the passage of this legislation the onus shifted, so that such people were legally entitled to be treated as any applicant: employers had to assume that an individual applying for a job did have the capacity to do that job's essential features even if that capacity could only be achieved by reasonable accommodations. Before the passage of ADA it was legal to deny individuals access to work because they could not do the auxiliary aspects of a job, even though they had the capacity to do a job's essential features. Thus, an applicant for a clerical position could be denied the job on the basis of an inability to make coffee, for example, even if he or she could use a computer and type. The ADA also ensures equal access to public services, housing, transportation, and systems of communication, all with the goal of improving the ability of people with disabling conditions to function in all aspects of daily life.

There is much question as to the vigor with which the ADA has been and will be enforced, but there is no question that if it is well enforced it will profoundly improve the prospects of people with disabling conditions for achieving a much fuller participation in society, in effect reducing the font of disability in work and every other domain of human activity.

Other public policies affect the extent to which the goals of the ADA will be achieved. The extent to which the built environment impedes people with disabling conditions is a function of public funds spent to make buildings and transportation systems accessible and public laws requiring the private sector to make these accommodations in nonpublic buildings. The extent to which people with impairments and functional limitations will participate in the labor force is a function of the funds spent in training programs, in the way that health care is financed, and in the ways that job accommodations are mandated and paid for. Similarly, for those with severe disabling conditions, access to personal assistance services may be required for participation in almost all activities, and such access is dependent on the availability of funding for such services through either direct payment or tax credits. A final example—one very germane to this report—of how public policy influences the extent to which people with disabling conditions will be able to function in everyday life is the level of public investment in research of all kinds, from discovering the mechanisms by which disabling pathologies arise through developing assistive technologies and finding out the best way of financing their distribution.

Thus, the potential mechanisms of public policy are diverse, ranging from the direct effects of funds from the public purse, to creating tax incentives so that private parties may finance efforts themselves, to the passage of civil rights legislation and providing adequate enforcement. The sum of the mechanisms used can and does have a profound impact on the functioning of people with disabling conditions.

Psychological Factors and Disability

This section focuses on the impact of psychological factors on how disability and disabling conditions are perceived and experienced. The argument in support of the influence of the psychological environment is congruent with the key assumption in this chapter that the physical and social environments are fundamentally important to the expression of disability.

Several constructs can be used to describe one's psychological environment, including personal resources, personality traits, and cognition. These constructs affect both the expression of disability and an individual's ability to adapt to and react to it. An exhaustive review of the literature on the impact of psychological factors on disability is beyond the scope of this chapter. However, for illustrative purposes four psychological constructs will be briefly discussed: three cognitive processes (self-efficacy beliefs, psychological control, and coping patterns) and one personality disposition (optimism). Each section provides examples illustrating the influence of these constructs on the experience of disability.

Social Cognitive Processes

Cognition consists of thoughts, feelings, beliefs, and ways of viewing the world, others, and ourselves. Three interrelated cognitive processes have been selected to illustrate the direct and interactive effects of cognition on disability. These are self-efficacy beliefs, psychological control, and coping patterns.

Self-Efficacy Beliefs Self-efficacy beliefs are concerned with whether or not a person believes that he or she can accomplish a desired outcome (Bandura, 1977, 1986). Beliefs about one's abilities affect what a person chooses to do, how much effort is put into a task, and how long an individual will endure when there are difficulties. Self-efficacy beliefs also affect the person's affective and emotional responses. Under conditions of high self-efficacy, a person's outlook and mental health status will remain positive even under stressful and aversive situations. Under conditions of low self-efficacy, mental health may suffer even when environmental conditions are favorable. The findings from several studies provide evidence of improved behavioral and functional outcomes under efficacious conditions for individuals with and without disabling conditions (Maddux, 1996).

How do self-efficacy beliefs affect disability? Following a stroke, for example, an individual with high self-efficacy beliefs will be more likely to feel and subsequently exert effort toward reducing the disability that could accompany any stroke-related impairment or functional limitation. The highly self-efficacious individual would work harder at tasks (i.e., in physical or speech therapy), be less likely to give up when there is a relapse (i.e., continue therapy sessions even when there is no immediate improvement), and in general, feel more confident and optimistic about recovery and rehabilitation. These self-efficacy beliefs will thus mediate the relationship between impairment and disability such that the individual would experience better functional outcomes and less disability.

Psychological Control Psychological control, or control beliefs, are akin to self-efficacy beliefs in that they are thoughts, feelings, and beliefs regarding one's ability to exert control or change a situation. A voluminous amount of literature has been written on the beneficial aspects of control and the need that people have for control over their lives. The research suggests that self-generated feelings of control improve outcomes for diverse groups of individuals with physical disabilities and chronic illnesses (Taylor et al., 1991).

The onset of a disabling condition is often followed by a loss or a potential loss of control. What is most critical for adaptive functioning is how a person responds to this and what efforts the person puts forth to regain control. Perceptions of control will influence whether a disabling condition is seen as stressful and consequently whether it becomes disabling.

Individuals with disabling conditions who perceive that they have control over the management of their health, rehabilitation, and related outcomes will fare better. Under conditions of perceived lack of control, people with disabling conditions are not likely to engage in behaviors (e.g., attend therapy or advocate for civil rights) to reduce disabling conditions and improve functional outcomes. Under these circumstances, the relationship between impairment and disability becomes circular. Once disability increases, so may the level of impairment and functional limitation as a result of not pursuing rehabilitation therapy. Conversely, under conditions of perceived control, a person is likely to engage in behaviors that will subsequently reduce disability. Once disability is reduced, one's level of impairment may subsequently be reduced.

Under conditions of perceived loss of control, the individual may actively cope to restore control through primary control efforts (e.g., engaging in behaviors directed at changing the external environment to fit the needs of the person) and secondary control efforts (e.g., engaging in thoughts and actions directed at changing one's views of self through mechanisms such as setting goals and adjusting expectations). An example of primary control would be a person with decreased mobility moving from a building with no elevators to a building with elevators. An example of secondary control would be when this individual changed his or her beliefs about the importance of mobility. What is relevant in this case is not whether the individual has actual control but whether the person perceives that he or she has control.

Coping Patterns Coping patterns refer to behavioral and cognitive efforts to manage specific internal or external demands that tax or exceed a person's resources to adjust (Lazarus and Folkman, 1984). Generally, coping has been studied within the context of stress (Young, 1992; Zautra and Manne, 1992). Having a disabling condition may create stress and demand additional efforts because of interpersonal or environmental conditions that are not supportive.

Several coping strategies may be used when a person confronts a stressful situation (Stewart and Knight, 1991; Affleck et al., 1992). These strategies may include the following: seeking information, cognitive restructuring, emotional expression, catastrophizing, wish-fulfilling fantasizing, threat minimization, relaxation, distraction, and self-blame.

The beneficial effects of certain coping efforts on adaptive and functional outcomes among individuals with disabling conditions have been demonstrated in several studies (Revenson and Felton, 1989; Kleinke, 1991; Affleck et al., 1992; Brown et al., 1993; Hanson et al., 1993; Zea et al., in press). In general, among people with disabling conditions, there is evidence that passive, avoidant, emotion-focused cognitive strategies (e.g., catastrophizing and wishful thinking) are associated with poorer outcomes, whereas active, problem-focused attempts to redefine thoughts to become more positive are associated with favorable outcomes (Affleck et al., 1992; Young, 1992; Zautra and Manne, 1992; Brown et al., 1993; Hanson et al., 1993). An adaptive coping pattern would involve the use of primary and secondary control strategies, as discussed earlier. What seems useful is the flexibility to change strategies and to have several strategies available (Stewart and Knight, 1991; Dunkel-Schetter et al., 1992).

In one study, Jarama (1996) investigated the role of active coping on mental health and vocational outcomes among people with diverse disabling conditions. The findings from that study indicated that active coping is a significant predictor of mental health and employment-related outcomes.

Under conditions in which individuals with disabling conditions use active and problem-solving coping strategies to manage their life circumstances, there will be better functional outcomes across several dimensions (e.g., activities of daily living, and employment) than when passive coping strategies are used.

An important component in the coping process is appraisal. Appraisals involve beliefs about one's ability to deal with a situation (Young, 1992; Zautra and Manne, 1992). Take, for example, two people with identical levels of impairment. The appraisal that the impairment is disabling will result in more disability than the appraisal that the impairment is not disabling, regardless of the objective type and level of impairment. Appraisal is related to self-efficacy in the sense that one's thoughts and cognition control how one reacts to a potentially negative situation. When a person feels that he or she can execute a desired outcome (e.g., learn how to use crutches for mobility), the person is more likely to do just that. Similarly, under conditions in which an individual appraises his or her disabling conditions and other life circumstances as manageable, the person will use coping strategies that will lead to a manageable life (i.e., better functional outcomes).

Personality Disposition

Optimism is a personality disposition that is included in this chapter as an example of a personality disposition or trait that can mediate how disabling conditions are experienced. Several other interrelated personality factors could be discussed (e.g., self-esteem, hostility, and Type A personality). Optimism (in contrast to pessimism) is used for illustrative purposes because it relates to many other personality traits. Optimism is the general tendency to view the world, others, and oneself favorably. People with an optimistic orientation rather than a pessimistic orientation fare better across several dimensions. Optimists tend to have better self-esteem and less hostility toward others and tend to use more adaptive coping strategies than pessimists.

In a study of patients who underwent coronary artery bypass surgery, Scheier at al. (1989) found that optimism was a significant predictor of coping efforts and of recovery from surgery. Individuals with optimistic orientations had a faster rate of recovery during hospitalization and a faster rate of return to normal life activities after discharge. There was also a strong relationship between optimism and postsurgical quality of life 6 months later, with optimists doing better than pessimists. Optimism may reduce symptoms and improve adjustment to illness, because it is associated with the use of effective coping strategies. This same analogy can be extended to impairment. Optimistic individuals are more likely to cope with an impairment by using the active adaptive coping strategies discussed earlier. These in turn will lead to reduced disability.

Summary Four constructs of the psychological environment (i.e., self-efficacy beliefs, psychological control, coping patterns, and optimism) were highlighted to illustrate the influence of these factors on disability and the enabling–disabling process. These psychological constructs are interrelated and are influenced to a large extent by the external social and physical environments. The reason for the inclusion of the psychological environment in this report is to assert that just as the physical and social environments can be changed to support people with disabling conditions, so can the psychological environment. In fact, voluminous empirical research supports the fact that psychological interventions directed at altering cognition lead to improved outcomes (i.e., achievement, interpersonal relationships, work productivity, and health) across diverse populations and dimensions. However, relatively little research has been directed at understanding the process by which the psychological environment can be enhanced for people with disabilities. This research is needed.

The Family and Disability

The family can be either an enabling or a disabling factor for a person with a disabling condition. Although most people have a wide network of friends, the networks of people with disabilities are more likely to be dominated by family members (Norris et al., 1990; Knox and Parmenter, 1993). Even among people with disabilities who maintain a large network of friends, family relationships often are most central and families often provide the main sources of support (Schultz and Decker, 1985; Brillhart, 1988). This support may be instrumental (errand-running), informational (providing advice or referrals), or emotional (giving love and support) (Clark and Rakowski, 1983; Croog et al., 1989; Norris et al., 1990).

Families can be enabling to people with functional limitations by providing such tangible services as housekeeping and transportation and by providing personal assistance in activities of daily living. Families can also provide economic support to help with the purchase of assistive technologies and to pay for personal assistance. Perhaps most importantly, they can provide emotional support. Emotional support is positively related to well-being across a number of conditions. In all of these areas, friends and neighbors can supplement the support provided by the family.

It is important to note, however, that families may also be disabling. Some families promote dependency. Others fatalistically accept functional limitations and conditions that are amenable to change with a supportive environment. In both of these situations, the person with the potentially disabling condition is not allowed to develop to his or her fullest potential. Families may also not provide needed environmental services and resources. For example, families of deaf children frequently do not learn to sign, in the process impeding their children's ability to communicate as effectively as possible. Similarly, some well-meaning families prematurely take over the household chores of people with angina, thereby limiting the opportunity for healthy exercise that can lead to recovery.

Current Research Efforts

As part of its general review and assessment of current rehabilitation-related research (e.g., abstracts from the various federal agencies, surveys

TABLE 6-4 Review of Abstracts Describing
"Disability" for How Environment Is Included
in Study Design: Summary of Findings

Focus of the Abstracts	Number of Abstracts
Research, environment as:	
Dependent	4
Independent	34
Unknown	29
Other	4
Neither	2
Assistive technology	41
Center grants, environment as:	
Dependent	1
Independent	13
Unknown	8
Other	8
Neither	0

of consumer groups, and focus groups), the committee made a concerted effort to identify and evaluate activities and areas of interest that focused on the environment as an independent variable, that is, where the focus is on the effects of the environment in causing disability.

Abstracts

Of the original sample of abstracts that were retrieved from Computer Retrieval of Information on Scientific Projects and from the other (non-Public Health Service) agencies and that were reviewed by the entire committee (a total of 388), 130 were identified as including some focus on "disability." These abstracts were subsequently reviewed further for their focus on the environment as a causal factor, that is, as an independent variable in a study that evaluated disability in some manner.

It was often difficult to assess the particular relevance of the environment in the individual studies. Those that did in fact seem to address the environment in some clear fashion were very small in number (see Table 6-4). The conclusion that can be drawn as a result of this qualitative assessment is that very little research focuses on the environment as an independent variable. Only 34 abstracts seemed to include any aspect of the environment as an independent variable.

CONCLUSIONS AND RECOMMENDATIONS

This chapter has suggested that the environment and characteristics of the individual conjointly determine disability. This chapter has cited numerous examples of how the natural and built environments, the culture of society and its social and economic structures, and the intrapersonal processes of the individual affect whether disability arises from any particular medical condition. Table 6-5 reviews some of this information. It indicates not only what is known about the contribution each makes to the enabling–disabling process, but also where there are gaps in our knowledge. It shows that much research is needed in order to specify ways in which different aspects of environments contribute to this process. The importance of the environment in increasing or decreasing the font of disability is reflected in such recent legislation as the ADA, which mandates equal opportunity to participate in all dimensions of life and which requires reasonable accommodation in the environment to achieve that goal. The importance of the environment is also reflected in the published guidelines for funding of the two major federal research organizations concerned with disability: the National Institute of Health's NCMRR and the U.S. Department of Education's NIDRR.

Despite the growing recognition of the importance of the environment in determining the prevalence of disability, the committee could find relatively little research that explicitly focuses on the impact of the environment on disability. Even though environmental variables do appear in the research, they are seldom the independent variable. Moreover, in much of the research included in the total number of abstracts, the environmental focus is only a small part of a larger project or center grant. Accordingly, the true magnitude of the effort spent on environmental research is much less than even the relatively small total would indicate.

Table 6-5 presents a summary of what is known and what is unknown and needed in the way of information with respect to cultural, psychological, political, and economic factors that affect disability. In addition, the committee offers the following specific recommendations:

Recommendation 6.1 In accordance with the current understanding of the importance of the environment in causing disability, more research is needed to elucidate and clarify that relationship. Such clarification will facilitate the development of more and improved intervention strategies, both preventive and rehabilitative. More specifically, research is needed to:

- *explicitly determine the relationships between the environment and disability where environmental factors are the independent variables, and disability, is the dependent variable,*

TABLE 6-5 Rehabilitation Science and Engineering Needs in Disability

Condition or Category	What Is Known or Available	What Needs to Be Known (unknown/needed)
Culture	Culture affects the acceptance of functional limitations	1. Are cultures more (or less) accepting of functional limitations? 2. What characteristics of U.S. culture are more or less accepting of different types of functional limitations? 3. What characteristics of other cultures make them more accepting of functional limitations? 4. What values and beliefs of subcultures in the United States affect how disability is perceived and ultimately experienced?
Psychology	Psychological factors (e.g, traits, beliefs, thoughts, and coping strategies) affect how limitations and disability are experienced	1. What is the relative contribution of different psychological factors on how disability is experienced? 2. How do psychological factors interact with culture to affect the experience of disability? 3. At what stage of the disabling–enabling process are psychological factors likely to have the greatest impact on how disability is experienced? 4. What is the differential impact of the type of psychological interventions on the experience of disability?
Economic factors	Economic factors affect the extent to which disability is experienced	1. To what extent do the economic resources of the person and family affect ability to purchase such services as personal assistance and assistive technology? 2. How do differences in the economic resources of adjoining communities affect the extent to which impairments and limitations will result in disability? 3. How do major differences in the economic resources of nations affect the extent to which impairments and limitations will result in disability?
Political factors	Public policy affects the objective and subjective experience of disability	1. Has the ADA affected the practices of hiring people with limitations? 2. To what extent are public and private entities improving accessibility to their facilities— either retrofitting old ones or making new ones that comply with architectural standards? 3. Have efforts to educate children with and without disabling conditions together decreased discriminatory attitudes and behaviors among those without disabling conditions 4. How do the different definitions of disability in such federal programs as Social Security, Vocational Rehabilitation, and Individuals with Disabilities Education Act affect the extent to which people with limitations participate in work or school?

- *identify critical factors in work, family, and community environments that enable people with functional limitations.*

Recommendation 6.2 The composition of study sections at NIH and other agencies that have relevance to disability issues should be broadened to include the expertise and awareness that is reflected in the model of disability that is described in this report.

7

Research on the Organization, Financing, and Delivery of Health Services

This chapter focuses on the current status and need for health services research (HSR) as it pertains to the delivery of health services and health-related support services for people with disabling conditions. As investigators continue to develop a better understanding of the pathology of physical impairments and how specific therapeutic interventions and advances in engineering assist in restoring and enhancing function, they must also learn how best to organize, deliver, and finance these interventions so that they can be readily accessed and effectively used by those who need them. This must be done, however, in an environment that continually challenges providers and insurers to contain costs and promote efficient use of limited resources.

The multidisciplinary field of health services research has been successful in developing approaches for studying the roles of organization, finance, personnel, technology, and prevention in the provision of health services and their impact on utilization, cost, and quality of care (Steinwachs, 1991). These methods have been applied across a broad range of populations and specific health conditions. There are limited examples, however, in which these methods have been specifically applied to evaluating the organization, financing, and delivery of services to people with disabling conditions. To the extent that HSR has included disability and rehabilitation in its agenda, it has focused primarily on issues regarding the care of children and the elderly; few studies have focused on the special needs of working-age adults with physical limitations (DeJong et al., 1989). Yet the number of working-age adults is growing faster than any other segment of the population with disabling conditions.

In general, there has been little interaction between the fields of HSR and rehabilitation science and engineering. In a review of articles published in 1986 in the *Archives of Physical Medicine and Rehabilitation*, Fuhrer (1988) found that only 6 percent were in the area of HSR. In 1995 this had increased to 22 percent—although nearly one half of these articles described the development or evaluation of functional outcome and disability measures without reference to the evaluation of services. Similarly, very few reports (less than 5 percent) in the major journals in HSR (e.g., Medical Care and Health Services Research) focus on issues of rehabilitation services delivery and outcomes.

HEALTH SERVICES RESEARCH AGENDA

Influencing Trends

The development of a more comprehensive HSR agenda in rehabilitation science and engineering will be heavily influenced by three important trends in the epidemiology of disability and in the way that health services are organized and delivered (Batavia and DeJong, 1990). First, as significant strides in the clinical management of disabling conditions continue to be made, there will be increasing numbers of people with disabling conditions who are living longer and more active lives. This trend underscores the need for research that incorporates a life-long perspective and that focuses attention on the special needs of people who are aging with a disabling condition. Of critical importance is the development and evaluation of health delivery models that integrate a health promotion strategy that facilitates greater individual control over the determinants of health (Wallerstein, 1992). Equally important, however, is the recognition that disabling conditions are not deficits, but rather conditions of life. The management of a medically stable disabling condition is a personal matter first and a medical matter second (DeJong, 1979). It will be important to evaluate the success of alternative health care delivery models in terms of these parameters.

Second, due in large part to the independent living movement, the expectations of people with disabling conditions have changed drastically and will continue to change in important ways. People with disabling conditions have determined that they are no longer willing to accept life-long dependent relationships, and they want to promote a view of disability as a socially constructed phenomenon. Independent living recognizes that people with disabling conditions are consumers of services rather than patients or clients. At the same time that the independent living movement is gaining momentum and increased acceptance and visibility, the U.S. society is witnessing a revolution in health care, that in general, places more emphasis on consumer preferences and expectations (Relman, 1988). Never before has the consumer's point of view of how well he or she is doing been so important. Their views and preferences are being used by clinicians in making treatment choices, by third-party payers in deciding what to pay for and what not to pay for, and by administrators and policy makers who are making difficult decisions regarding the allocation of expensive resources at the level of the individual practice as well as across society as a whole (Ellwood, 1988; Epstein, 1990). These similar perspectives on the important role of the consumer provide a unique opportunity for the fields of rehabilitation science and engineering and HSR to work together closely in the development and evaluation of health care delivery models that incorporate a consumer orientation toward the identification of needs and appropriate strategies for meeting those needs.

A third and important trend that will influence the agenda of HSR in rehabilitation science and engineering is the continued interest in health care reform with an emphasis on cost-containment and value. New and innovative approaches to the organization, financing, and delivery of health services are being proposed. It is imperative that the rehabilitation field take aggressive and proactive steps toward evaluating the potential impacts of these changes on access, quality, and outcomes of services for people with disabling conditions.

Priorities

The following pages summarize the major HSR issues that need to be addressed over the next decade. These issues have been identified through a review of several major publications that have documented the need for and current deficiencies in the current HSR agenda as it pertains to people with disabling conditions. This review is followed by a discussion of alternative strategies for improving the interface between the fields of HSR and rehabilitation science and engineering.

Before proceeding, however, it is important to point out two caveats to the discussion. First, the committee chose to focus on the current status and needs for HSR as it pertains to the delivery of health services and health-related support services only. These services have been defined as encompassing (1) medical rehabilitation services required for improving and maintaining function, (2) primary health care services for health maintenance and the prevention of secondary conditions, (3) long-term institutional care for those unable to live in the community, and (4) support services including personal assistance services and assistive technologies to assist people with disabling conditions (Batavia and DeJong, 1990). In limiting the discussion to these services only, the discussion will not directly address the organization, financing, and delivery of social and vocational services that, although important to the enabling process, are not traditionally thought of as part of the health care system. However, it is important to underscore the need to develop and evaluate better mechanisms of integrating the delivery of health and social-vocational services; the existing fragmentation of these services is of major concern.

Second, this chapter primarily focuses on the organization, financing, and delivery of *post-acute* care services. The committee recognizes the important role that access to quality care in the acute clinical care setting plays in minimizing the life-long consequences of disabling injuries and illness. It also recognizes that although a growing literature exists on the clinical effectiveness of acute care interventions, much of this literature falls short in identifying the impact of alternative treatment strategies on long-term functional outcomes and quality of life. The needs for research in this area, although not detailed in this chapter, are critical to an overall strategy of improving and enhancing life following major illness or injury.

Several landmark publications have discussed HSR priorities in rehabilitation and engineering (DeJong et al., 1989; Batavia et al., 1991; U.S. Department of Health and Human Services, 1995) The agenda for research encompasses a broad range of substantive and methodological issues; the committee chose to focus on three areas in which more research is particularly important if society is to better ensure that people with disabling conditions have access to the best possible care at costs that are affordable to the individual consumer and to society as a whole. They are as follows:

• Demonstrating the cost-effectiveness of clinical interventions and alternative service delivery models. This research must incorporate a broad range of outcomes, including impairment, functional status, and quality of life, as measures of effectiveness.

• Evaluating how primary health care and long-term support services are accessed, organized, and delivered for people with disabling conditions. The impacts of these services on the prevention of secondary conditions and promotion of well-being over the lifecourse should be given the highest priority.

• Evaluating the impact of managed care delivery systems on access to and use of services, quality of care, costs, and outcomes. This work should extend beyond the evaluation of Medicaid and Medicare programs to include assessments of innovative programs targeted at working adults with disabling conditions.

Cost-Effectiveness Research

Perhaps most important to the HSR agenda in rehabilitation science and engineering is an urgent need for a comprehensive program in clinical effectiveness and outcomes research. Outcomes research is not new to the field of rehabilitation. Yet, the breadth and rigor of the research are not sufficient for serving as a basis for shaping policy, defining treatment services guidelines, developing quality of care criteria, or developing innovative delivery models with greater integration of services.

It is already known that people with disabling conditions use a disproportionate share of health care resources compared to those without disabling conditions. Trupin and colleagues estimate that approximately 17 percent of the population with an activity limitation account for 47 percent of total medical care expenditures (Trupin and Rice, 1996). These individuals incur medical care costs four times as great as people without disabling conditions. Overall, people with disabling conditions account for an estimated $282 billion (in 1993 dollars) in health care expenditures, or 3.1 percent of the gross domestic product (GDP). These figures are only likely to increase given the growing number of people with chronic diseases and disabling conditions, improved availability and access to services, and the proliferation of high-cost technologies. The investment in these expenditures is expected to be outweighed by the economic, social, and personal benefits accrued from getting people back to work or school and living independently. Unfortunately, very few studies have adequately examined the extent to which rehabilitation achieves these goals—and the relationship of achieving these goals to costs. In today's climate of rising health care expenditures and emphasis on cost-containment, it is incumbent upon the rehabilitation community to demonstrate what works best and at what cost. If something costs less, rehabilitation professionals need to make sure it is of comparable value, and if more is to be spent, there should be measurable benefits. Rehabilitation services and outcomes studies should not only focus on the cost-effectiveness of specific treatments and therapies, as discussed in Chapter 4, but should also address the costs and benefits of innovative models and systems for delivering care.

HSR has long recognized that the area of clinical effectiveness and outcomes research is central to its agenda. In the past several years, however, outcomes research has received increased attention from the public and private sectors because of its potential for providing scientific information on which to base decisions (embodied in practice guidelines, insurance coverage, and payment policies) regarding the delivery of cost-effective and efficient health care. Through its multidisciplinary approach to the study of the organization, financing, and delivery of care, HSR has developed new (and has refined existing) paradigms and methodological approaches for examining the relationship between quality of care, costs, and health outcomes (Foundation for Health Services Research, 1991; Grady, 1992; Maklan, Greene, and Cummings, 1994). These approaches to outcomes research have been successfully used in evaluating the cost-effectiveness of specific surgical procedures and alternative approaches to managing acute medical conditions. The results are being effectively communicated among providers and policy makers and are significantly influencing the practice of medical care.

There are very few examples, however, in which HSR methods have been applied to evaluating the effectiveness of rehabilitation services. Yet it is known that substantial variations in practice patterns exist. Variations in the clinical management of disabling conditions and the implications of these variations on outcome were discussed in Chapter 4. In addition to examining the relative effectiveness of specific clinical interventions, attention must also be focused on how services are organized and delivered across different settings and by different types of providers.

Rehabilitation services remain one of the fastest-growing sectors of the health care industry. The characteristics of its growth, however, have changed dramatically over the past several years due to an increased emphasis on managed care as well as changing expectations of providers and consumers. In the 10 years between 1985 and 1994, the number of freestanding rehabilitation hospitals increased from 68 to 187 hospitals (175 percent), and the number of rehabilitation units in acute care hospitals increased from 386 to 804 (118 percent) (DeJong and Sutton, 1994; Wolk and Blair, 1994). With the more recent and growing emphasis on managed care and cost-containment, however, increased emphasis is being placed on lower-cost alternatives to traditional (specialized) inpatient rehabilitation (DeJong et al., 1996). In a study of three advanced managed care markets (San Diego, California; Minneapolis-St. Paul, Minnesota; and Worcester, Massachusetts) DeJong et al. (1996) reported a decline in occupancy rates in rehabilitation hospitals of up to 40 percent; the average length of stay declined from 30 to 35 days to 20 days. Inpatient rehabilitation is now often reserved for individuals with only a handful of conditions.

An increasing number of individuals who were traditionally discharged to inpatient rehabilitation are now being referred for subacute care. Subacute care generally refers to a broad range of medical and rehabilitation services and settings that provide care to post acute patients (Lewin-VHI, 1995). These services are being offered in a variety of settings, including (1) traditional inpatient rehabilitation providers who have diversified and are offering subacute care alternatives, (2) skilled nursing facilities that have added a rehabilitation component, and (3) a growing number of national for-profit chains of providers specifically focused on the delivery of subacute care. Since subacute care day rates are generally half those of inpatient rehabilitation ($500 versus $1,000), substantial cost savings are potentially realized by substituting subacute care for conventional inpatient rehabilitation. These cost savings are generally realized by providing less intensive services (Keith et al., 1995). Very little is known, however, about the comparative merits of these alternative approaches to rehabilitation. It will be important to look at the quality of rehabilitation services provided by subacute care facilities and to compare outcomes for patients treated in subacute care versus conventional inpatient rehabilitation settings. Critical to such a comparison will be adequate control for differences in the casemix of patients treated in alternative settings. In addition, given the diversity in quantity and type of services provided by both subacute care as well as rehabilitation units, it will be important to characterize the mix of services provided within any given setting and to correlate the mix of services with patient outcomes.

As mentioned above, outcomes research is by no means new to the field of rehabilitation. Indeed, some of the earliest contributions to the literature on functional outcomes assessment were made by rehabilitation specialists (Mahoney and Barthel, 1965; Granger et al., 1979). The Functional Independence Measure (FIM) evolved from this early work and is now widely recognized and used as a standard measure of outcomes in medical rehabilitation (Keith et al., 1987). Although further testing of FIM is warranted, it holds promise as an effective tool for routine outcomes assessment for inpatient medical rehabilitation. As discussed in more detail below, however, FIM does not encompass broader issues of outcome such as role activity, psychological well-being, and general health perceptions. It has also been criticized for its lack of sensitivity to the range of disabling conditions associated with traumatic brain injury and other conditions associated with cognitive impairment.

Despite these major advances in outcomes measurement, most experts in the field would agree that a large share of the rehabilitation services delivery and outcomes research being conducted today is deficient in both scope and scientific rigor. Major deficiencies are summarized below.

Measuring Outcome When evaluating the effectiveness of comprehensive rehabilitation services and programs of care, it is important to move beyond the use of narrowly defined measures of morbidity, impairment, and ADL and IADL performance to include more global measures of health status and health-related quality of life (HRQL) (Fawcett et al.,

1993; Ware, 1995). Examples of these types of measures include the Sickness Impact Profile, the Short Form of the Health Status Questionnaire (SF-36), the Child Health Questionnaire, the Functional Status Questionnaire, the Quality of Life Survey and the Quality of Well-Being Scale (Bergner et al., 1985; Jette et al., 1986; Kaplan et al., 1989; Ware and Sherbourne, 1992; Landgraf et al., 1996). Although these measures vary in form and content, they all share two important characteristics in common which distinguish them from measures like FIM. First, they measure function across several domains, including not only physical health, cognitive and mental health, and social function, but also role function and general health perceptions. Perhaps most important, health status and HRQL measures assess outcomes from the consumer's point of view through the use of consumer questionnaires.

It is important to emphasize that HRQL measures should not replace the more traditional measures of impairment, functional capacity, and performance. Rather, they should complement these measures in an attempt to better elucidate the relationships between impairment, functional limitation, disability, and quality of life. An important challenge in outcomes research is choosing an appropriate measure that is meaningful in a clinical or policy context but that is also sensitive enough to detect important differences or changes in outcome.

It is also important to note that these broader measures of outcome and effectiveness greatly expand the power of evaluation research. With these broader measures that are applicable across types of disabilities and programs, it becomes possible to compare evaluation results across types of programs. This is critically needed for addressing resource allocation questions in a time of constrained funding for services (Patrick and Erickson, 1993).

Lack of Comparison Groups A common methodologic deficiency in rehabilitation services and outcomes research is the infrequent use of comparison groups; the use of randomized controlled trials (RCT) is almost nonexistent. In many instances, one can appropriately argue that a RCT is not feasible, too costly, or unethical. However, well-conceived and executed nonrandomized, or quasiexperimental studies that incorporate appropriate, although not randomized, comparisons can provide critically important and often compelling inference. Increasingly, nonexperimental data are being used to guide program and policy decisions. HSR has played an important role in improving the collection, interpretation, and communication of nonexperimental data (Fowler, 1989; Sechrest et al., 1990). These methods, although challenging, must be more widely applied to the evaluation of rehabilitation services and programs.

Need for Conceptual Framework and Longitudinal Designs In addition to incorporating appropriate comparison groups, priority should be given to longitudinal studies of outcome. Both the disabling and enabling processes are complex and longitudinal. To better understand the course of disability, the role of multiple risk factors, and the opportunity for intervention, it is essential that a "lifecourse" perspective be given more attention in research. This research, however, must be undertaken within a theoretical or conceptual framework that emphasizes the important role of nonmedical factors in influencing outcomes. Individuals vary greatly in their ability to adapt to an impairment or functional limitation (Yelin, 1989; Wilson and Cleary, 1995). Variability in outcome depends on a host of personal, social, and environmental factors, many of which are not addressed adequately in rehabilitation services and outcomes research.

Some might argue that such studies do not fall strictly under the purview of health services and outcomes research since many of the services aimed at getting people back to work are focused on educational and training interventions and relate to broader social issues. Yet it is apparent that many of the failures in getting people back to work after the onset of a disabling condition (and keeping them employed) are due to the fragmented nature of the services provided and the lack of communication between the providers of health services on the one hand and psychosocial and vocational services on the other. Better ways to integrate these services are needed. Outcomes studies must take a broad perspective in looking at the multiple determinants of recovery so that appropriate interventions can be identified and effectively targeted. A major challenge of rehabilitation services research is defining and improving the interface between the traditional health care system and the social and vocational services system.

Application of CBA/CEA Cost-benefit analysis and cost-effectiveness analysis (CBA/CEA) of rehabilitation services can be greatly strengthened by incorporating a broader scope of outcome measures. More global measures can facilitate comparison and integration of results across types of disabilities and programs and thereby enhance the power of the analysis. Efforts to incorporate outcomes measures based on consumer input are also important. To date, CBA/CEA studies that value outcomes have tended to focus on measures such as increases in earnings or reduced costs of related public services. The consumer's own valuations of greater community integration, improved quality of life, and increased independence have not been factored into the CBA/CEA calculations. Thus, CBA/CEA have omitted major aspects of program effectiveness that should be recognized if the full value of rehabilitation service programs is to be reckoned.

In the broader health services literature on CBA/CEA, more global outcomes measures based on consumer input and valuation have only recently become widely recognized. The use of these measures has become the focus of a new subfield within health services CBA/CEA, commonly referred to as "cost-utility" analysis (Russell et al., 1996). Extending this cost-utility literature to rehabilitation services is an important research priority.

Broad Framework of Health Systems Finally, it is important that the effectiveness of rehabilitation services and programs be examined within the broad context of the entire health care system. J. Paul Thomas (p. 36) points to the lack of this broader perspective as a serious deficit in rehabilitation services research and training: "It fails to impart an adequate understanding of the larger American health care system of which we are all a part. If we evaluate the efficacy of our clinical efforts without considering the larger health care system, much of our work may become irrelevant and of little use to our clientele" (Batavia et al., 1991).

In an effort to reduce the lengths of stay for hospitalization, for acute care, patients are being discharged earlier, often with a poorer functional status. This approach to cost-containment for hospitalization for acute care is likely to increase the demand for and expenditures associated with outpatient rehabilitation. In the long run, however, overall costs for achieving equivalent, if not better, outcomes may be lowered. It may well be that in an effort to reduce overall costs of health care, the volume and total expenditures for rehabilitation may, in fact, increase (or remain stable). The appropriate timing, intensity, and mix of rehabilitation services may accelerate the recovery process as well as decrease the long-term demand for acute care services for secondary conditions. Thus, the development and application of an "episode approach" to examining the relationship between the use and costs of services (both acute health care and rehabilitation) and outcomes should be given high priority.

It is also important to emphasize that many of the problems associated with poor outcomes in rehabilitation relate back to problems of access to services and its relationship to health insurance and employment (National Council on Disability, 1993). Clearly, these issues are prominent in the national debate on health care reform. Therefore, any studies of access and its relation to outcome must be undertaken in the context of this debate.

Assessing and Meeting the Primary Health Care and Long-Term Support Needs of People with Disabling Conditions

A much-neglected HSR issue in rehabilitation and engineering is the organization, delivery, and cost-effectiveness of services aimed at the primary health care and long-term support needs of people with disabling conditions (Batavia and DeJong, 1990). These services are critical to the prevention of secondary conditions and to the maintenance and improvement of function and well-being over the lifecourse. Yet little attention has been paid to the development of a coherent policy on the provision of these services for people with physical limitations. The committee has identified three broad areas of research that should be given high priority to ensure that people with disabling conditions receive the appropriate primary care and support services they need and are afforded every opportunity to achieve independence, equality, full participation, and economic self-sufficiency. These areas are consistent with the research priorities established at a national consensus conference focused on the primary health care needs of people with physical disabilities (DeJong et al., 1989; Burns et al., 1990).

Primary Health Care Needs and Impediments to Access to Services First, it is important that a better understanding of the primary health care needs of people with disabling conditions and the barriers that impede access to appropriate services be developed. Intrinsic to primary care practice is the promotion of health and the prevention of disease through a sustained partnership between patients and clinicians and within the context of family and community (Institute of Medicine, 1996). In this regard, access to appropriate primary health care is as important to people with disabling conditions as quality medical rehabilitation aimed at restoring function. People with disabling conditions are not only susceptible to acute and chronic health conditions that are typically associated with aging or exposure to environmental hazards or unhealthy lifestyles, but they are also at risk of secondary conditions directly related to their primary condition. It is well known that people with disabling conditions are particularly vulnerable to acute health problems such as decubitus ulcers, urinary tract infections, and contractures. The Centers for Disease Control and Prevention (CDC) through their community based surveillance and prevention programs have fostered the wide recognition of secondary conditions as a significant health problem among persons with disabilities (Graitcer and Maynard, 1990; Toal et al., 1993). These problems not only affect individual quality of life but are also associated with high health care costs, often paid for by public sources. Although a better understanding of the factors related to their incidence is still needed, there is substantial evidence to suggest that many of these problems are avoidable through the promotion of self-care and counseling, screening for early detection, appropriate and timely treatment, and early recognition and reduction of known risk factors (Marge, 1988; Institute of Medicine, 1991; Toal et al., 1993).

Somewhat less is known about patterns in incidence of chronic health problems among people with disabling conditions. There is some evidence to suggest, however, that because of their low margin of health, people with disabling conditions are at risk of developing common chronic health problems such as heart disease and arthritis at an earlier age than the general population (Burns et al., 1990). Furthermore, the impacts of these problems on the individual are often magnified due to the presence of the underlying limitation or disability. More work is needed to better understand the risk of chronic disease among people with disabling conditions. Even more important, however, is research on effective ways of reducing known risks or ameliorating the consequences of common chronic conditions among people with disabling conditions. Much attention has been focused in recent years on the development and evaluation of effective health promotion and disease prevention strategies for reducing an individual's risk of chronic conditions (U.S. Preventive Task Force, 1989). These strategies include protocols for weight reduction, regular exercise, reducing substance abuse, as well as ensuring access to and use of screening protocols for heart disease, cancer, and diabetes. Although some of these strategies may be directly transferable to people with physical limitations, many are not (De Jong et al., 1989; Patrick et al., 1994).

Although one can effectively argue for the importance of primary care services for people with disabling conditions, little is known about how they are accessed and used and even less is known about their quality and impact on well-being and costs. What is known is that existing services are fragmented and often inadequate in addressing (in a timely and cost-effective manner) the constellation of health problems experienced by people with disabling conditions once they are discharged from rehabilitation. Primary care providers are not typically trained to recognize the general health care needs of people with disabling conditions. In the absence of this training, they too often focus on the specific limitation and underlying physical and cognitive impairment and not on the individual's increased susceptibility to acute and chronic health conditions. It also happens that primary care providers who are ill-equipped to address the multiple health problems of a person with a disabling condition inappropriately make referrals to multiple specialty care providers, often resulting in delayed treatment and high health care costs (DeJong et al., 1989). More research is needed to define indicators of quality primary health care for people with disabling conditions and the factors that impede access to appropriate use. This research should refine existing frameworks that have been developed for looking at access, use of and quality of primary health care, and incorporating parameters that are particularly relevant for people with disabling conditions (IOM, 1993, 1996). In identifying factors related to the use of services, for instance, existing frameworks often underemphasize the role that unrecognized need and provider attitudes and perceptions play in accessing and using services. Furthermore, quality indicators do not typically address issues of consumer empowerment and the important role that nonmedical support services play in maintaining health and avoiding hospitalizations (Burns et al., 1990).

Access to Use and Quality of Long-Term Support Services Related to issues of access to and quality of primary health care are issues related to the access, use, and quality of long-term support services. The need for long-term support services to assist people with a disabling condition compensate for a functional limitation is well recognized. These services generally consist of attendant or personal assistance services, assistive technology, as well as institutional care for people with very severe limitations that require daily assistance from medical personnel. Not only do these services help the person with a disabling condition maintain his or her health, but they are also often required for performing activities of daily living comfortably and safely. In many cases, adequate attendant services and assistive technology provide an effective alternative to institutional care. There are very few published studies, however, that scientifically demonstrate the value of these services in improving health and well-being while reducing overall costs to the health care system and society at large (Nosek, 1993). The conduct of these studies will be critical in arguing for adequate coverage of these services by insurers and managed care organizations.

The importance of research on the access to and cost-effectiveness of support services was highlighted at the consensus conference on research priorities in the area of primary health care needs of people with disabling conditions mentioned above (Burns et al., 1990). Developing a better understanding of how personal attendant services are used and financed and their impact on the health and well-being of people with disabling conditions was consistently ranked among the highest priorities. Of particular note is that conference participants ranked access to appropriate attendant services as the number one issue to be addressed in reducing the high rate of rehospitalization among people with disabling conditions. Quantitative research is needed to establish the extent and nature of the relationship between personal assistance and health.

It is important that research focused on the use of and value of long-term support services recognize the critical role of the consumer in framing appropriate research questions and developing appropriate indicators of access and quality (Williams, 1994). Often, too little attention is paid to the needs and preferences of the consumer, leading to dissatisfaction with services, and the disuse and abandonment of technologies. In a review of the literature on the use of prosthetic devices by lower limb amputees, Grisé and colleagues (1993) found that rates varied considerably from 47 to 96 percent. They attribute these differences to variable case definitions as well as to inconsistencies in the definition of "successful prosthetic use." The studies reviewed were even less consistent regarding the factors that influence use and typically did not relate use to functional outcomes and quality of life. Some effort has been directed, however, in developing useful frameworks for looking at these issues. Grisé developed a framework for identifying the predisposing, enabling, and reinforcing factors that are likely to influence use of prosthetic devices. Batavia and Hammer (1990) used a small focus group to develop consumer-based criteria for the evaluation of the quality of assistive technologies (Batavia and Hammer, 1990). Similar efforts are needed to assist in the evaluation of personal assistance services (Ratzka, 1986; Nosek, 1993).

Organization and Financing of Primary Health Care and Long-Term Support Services A third critical area for future research pertains to the organization and financing of both primary health care and long-term support services for persons with disabilities. A major (although clearly not the only) barrier to accessing and appropriately using primary care and long-term support services relates to how these services are organized within the current health care system and how they are financed. The coordination of these services together with more traditional medical rehabilitation services is critical for ensuring life-long continuity of care. The role of innovative approaches to the organization and financing of these services to ensure this coordination and integration should be given high priority in the HSR agenda for rehabilitation and engineering. The issues that need to be addressed in the context of this agenda are discussed in more detail below.

It should be emphasized here that in studying how support services, in particular, are organized and financed, it is critical that a better understanding of the appropriate role of the informal caregiver be developed. Recent reports indicate that only a small proportion of those needing these services are receiving them from formal caregivers (Nosek, 1993; Ratzka, 1986). In most cases family members are providing the assistance. Although research is limited regarding the impact of these arrangements on the family environment, there is sufficient evidence to raise serious questions about the wisdom of this approach in many cases. At the same time there is also evidence to suggest that the care rendered by informal caregivers is not always as effective as the care provided by paid, non-family members. More research is needed to better understand the trade-offs involved in providing personal assistance through formal versus informal caregivers. In doing so, it will be important to develop adequate measures of the quantity and quality of service use. Also, when comparing costs of formal versus informal assistance, both direct expenditures as well as indirect costs accruing to family members should be examined.

Impact of Managed Care

The increasing trend toward managed care in both the public and the private sectors will no doubt have a significant impact on people with disabling conditions. Although good information is lacking regarding the participation of people with disabling conditions in managed care plans, there is evidence to suggest that the percent who are enrolled in some type of managed care organizations (MCO) is similar to that estimated for people without disabling conditions (DHHS, 1995). It will be important for the field of rehabilitation science and engineering to work closely with health services researchers to proactively evaluate the potential impacts of various models of managed care on access to and use of services, quality of care, costs, and outcomes.

The term *managed care* has been used to describe a diversity of integrated service delivery models proposed as alternatives to the traditional fee-for-service indemnity health insurance plan (Weiner and de Lissovoy, 1993). These alternative delivery systems range from managed indemnity plans in which the insurer uses a variety of utilization controls to manage the practices of its providers (who are still paid on a fee-for-service basis) to health maintenance organization (HMOs) or prepaid organized delivery systems where physicians are typically paid on a capitation basis but have financial incentives linked to productivity and efficiency. What these models have in common is an integrated approach to managing service delivery for an enrolled population.

The goal of managed care is to "control health care costs and improve access to and continuity and coordination across a continuum of services." (DHHS, 1995). If this goal were truly realized, a managed care approach to the delivery of health services and health-related services for people with disabling conditions would hold great promise. At present there is little evidence to judge whether or under what conditions these goals can in fact be met. The disability community, however, remains skeptical about the potential success of managed care in meeting its present and evolving needs (see Focus Group discussion in Appendix A). This skepticism is largely based on a lack of information and meaningful evaluation of currently proposed service delivery models. Most of the research and evaluation to date on the impact of managed care for people with disabling conditions has focused on elderly people (DHHS, 1995). A variety of demonstrations have been mounted with funding from the public and private sectors. These include the Social Health Maintenance Organizations (SHMOs), the Program of All Inclusive Care for the Elderly (PACE), and HMOs established under the Medicare Risk Program (and implemented under the Tax Equity and Responsibility Act or TEFRA). These programs have met with varying success; a largely unanswered question is the extent to which they can be successfully extended to younger populations (DHHS, 1995).

The Office of Disability, Aging and Long-Term Care Policy (of the Office of the Assistant Secretary for Planning and Evaluation, U.S. Department of Health and Human Services) has developed a comprehensive research agenda on managed care and disability. The committee endorses this agenda and recommends that federal and private funding agencies use it as a template for establishing their individual priorities in this important area of research. Some of the critical research questions identified in the report include the following:

• What is the impact of different managed care models on access to and use of rehabilitation professionals such as occupational therapy, physical therapy, speech-language therapy, audiology, cognitive therapy, and assistive technologies? If MCO case managers have a good understanding of the service needs and preferences of people with disabling conditions, one can envision systems in which increased access to an appropriate mix of services (i.e., preventive versus curative services and community-based versus institutional care) may result in lower overall costs, increased consumer satisfaction, and better outcomes. Most of the documented and anecdotal evidence accumulated to date, however, suggests that MCOs (particularly private MCOs) are increasingly restricting access to and use of rehabilitation services primarily through the imposition of annual or lifetime caps on use (DHHS, 1995). The impact of these restrictions on consumer outcomes has not been adequately evaluated. Better classification systems and casemix measures are needed to prospectively estimate the services and resources needed to care for people with disabling conditions within an MCO environment. There has been limited success in developing such systems and measures for use in setting hospital reimbursement rates for people with physically disabling conditions. The extent to which these approaches can be used in the context of an MCO has not been evaluated but may hold some promise (Wilkerson et al., 1992; Harada et al., 1993; Stineman et al., 1994). Further research is also needed to evaluate the widely held belief that if MCOs covered needed services on a long-term and ongoing basis that secondary conditions would be avoided and costs savings would be realized through a decrease in hospitalizations

• To what extent and how should both acute care and long-term support services be integrated into a single, consolidated managed care arrangement? What models of integration are most promising? As described above, personal assistance services are critically important to the enabling process. Integrated service delivery models that offer and coordinate long-term care and support services in addition to acute care have the potential of reducing overall health care costs while improving consumer health status and quality of life. Substantial cost savings can be realized since personal assistance and support services are often a less expensive alternative to institutional care. Integrated systems range in character from vertical integration in which all services are provided under a capitated arrangement and within a single delivery system to network arrangements in which providers coordinate services across a wide range of settings (Weiner and de Lissovoy, 1993). A limited amount of research has been focused on the success of these alternative models for integrating services. Again, most of this research has focused on frail elderly people and is process as opposed to outcomes oriented. One exception to this rule has been the evaluation of Boston's Community Medical Alliance (CMA), which is one of the first MCOs to target services exclusively to adults with severe disabling conditions (Meyers and Masters, 1989). Limited evaluation of this program suggests both cost savings and quality care. Critical to this area of research is the development of metrics for assessing the degree of integration.

• What are the advantages and disadvantages of designing and implementing specialized managed care systems for people with disabling conditions (so-called targeted MCOs) versus models that include people with disabling conditions along with the general population? A related question is whether it is more effective and efficient for a targeted MCO to address the needs of all people with potentially disabling conditions versus those of one particular subpopulation (e.g., people with spinal cord injuries)? Although there would appear to be several advantages to MCOs that specialize in managing service delivery for people with disabling conditions, there are major concerns regarding the fiscal viability of such programs. Further concern is raised about the potential for developing a separate but unequal health care system for people with disabling conditions that is constrained in its practice because of limited resources, thereby resulting in inferior care. Although several plans with a targeted focus on delivering care to people with disabling conditions have been implemented, their evaluation has been limited or absent. More research focused on this critical element in the design of MCOs should be given high priority.

• What are the advantages and disadvantages of various risk-sharing arrangements and risk adjustment methods to MCOs? There are few if any financial incentives that presently encourage MCOs to include people with disabling conditions in their practice plans. Given current knowledge, it is exceedingly difficult to predict the costs associated with serving a population with disabling conditions, making it difficult for MCOs to set reasonable and realistic rates. Moreover, if higher premiums are charged, healthier, low-risk participants are likely to disenroll in favor of lower-cost plans. It is critical that more effective strategies for spreading financial risk between payers and providers and between providers and plans be developed and evaluated. For instance, partially capitated or specialty carve-out programs that incorporate reinsurance or stop-loss provisions are used by many states to encourage MCOs to serve high-risk populations. The success to which these programs can effectively serve the needs of people with disabling conditions while ensuring that providers are protected from large financial losses must be examined.

Another important focus of research efforts should be the development of improved methods of risk adjustment. The development of effective adjustment methods has been difficult due to the wide variability in service needs and utilization among people with disabling conditions as well as the disproportionately high use by a small and unpredictable subgroup of the population. For the most part MCOs currently rely on prior utilization and cost data to forecast expected expenditures. There is a growing consensus, however, that effective risk adjustment methods must incorporate appropriate measures of functional status to better predict potential resource utilization and costs (Wilkerson et al., 1992; DeJong and Sutton, 1994; Heinemann et al., 1994, Stineman, 1995).

In summary, much work is needed to better understand the advantages and disadvantages of various managed care models of service delivery. In conducting this research it will be important to carefully distinguish among the range of managed care arrangements and practices and to determine what aspects of each are associated not only with lower costs but also with improved outcomes and consumer satisfaction. To do this, the field of rehabilitation science and engineering must develop appropriate measures of quality of care that are relevant to the ongoing and lifelong needs of people with disabling conditions. It will also be important to examine the impact of managed care for people across the broad spectrum of types and levels of disabling conditions since service needs and effective strategies for addressing these needs may vary substantially. **Finally, the needs of the working age population need to be of higher priority in the development and evaluation of new strategies to provide sufficient care.**

Summary

This chapter has attempted to summarize some of the health services research issues in rehabilitation and engineering that deserve priority attention. It is clear that what is needed to address each of these issues is better data and access to information systems that can be used to identify needs and evaluate access, use, quality, outcomes, and costs of services to address these needs. The Interagency Committee on Disability Research through its Disability Statistics Subcommittee has reviewed in detail the federal databases that include information about disabling conditions. They point to several inadequacies of these databases, including lack of uniform definitions of disability, a lack of attention to the needs of children and working age people with disabling conditions, limited measures of disability that do not encompass dimensions of health beyond activities of daily living, as well as the decentralization of many data systems. In addition, there exist no longitudinal or panel data maintained on a national level to track the needs of people with disabling conditions over the lifecourse. The 1994–1995 Disability Supplement to the National Health Interview Survey (NHIS) was the first exhaustive survey on disabling conditions undertaken since 1978 (see Chapter 2). It holds great promise as a rich source of data on many issues important to the agenda in HSR research in rehabilitation science and engineering. Unfortunately, the 1994–1995 Disability Survey is currently planned as a one-time supplement to the NHIS. Developing the supplement into a panel study would be of enormous value to the research community.

DEVELOPING A HEALTH SERVICES RESEARCH CAPACITY IN REHABILITATION SCIENCE AND ENGINEERING

To address the research agenda discussed above adequately, it will be important to develop a stronger HSR capacity in the field of rehabilitation science and engineering. As previously discussed, there is little interaction between traditional rehabilitation researchers on the one hand and health services researchers on the other. Few providers of rehabilitation have been adequately trained in the methods needed in HSR. At the same time, few health services researchers have focused their work on issues related to the organization, delivery, financing, and quality of services for people with disabling conditions. The field of aging research has established an extensive HSR agenda focused on elderly people with disabling conditions. Yet there is still very limited interaction between this field and the disability and rehabilitation research community. Often, the two fields speak different languages and espouse different paradigms for examining similar issues. The values and perspectives of both are important and should be better integrated to address the multiplicity of issues in ensuring that services to people with disabling conditions of all ages are provided in a cost-effective and cost-efficient manner.

The committee recommends two approaches to facilitate the development of a broader HSR capacity in rehabilitation science and engineering. First, it recommends that transdisciplinary doctoral and postdoctoral training programs be developed in HSR with a concentration in rehabilitation science and engineering. These programs should be designed both for clinicians who require additional training in the issues and techniques of HSR as well as for health services researchers who are interested in applying their knowledge and skills to the study of rehabilitation service delivery. The training programs should emphasize the cross-disciplinary and interdisciplinary nature of the field. Several federal programs have endorsed the establishment of training programs as a high priority. Often, however, these priorities are not translated into appropriations of sufficient funds. Furthermore, few opportunities exist for training specific to HSR.

A second strategy for developing the HSR capacity is the establishment of Centers for the Organization, Delivery, and Financing of Health and Health-Related Services to People with Disabilities. These centers should be collaborative ventures across departments and schools in a university setting that has well-established programs in both rehabilitation science and engineering as well as health services research. One possible model that can be used in establishing these centers is the one used by the National Institute of Mental Health to establish its Centers on the Organization and Financing of Care to People with Severe Mental Illness. These centers have been very successful in forwarding the agenda in HSR and mental health through the establishment of transdisciplinary research collaborations and training and the creation of a sustaining environment to support researchers and research. The Injury Prevention and Research Centers funded by the National Center for Injury Control and Prevention at the CDC have also been successful in forwarding the research agenda needed to reduce the incidence and impact of traumatic injuries. These centers, which currently number 10, are specifically designed to integrate multiple disciplines in addressing the prevention and control of injuries. They have successfully stimulated the development of new teams of injury researchers that have been critical to the development of the science of injury control.

RECOMMENDATIONS

Recommendation 7.1 Highest priority should be given to research in the following three areas:

- *Cost-effectiveness of specific clinical interventions and service delivery systems. This research should incorporate a broad range of outcomes including impairment, functional status, and quality of life as measures of clinical and program effectiveness.*

- *Access to and organization and delivery of services that address the primary health care and long-term support needs of people with disabling conditions. The impacts of these services on the prevention of secondary conditions and promotion of well-being over the lifecourse should be given the highest priority.*

- *The impact of managed care on access to and use of services, quality of care, cost, and outcomes. This work should extend beyond the evaluation of Medicaid and Medicare programs to include assessment of innovative programs targeted at working-age adults. Add-ons to major demonstrations of managed care delivery systems should be funded. These add-ons should specifically examine the impact of managed care on people with disabling conditions.*

Recommendation 7.2 Establish Centers for the Organization, Delivery, and Financing of Health and Health-Related Services to People with Disabilities. These centers should be collaborative ventures across departments and schools in a university setting and should incorporate components of research, teaching, and community outreach service.

Recommendation 7.3 Develop transdisciplinary doctoral and postdoctoral training programs in health services research with an emphasis in rehabilitation and engineering. These programs should be designed for both clinicians and nonclinicians and emphasize the cross-disciplinary and interdisciplinary nature of the field. Special efforts should be made to encourage and facilitate such training among persons with disabilities. Additional funding would be required to support this activity.

Recommendation 7.4 Develop and maintain longitudinal databases that track the health care needs of people with disabling conditions, their use of services, and outcomes or health status. Specifically, the 1994–1995 Disability Supplement to the NHIS should be developed into a panel study and supported over time to perform maintenance and analysis activities. Additional funding would be required to support this activity.

8

Translating Research into Practical Applications

Scientific discoveries must be translated into clinical practice to benefit humanity. *Technology transfer* is the transmittal of developed ideas, products, or techniques from a research environment to one of practical application, and thus is an important component of rehabilitation science and engineering. By disseminating the knowledge and products that researchers have developed, their science attracts more attention and success and has value to society by improving the health and quality of life of those who ultimately benefit from the knowledge. No topic is likely the focus of more discussion but less productive action than technology transfer. The reason is simple: technology transfer is difficult and problematic. Rogers (1983, p. 1), in *Diffusion of Innovations*, says, "One reason why there is so much interest in the diffusion of innovations is because getting a new idea adopted, even when it has obvious advantages, is often very difficult."

In the context of governmental agency support for research, the idea of technology transfer usually means moving the results of government-sponsored research and development (R&D) out of laboratories and into practical application. With companies, it means developing or obtaining new technologies for their business enterprises. The technology may be products or devices, procedures, techniques, processes, software, knowledge, concepts, and so forth. Once the technology or knowledge is available, the issue becomes how it should be diffused throughout society. For purposes of this discussion it is assumed that technology transfer represents positive action for society.

THE CURRENT STATE OF TECHNOLOGY
TRANSFER IN REHABILITATION

This definition of technology transfer has application for rehabilitation science: the biomedical and engineering applications of rehabilitation research can follow some, but not all, of the traditional technology transfer mechanisms. Rehabilitation research does pose a new challenge that requires additional mechanisms for transfer, because much of the research results in therapeutic interventions that are applied in exercise techniques and educational strategies by professionals, not through the use of drugs or equipment.

In traditional pharmaceutical clinical research, after a drug is synthesized in the laboratory and tested with animal models or after the device is developed and bench tested, it is subjected to clinical (phase I to IV) trials—research studies designed to address specific questions about the safety and effectiveness of new methods or tools in prevention or treatment—supervised by the U.S. Food and Drug Administration (FDA). Phase I trials focus on safety and usually involve small samples (20 to 100) of healthy volunteers. Phase II trials test the efficacy of the drug, usually in studies with dozens or hundreds of patients and often in randomized controlled trials. Phase III trials test the safety, efficacy, and possible adverse reactions, usually in multicenter, randomized, and blinded trials. Phase IV studies usually compare the new therapy with the available alternative interventions and determine its long-term effectiveness and side effects and the cost-effectiveness of the intervention(s) (Pocock, 1987). Most clinical research is funded by private industry (biotechnology or pharmaceutical companies) or the federal government (e.g., the National Institutes of Health [NIH], the National Science Foundation, the Centers for Disease Control and Prevention, or the National Institute on Disability and Rehabilitation Research [NIDRR]).

The successful transfer of rehabilitation interventions such as therapeutic exercise and physical modalities from research to practice poses a different set of problems than the transfer of drugs. Drugs are discrete entities and are thus easily regulated by the federal government, but rehabilitation interventions are more generic and are less amenable to FDA regulation. Indeed, most such interventions would be "grandfathered" because despite subtle differences in approach, practice regimen, and other details, most rehabilitation interventions would still be "exercise" and thus not subject to regulation. Nonetheless, initiatives such as the stroke care guidelines of the Agency for Health Care Policy and Research provide valuable federal guidance to local practitioners (Gresham et al., 1995) by offering structure to the best and evidence-based practices that should result in comparable care for individuals following a stroke. Rehabilitation relies at least in part on methods such as this for the dissemination of interventions proven to be effective by research.

Those who require access to information generated from rehabilitation research include professionals in practice and in training, rehabilitation scientists, people with disabling conditions and their families, architects, and policy makers including elected officials, insurers, and administrators. Research findings should foster high-quality care and services for people with disabling conditions, enable better disability prevention, build community networks of care to guide the development of effective and efficient rehabilitation services, and stimulate further research efforts.

No organized mechanism for the development of rehabilitation science exists, however, nor does a formal mechanism for distributing the findings of rehabilitation science to those providing services. Few journals focus on interdisciplinary research. Although the U.S. Department of Veterans Affairs (VA) publishes and distributes free for the asking *The Journal of Rehabilitation Research and Development*, VA does not presume that it publishes all the information that the federal government should disseminate. In part because the journal is chronically underfunded, the delay between the time of submission and the time of publication is, on average, longer than 1 year, and the journal is not widely distributed, so it lacks the prestige of major journals. More funding would help to improve the turnaround time for articles in this journal and to improve the prestige of this journal and others like it. An additional dissemination problem results from the fact that rehabilitation professionals are taught according to an individual profession's criteria and traditions; few opportunities for cross-disciplinary interaction are available and the professions are not knowledgeable about the science of the other professions.

Models are needed to increase cross-disciplinary communication. Rehabilitation is an interdisciplinary field and ultimately patients will only benefit when professionals have access to information that will support their patients through their recovery and re-entry to their family, work, and community lives. One such model for rehabilitation science and engineering to consider for dissemination is the extension model used by the U.S. Department of Agriculture (USDA). This model allows physicians, farmers, homemakers, and scientists alike to obtain state-of-the-art information from USDA county extension agents, pamphlets, and from USDA-sponsored information services. The Administration on Disability and Rehabilitation Research could facilitate transfer of information among (See Chapter 10), to give nurses, therapists and physicians access to information that would support organizations, professions, consumer groups, providers, and others access to accurate, evidence-based rehabilitation information. Just as USDA's sponsorship of home economics classes encouraged better nutrition nationwide, similar encouragement related to disability prevention and the adaptation of a healthy lifestyle could be provided if information were readily available.

Perhaps the proposed Administration on Disability and Rehabilitation Research could foster the development of dissemination centers to address the regional needs of rehabilitation providers. A model such as the *Dartmouth Atlas of Health Care* (Center for the Evaluative Clinical Sciences, Dartmouth Medical School, 1996) documents a substantial nationwide variability in many health care interventions and there is no reason to believe that rehabilitation interventions would be more homogeneous nationwide. Therefore, the federal government through the ADRR could facilitate the provision of information on scientifically based practices to all locales to prevent the selective implementation on the basis of the specific characteristics of a locale.

PRESUPPOSITIONS FOR TECHNOLOGY TRANSFER

Technology transfer presupposes several conditions; otherwise, it cannot come about. Some of the presuppositions are described in the following sections.

A Technology Must Exist

Technologies must exist to be transferred. This seems obvious, but technologies do not appear de novo. Someone must bring them into existence. Usually, new technologies come from R&D programs, although a limited number of technologies may result from innovation or invention processes that may not be strictly classified as R&D. For much technology transfer to come about, sponsored R&D projects, public or private, need to exist. There will not be much technology transfer if there is not strong, productive research, and funds must be available for R&D efforts. A supply of competent and creative researchers must also exist. The existence of productive scientists and engineers in laboratories presupposes that good educational programs exist. The preparation of people for careers in R&D is fundamental to new technology development. In short, a strong R&D effort and infrastructure for technological development must exist before technology can be transferred.

Organizational Structures and Mechanisms

Organizational structures and mechanisms that can foster technology transfer need to exist. A structured method or mechanism is needed to promote the process of technology transfer and to help eliminate barriers to the transfer process. People involved in R&D frequently do not want or have the skills required for technology transfer. Technology transfer officers facilitate the process in some research organizations. Unless someone or some group accepts responsibility for the transfer process, it is likely to wither and stop. Even if assistance is available, the process often halts after the demonstration of concept.

Even if transfer to commercialization takes place, the technology still needs to be diffused into society. Rogers (1983, p. 5) says, "Diffusion is the process by which an innovation is communicated through certain channels over time among the members of a social system." For example, VA has a Technology Transfer Section within its Rehabilitation Research and Development Program that attempts to transfer technology developed through VA-sponsored rehabilitation research. This unit has the capacity to fund technology transfer by soliciting the manufacture of prototype devices from manufacturers and by evaluating the prototypes in VA medical centers. Positive evaluation leads to VA approval of the technology for purchase. This process stimulates the commercialization of the product. The Small Business Innovative Research (SBIR) process is a mechanism that the U.S. Congress set up to stimulate technology transfer by providing start-up funding to small companies that develop technologies that may come out of agency-funded research. NIDRR funds a center that has the mission of fostering technology transfer. From about 1950 to 1975 the Committee on Prosthetics Research and Development of the National Research Council coordinated prosthetics research efforts and conducted evaluation studies, which often resulted in technology transfer.

Private companies encourage technology transfer by two primary means. First, some of them conduct in-house R&D and transfer the technology directly. Second, large companies often purchase small companies to obtain the technologies that they want. This purchasing technique is an efficient means of obtaining technologies that are desirable, and it has become a prevalent method as companies have decreased their own involvement in R&D. Because rehabilitation is generally a service rather than a product, the purchasing method is not a viable option unless health systems have an incentive to develop the service as a product.

Wherever technology transfer occurs, it often involves the patent process, trade secrets, licensing arrangements, and other legal matters. A number of laws concerning technology transfer have been passed by Congress. Many believe that the Technology Transfer Act of 1986 (Public Law 99-502), which amends the Stevenson-Wydler Act of 1980, is the most significant, particularly with respect to government laboratories and private organizations.

Rogers (1983, p. 159) believes that the agricultural extension model, which involves a research system, county extension agents, and state extension specialists, has been the most successful federal agency model in securing users' adoption of research results, although not everyone shares his viewpoint. He points out that the extension program spends about the same amount on technology transfer that is spent on agricultural research. Most federal agencies apparently spend only about 4 to 5 percent of their research funding on transfer and diffusion activities, which is nowhere near the amount spent in the agricultural extension model. Several government agencies, such as the National Cancer Institute's Community Clinical Oncology Program, have tried to copy the agricultural extension model with mixed success. It is clear that dissemination requires a commitment of resources that must be built into the mission of the agency and must be funded.

Promoters and Champions of Technology

Intelligent decision makers and promoters need to exist. It appears that few technologies are ever transferred without a person or groups of people to champion their cause, sometimes over a long period of time (see Box 8-1). This person may be a technology transfer officer, the developer(s), or some other interested party. It is clear that considerable effort and perseverance are needed by this advocate if the technology transfer is to come about. The supporter often is someone who has a vision of what the technology can become. In this respect, champions for technology transfers are like good scientists; they have intuition concerning what technologies should be pushed for transfer and what should be left alone. They may have administrative acumen, and good administrators may know how to cut through red tape and bureaucratic delay. Few experts on technology transfer exist, however, and the field is not systematized. Market research can help, but it is not a complete answer. Consumers do not always know what they need or what they would purchase. Marketing managers in companies regularly launch new products, some of which have gone through extensive marketing surveys, but according to Rogers (1983, p. 74), only 1 of every 540 ideas results in a successful product and only 8 percent of the approximately 6,000 new consumer items introduced each year have a life expectancy of 1 year or longer.

Although intelligence and experience are needed in the technology transfer process, they do not ensure success. Even products or ideas that are clearly superior to those that already exist are not always successful. For example, from an ergonomic viewpoint, the Dvorak keyboard for typewriters and computers is clearly advantageous over the commonly used QWERTY arrangement. Nevertheless, even though a conversion would be technically very simple today

---

BOX 8-1
Technology Transfer: A Sometimes Lengthy Process

Although success stories in research and development and in technology transfer abound, one seldom knows about the tortuous path, effort, and time associated with a transfer. Likewise, one is seldom aware of the research and development work that does not pan out or that for some reason does not reach users. Only a small amount of research and development work is successful all the way to technology transfer. That does not mean that most research and development is not vital. It is as important to find out what does not work as to find what does, and even perhaps more so. In the long run, negative results may help science and engineering more than positive results, because research—whether it results in positive or negative results—advances knowledge and knowledge is the foundation on which all further advances are based.

For example, blood substitutes that can be stored for long periods of time, that do not have to be Rh matched to recipients, and that can be made free of pathogens will soon be available for clinical use. This new product of research and development is predicted to save thousands of lives annually in trauma management alone. By the time commercial production begins and the product is available in the United States, probably in 1998, 14 years will have elapsed since the substitute's active components, stitched hemoglobin molecules, were demonstrated in a University of Iowa laboratory. This example illustrates that even discoveries of great medical importance and high potential profit often take a long time to be transferred from the bench to the bedside. Technology transfer is seldom rapid and often takes longer than the research itself. Therefore, the research team that made the discovery usually moves on to other important research work, and rightly so. Only when the product or technique has someone who serves as its champion or when there are excellent possibilities for financial profits does the technology have much chance of being transferred.

Technology transfer out of federal agency-backed research programs is arduous, but similar difficulties exist even when the product is developed by a private company's own research laboratories. For example, it is well known that scientists and engineers at Xerox Corporation's Palo Alto Research Center developed the precursors of today's personal computers, with mice and graphical user interfaces, 10 to 12 years before the Apple Corporation introduced the Macintosh and more than 20 years ahead of Windows 95. The technology was there, but its importance was initially not understood or acted upon. Consequently, technology transfer did not occur. This kind of difficulty with technology transfer is more common than might be expected by those who have not had experience with the process.

---

with computers, involving only some software changes, there has yet been no movement to the Dvorak system.

Goal-directed R&D is effective if knowledge concerning what is needed exists and if the technology to produce what is needed exists. In rehabilitation research, the application must be of use to people with disabling conditions. Thus, the research process requires consumer involvement in the design and implementation of studies if the results are to have wide applicability. Basic research often creates the knowledge concerning what needs to be done. It also often creates the knowledge necessary to produce the needed technology. Basic research and goal-directed research are both important. Technology transfer withers if either is missing for a period of time.

The Market

A market must exist for innovations. Technology transfer and diffusion cannot proceed without customers. Even though there are millions of people with disabling conditions, their problems are individual and their resources for technology are limited, so markets are generally small and the products needed are extremely varied. There is no mass market, but the needs are nevertheless great. Some of the markets are similar to "orphan drug" markets and might be called "orphan product" markets. Societal assistance may be necessary to meet some needs for orphan products in rehabilitation. Other needs are frequently met by small companies that can be effective in niche markets. Mass-produced products of major companies can often be modified to effectively meet rehabilitation needs, and rehabilitation engineers have taken the lead with such modifications. The concept of universal design is generally a good one for the design of products. Often, small modifications can make major products accessible to almost everyone. Design of this nature can come about naturally through communications with companies about the need for universal design; however, laws concerning access can also be effective in bringing about design that permits access by as many people as reasonably possible.

The Role of Federal Agencies

Agencies must want the innovations that they research to be transferred. Most universities have technology transfer officers and incubation facilities for small companies, some started with SBIR funding. In rehabilitation, the Committee on Prosthetics Research and Development of the National Research Council was effective in research coordination and technology transfer during a previous era. Whether the R&D milieu in Washington, D.C., permits such action today is questionable. The SBIR process apparently seems to be working well in some areas of medicine, but its influence on rehabilitation product transfer remains undetermined. The Technology Transfer Section of the Rehabilitation R&D Program in VA has been successful in technology transfer, and although it is limited to developments made by VA medical centers, its organizational and functional structure can be applauded. The NIDRR model, which uses a center to advance technology transfer matters, has yet to be scientifically evaluated.

NIH has the Office of Technology Transfer (OTT), but it apparently does not involve rehabilitation science and engineering. Each of the institutes, centers, and divisions within NIH conducts its own dissemination and technology transfer activities. NIH as a whole uses OTT as a focal point for coordinated technology transfer in the planning stages of the research process. This office uses Cooperative Research and Development Agreements to forge joint government–industry research projects and Material Transfer Agreements to facilitate the exchange of research materials. OTT also handles the intellectual property portfolio, which includes patenting, for NIH scientists and research.

The National Cancer Institute (NCI), through its Community Clinical Oncology Program (CCOP), has been particularly successful at technology transfer by providing patients access to state-of-the-art care. Established in 1983, the program focuses on clinical trials as its primary vehicle for dissemination. Central to the success of this program is the linkage of patients and providers, each with their own incentives. By increasing the number of patients and physicians who can participate in clinical trials, CCOP hopes to bring the latest techniques and technologies to a larger number of people at the community level while increasing the knowledge base of cancer treatment research as a whole.

Because, as noted earlier, most rehabilitation interventions do not require FDA approval, the federal control exerted in a program such as CCOP alone cannot work in transfer of rehabilitation technology. Controlling access to powerful anticancer drugs gives the government a lever to encourage patients to enroll in clinical trials; only in trials involving a medical device (e.g., prosthetic and orthotic) would this encouragement be apt. To be done properly, strong federal support is required, but occasionally, innovative individuals can generate important new contributions to the science. Therefore, the committee does not recommend that a restrictive system such as CCOP be adopted to enhance rehabilitation technology transfer. The CCOP system could, however, be adapted to the rehabilitation science and engineering environment to encourage multicenter trials. As such, a system coordinated by the ADRR would need to be developed with the expressed mission to:

- improve quality of care;
- serve as continuing education for physicians and other health professionals;
- support a diversified research agenda spanning many scientific disciplines and foster interdisciplinary efforts;

- provide a mechanism for the linkage and participation of basic, clinical, behavioral, and social scientists;
- serve as an umbrella for fundamental as well as applied research, thus enhancing the activities of the investigators;
- create bridging mechanisms to link prevention and clinical studies with ongoing research activities;
- provide a mechanism to manage the explosion of new information and assimilate new information into clinically meaningful concepts for dissemination to practicing clinicians;
- support broad social policy to spread the benefits of treatment of the population to control research;
- create a spirit of cooperation both within the institution and among institutions working on the same disease or disorder;
- be cost-effective by reducing the need for repetitive samples, (studies at multiple centers allow for multiple analyses); and
- allow for the timely accomplishment of an effort.

Two additional benefits could be achieved by having a technology transfer mechanism:

- individuals with disabling conditions can function as consultants to centers to bring validity to the questions and methods used to identify and study the constructs, and
- a registry of people involved in studies will bring together resources for long term follow-up and analysis.

As noted at the beginning of this chapter, technology transfer is difficult and complicated. It is an important human process, however, that is chaotic, unstructured, and problematic. It is also full of promise, opportunity, and excitement.

BARRIERS TO INFORMATION TRANSFER

The barriers to translating rehabilitation research into clinical practice are rooted in limited mechanisms to transfer the research. Clinical rehabilitation research is severely underfunded and thus is still in its early stage. Likewise, because several disciplines are involved, little formal theory has emerged across the disciplines and formal mechanisms for transferring knowledge are limited. More research in rehabilitation science and engineering would likely change this situation. However, more research requires formal mechanisms for transferring knowledge to multiple disciples. There currently is not a joint journal or conference to facilitate communication among the rehabilitation sciences like the Gerontology Society which has a medical science, behavioral science and social science division.

Because few rehabilitation procedures have undergone rigorous clinical trials, treatments are based on theoretical rationale rather than data from tests with people with disabling conditions. Most rehabilitation research to date has been focused at the pathology and impairment levels and not at the levels that relate to functional limitation and how people with disabling conditions interact with the environment (see Chapter 4 of this report) (Jette, 1995). For example, no randomized prospective trials on even the most frequently used rehabilitation treatments, such as postcruciate ligament repair surgery, have been conducted. Few models exist that bring the patient, the physician(s), therapists, scientist, engineers, and communities together to solve problems that limit disabilities. One of the first issues that the federal effort in rehabilitation research needs to address is this shortage of knowledge.

Limited funding for rehabilitation research also limits the number of trained and experienced researchers and artificially lowers the demand for training in clinical research. At this time, only a few universities offer formal degree-granting programs in clinical investigations. With increased funding, rehabilitation could develop a cadre of researchers who could establish formal theories that would drive future rehabilitation science and engineering.

Finally, formal mechanisms of knowledge transfer are not well developed in rehabilitation science. The availability of as well as access to properly controlled outcomes research is very limited. To build the most effective mechanisms for the transfer of products of research, a partnership among the researchers, the government programs that fund the research, educators, health service providers, and consumers will be required. To increase the likelihood of successful technology transfer, rehabilitation research needs a market link. This involves tying the products of R&D to the market economy and increasing the knowledge available to the consumers of rehabilitation products to increase market demand. This will strengthen the interest of people with disabling conditions who have needs that can only be served by knowledgeable professional and private enterprise. The demands should invigorate research and technology transfer, similar to the relationship that research now has with drug companies, which fund the majority of clinical trials.

TECHNOLOGY TRANSFER MECHANISMS
IN THE PRACTICE PROFESSIONS

Traditional mechanisms intended to engender evidence-based clinical practice are largely untested. It is widely assumed that clinicians read and update their fund of knowledge from peer-reviewed research articles, review articles based on the these research articles, and textbooks. The quality of review articles varies substantially, from those that are based on studies performed by controlled, scientific approaches to those with clearly biased perspectives. The Cochrane Collaboration is an ongoing effort to assemble and disseminate clinical research evidence pertinent to best clinical practices (Silagy and Lancaster, 1995). The Cochrane Collaboration has volunteers reviewing "every trial of a medical treatment ever done," most of which "have been either forgotten or simply lost" (Taubes, 1996). This "diffusion gradient" approach, however, assumes that clinicians simply need access to sufficient quantities of relevant research to change their beliefs and practice habits. No such collaboration exists in rehabilitation. Moreover, not all clinical research is equally valid. As many as half of the published randomized, blinded clinical trials may have been inadvertently unblinded by inadequate concealment (Schulz et al., 1994, 1995). Instead, clinicians apparently demand that all new ideas look like old ideas: "Proposed changes in practice are much more likely to succeed when they are compatible with existing beliefs" (Graham, 1996).

Continuing education programs also stimulate change in practice behaviors. Practicing clinicians either spend their own money or decide to use a continuing education allocation for a given continuing education offering and therefore have a strong incentive to implement the findings described during a continuing education course. In rehabilitation in particular, continuing education courses are most often taught not by scientists or clinical researchers who have published peer-reviewed research articles, but by clinicians who often offer charismatic presentations based on dogma and their own anecdotal experience. Indeed, so little clinical research is conducted in rehabilitation that charisma and persuasive rhetoric are often the main criteria on which professionals can judge continuing education courses; course content is almost never based on outcomes research or other forms of clinical investigation, and thus is forced to rely on anecdotal experience (Rothstein, 1992).

Finally, peer, consumer, and payer pressures shape some aspects of clinical decision-making in rehabilitation. If the community standard is to provide myofascial release or trigger point therapy for back pain, then the local physiatrist and therapist will be expected to offer this modality, irrespective of its basis in science or logical rationality. In fact, a number of MCOs are beginning to recognize and pay for methods of rehabilitation services that have not been tested scientifically. Clearly, some better mechanisms need to be put in place to offer accountability to consumers who have disabling conditions that require management and may benefit from a much more comprehensive approach that considers the factor that will contribute to their return to family, work, and community life.

Clinical Research Evidence

U.S. health care practice, and rehabilitation practice in particular, is not now bound by patient-oriented research evidence. It could, however, reasonably be guided by clinical research evidence. At least three impediments now exist: (1) lack of evidence pertinent to the clinical decision, (2) paucity of training and techniques for effectively transferring the evidence that does exist to the practicing clinician and to the rehabilitation consumer, and (3) lack of incentives and inappropriate priorities that can be used to guide clinicians in implementing their existing knowledge of best practices.

Lack of Clinical Research

Evidence-based health care practices are not the norm, particularly in rehabilitation (Benjamin, 1995; Taubes, 1996). The first barrier to conforming to best practices-based clinical care is the extreme paucity of clinical effectiveness research. Few data documenting controlled randomized trials of even the most common interventions and procedures in rehabilitation exist, primarily because of a lack of direct institutional and federal support for resource and incentive structuring of strong research and training programs in rehabilitation (Selker, 1994).

Clinical or patient-oriented research is defined as the type of research performed while the patient and clinician or care provider are in direct contact. Clinical research is chiefly oriented toward determining what works rather than the cellular or detailed mechanisms by which an intervention is effective. However, properly controlled clinical research provides insight into treatment mechanics and will guide future research by helping to generate theoretical explanations for what works (Gresham et al., 1995).

Rehabilitation has a limited tradition of clinical research. Only a few residency programs and entry-level therapist programs train clinicians in data collection and research designs that are congenial to rehabilitation research in clinical settings (Selker, 1994). Traditional research design classes assume that research in phase I to IV trials is the norm in the clinic when in fact few rehabilitation practitioners have any hope of applying such designs in the clinical setting. Clinical research can be divided into outcomes and translational research. Outcomes research usually encompasses treatment effectiveness and, in some cases, cost-effectiveness. Because so little effectiveness research is done, cost-effectiveness research is largely conjecture and is based on estimates of indirect benefits.

Translational research takes bench research directly to the bedside, usually when the risks are small or the benefit could be overwhelming. For example, there is little risk in translating orthotic materials research directly from improved metal alloys to use of the alloys in improved leg braces. Greater risk may be acceptable when the disease will surely and swiftly lead to death; gene therapy, in such cases, may be an attractive, albeit little tested, alternative. Gene therapy offers another example of a new means of intervening in many genetically induced, chronic illnesses, including cystic fibrosis, Tay-Sachs disease, and many other inherited diseases. Although such therapy may well obviate cystic fibrosis in the future, similar to the way that vaccinations against polio virus eradicated polio and changed the rehabilitation needs of people who had polio. However, the consequences of polio in an aging population remain untested and the side effects will remain unknown until large-scale studies, including phase I to IV clinical trials, are complete (Blaese et al., 1995).

Such bench-to-bedside translational research may bring a revolution to rehabilitation if familial diseases can be eradicated or ameliorated, but it is too soon to know the impact of such "cure" research. For example, if congenital limb deformities can be prevented, pediatric upper limb prosthetics will be essentially unneeded unless they are needed as a result of, for example, farm injuries (Krebs and Fishman, 1984). Translational research can also take observations from the bedside, that is, from direct patient observation, to the laboratory, where disease mechanisms can be investigated in reductionistic cell or animal models with the ultimate purpose of better understanding the fundamental nature of the disease process.

Translational research can also benefit tradition rehabilitation "care" research. Anatomy laboratory observations of joint arthrokinematics translate into the now commonly accepted practice of joint mobilization— the practice of applying linear motions (e.g., distraction and gliding) to increase angular range of motion, rather than simply forcibly flexing or extending a stiff extremity or spinal joint.

It is also notable that surgical interventions are largely immune from control, in the manner of pharmaceutical interventions. A surgeon desiring to take a posterior rather than a lateral approach to, for example, femoral neck fractures, need not complete FDA-supervised clinical trials before doing so. Similarly, most rehabilitation interventions are not regulated by FDA, as discussed earlier. The lack of clinical outcomes research over the short term, however, can lead to nonbeneficial, costly expenditures on interventions and devices. For example, Salter's continuous passive motion machines were beneficial to postcasting and postsurgical rabbit knees, but continuous passive motion has yet to be shown to be effective in humans, even though it is widely used.

Perhaps the most important conclusion to be drawn from the evidence presented is that more experiments that explicitly and empirically determine the best approaches to encouraging clinicians to implement results from clinical research are needed. Training and incentives provided by the federal government are lacking, but a fuller understanding of clinicians' beliefs and how they can be modified cannot be attained without systematic federally sponsored research (Graham, 1996).

Clinical research is more expensive than bench research because the researcher must control not only the intervention but also the environmental influences that are different for people who are outside the laboratory. NIH, notwithstanding the limited budget of the National Center for Medical and Rehabilitation Research ($15 million), could fund such multicenter, human research. Because of competing priorities and study sections' insistence on applying animal-model standards to human research if more money was available, however, clinical research is being performed on only a few of the most prevalent diseases, such as heart disease, which has also received attention from NIH.

A recent trend shows Medicare, Medicaid, and many managed care organizations (MCOs) now instituting an anti-research treatment reimbursement. That is, if any part of the patient's care is experimental, then the entire costs of the hospitalization must be borne by the research protocol, making clinical research even more expensive and impractical. For example, if a patient is hospitalized for amputation and he or she were offered an experimental direct attachment (Branemark) prosthesis, the costs of amputation, medications, and rehabilitation and all other charges would accrue to the experimental protocol. Such direct attachment devices have been used in Sweden since the early 1990s, but they have yet to debut in the United States. More clinical research is needed to build first-class rehabilitation science that can guide practice and that is equivalent in rigor, prestige, and funding to basic and other medical sciences. Some of this research can be conducted in the course of care, but only if mechanisms for payment allow it.

Incentives and opportunities for the insurance and MCO industries must be changed to require that best practices be offered to rehabilitation consumers. Currently, short-term costs are the dominant concern of provider organizations and the insurance industry, but rehabilitation is not a short-term problem. Long-term or lifetime costs should be the dominant concern because of the prevalence of secondary conditions that emerge when patients are not encouraged to learn skills or adopt practices that will achieve a healthful management strategy to avoid the secondary conditions. This approach requires a life-long management strategy. In addition, public education and increasing consumer demand for the clinical research product might provide market-driven incentives. To effect this shift in incentives, more federally funded model care centers (such as NIDRR's Rehabilitation Engineering Research Centers) should be funded to provide clinical research and transfer its findings to consumers by providing the best possible care. Models such as these could be coordinated by the proposed Administration on Disability and Rehabilitation Research. Finally, best practices should be widely disseminated through various public media, including television "health news" reports, the World Wide Web, and newspapers (such as the technique used by the *Journal of the American Medical Association* and the *New England Journal of Medicine*, which de facto requires that physicians read the latest research from those journals to be able to answer their patients' questions the next day).

Lack of Training and Techniques to Transfer Existing Evidence to Practice

Despite the importance of clinical investigations, current rehabilitation education opportunities for physicians and other clinicians are inadequate. There are only a few formal degree-granting programs in "Clinical Investigations." The Institute of Medicine has written persuasively that training in and support of clinical investigation is "fragmented, frequently undervalued, and potentially underfunded" (Kelley and Randolph, 1994). So few investigators with formal training exist that currently, most clinical investigators obtain their training via informal postdoctoral experiences or by apprenticing themselves to someone who also has no formal training as a clinical investigator. Formal training in clinical investigation should become a requisite for both doctorally prepared principal investigators and nondoctorally prepared study coordinators and other team members.

The lack of funded mentors with training in clinical investigation is a great impediment to future rehabilitation treatment efficacy research. Because the federal government has neglected clinical investigations in rehabilitation for so long, some private foundations (e.g., the American Occupational Therapy Foundation) have developed mentored rehabilitation research funds and, indeed, NIH-like program project grants and clinical research centers (Foundation for Physical Therapy, 1994). The apparent motivation of these private foundations is to generate sufficient treatment outcomes evidence to prevent denial of services in an increasingly competitive environment. A more sagacious approach would be for the federal government, probably through NIDRR or NIH, to assemble disinterested parties to assess treatment outcomes as impartially as possible, but subjecting the treatments to usual standards of scientific inquiry. Moreover, such an approach might be more likely to generate a new treatment paradigm rather than simply test the custom-based paradigms currently taught in rehabilitation.

Incentives and Priorities

Despite years of clinical research, federal incentives to change the practice habits of health care providers remain insufficient. Several mainstream-medically oriented examples exist: for two decades it has been clear the tourniquet applied to maintain a blood-free operative field during knee surgery causes 30 to 60 percent of the subjects to have frank neuropathy (Krebs, 1982, 1989); nonetheless tourniquets continue to be used in virtually all limb surgery, in part because the neuropathies usually resolve spontaneously (Krebs, 1982). Moreover, thirty percent of durable medical equipment used for rehabilitation is thrown out by the first month following its issue to the patient. (For further evidence, one need only think of all the walkers, canes, and crutches in one's own basement! The basements of persons with permanent functional limitations are often more stalwart silent sentinels to insufficient technology matching.) The former example clearly demonstrates the extraordinarily slow process of technology transfer (or the transfer of ideas in this case) from research to implementation in clinical practice; the latter demonstrates how better treatment guidelines could save money, which could help fund best practice guidelines research. Currently, MCOs' interests may seem to be best served by playing Old Maid (a children's card game whose objective is to entice the competition to take the unwanted card) with people with disabling conditions; MCOs can lower their short-term costs by reducing or denying care (Ware et al., 1996). If federal regulations required MCOs to provide the best care possible to people with disabling conditions, long-term MCO incentives would change to incorporate prevention and advances in health science at all levels (Rubin, 1996).

Saving money alone cannot be an ethical health care goal. Indeed, efficiency is an institutional value; individuals, by contrast, value access to care, quality of care, health-related quality of life, and treatment effectiveness. The necessary tension between collective and individual goals in an MCO has led to some disability rights groups considering class-action suits to better balance the needs of corporations and individuals (Hadorn, 1992). Recent evidence indicates that at least some MCOs deny care to people with chronic illnesses, resulting in poorer outcomes than those for patients who have less restricted, fee-for-service access to care (Ware et al., 1996).

Technology transfer incentives need federal attention not just among clinicians and patients but also among engineers, architects, and politicians. Until the 1990s building designers informally consulted friends who might be rehabilitation professionals or consumers to determine the widths of accessible ramps, restrooms, and doors to make buildings accessible to people with potentially disabling conditions. After passage of the Americans with Disabilities Act of 1990 (ADA), many architects established formal guidelines for acceptable barrier reduction. Such guidelines however, are not comprehensive, for example, retrofitting to make existing buildings accessible. It is the federal government's role to set national standards, which has begun in part because of the guidelines set forth in ADA. Much remains to be done, however, from the prosaic, such as ensuring that all city crosswalks have audible cues, curb cuts, and sufficiently long Walk/Don't Walk ratios, to the more exotic, such as determining Social Security Insurance disability standards that correctly separate "can't work" from "won't work." Transferring research findings into clinical and societal practice cannot occur if only the short-term cost to the builder or care provider is at stake. The federal government's interest in enhancing work opportunities for all Americans must be crafted into incentives that require people with disabling conditions to participate at all levels of society.

Clinical Practice Guidelines

Clinical practice guidelines, defined as "systematically developed statements to assist practitioner and patient decisions about appropriate health care for specific clinical circumstances," can be an integral part of technology transfer (Institute of Medicine, 1990, p. 38). Guidelines, usually constructed through informal consensus development, refine the clinical question and balance trade-offs, attempt to address issues relevant to the decision, emphasize clinical contexts, and usually make specific recommendations (Hayward et al., 1995). To be useful in the technology transfer process, clinical practice guidelines include rigorous science-based procedures as part of their development, focus on specific clinical circumstances, and must be practical and definite (Lohr, 1995). Clinical practice guidelines are therefore expected to achieve a number of goals, including improving the quality of health care, protecting professional autonomy, reducing litigation risk, minimizing practice variation, providing standards for auditing medical records, reducing health care costs (and therefore health care premiums), defining areas of practice, improving the efficiency of practice, and identifying inappropriate care (Woolf, 1990).

Clinical practice guidelines can be instrumental in verifying the results of new or innovative research. Also, by exposing the results to scrutiny by different types of specialists, the intervention or procedure gains credibility and exposure to the professional community. As such, the guidelines can then serve their clear purpose: to guide the practice of rehabilitation. If practitioners can access and correctly implement the guidelines, then the process has effectively transferred newly researched ideas to the care of individuals with disabling conditions.

Clinical practice guidelines can have positive and negative impacts on patient care. By using currently synthesized scientific information and expert opinion, properly developed guidelines can provide clear information regarding clinical decisions. However, if recommendations are impractical, poorly justified, biased, or otherwise flawed, rigid enforcement could interfere with appropriate health care decision making. A clinician must be able to review and evaluate the usefulness of clinical practice guidelines in daily practice situations (Hayward et al., 1995).

The larger issue, however, is the impact of the guidelines. With regard to physician practices, expanding medical knowledge is the most likely outcome, as opposed to changing attitudes or behaviors, in part because of the varied quality of the present practice guidelines or the scientific evidence on which they are based (Woolf, 1993). Disclosure of the process and methodology used to develop guidelines is an initial step in allowing clinicians, policy makers, and others to make informed choices about the quality of the guidelines and how they should be used (Woolf, 1993). Physicians continue to express concern about "cookbook medicine" approaches to patient management and possible effects on autonomy of practice (Harding, 1994). Issues of implementation and enforcement have yet to be clarified. Guidelines, pathways, and audits have been used for quality assessment and physician performance measures in a variety of ways (Parker, 1995; AMA report, 1995). Implementation strategies have been directed at the local, regional, state, and national levels (Woolf, 1993; Gates, 1995; Kalunzy et al., 1995). Most success has been made locally or as a part of MCOs. What has become clear is that guidelines must be translated to the local environment to be accepted and effective. Support from the health care system is also important for making changes in behavior.

Conducting symposia that facilitate the development of clinical practice guidelines should be a priority of the agencies sponsoring rehabilitation research. A program that does this is the Consensus Development Program of NIH's Office of Medical Applications of Research. Convening an expert panel to review recent research results can heighten the scientific community's awareness of the agency's activities and the professional community's awareness of the agency's results. By funding conferences or seminars to this end, the agency would disseminate the results of the research, and therefore increase the effectiveness of its research budget.

Participatory Action Research

People with disabling conditions can play a vital role in technology transfer as consumers. Unfortunately, they are often viewed as passive individuals whose only role is to reap the benefits from newly developed technologies. Contrasting this dated notion is the increasing attention that is given to a more active role for consumers. Increasing attention is being given to the philosophy and practice of participatory action research, which is described below.

The spirit of collaboration that is the heart of participatory action research (Whyte, 1991) calls for the involvement of participants as active partners in the process of research and the dissemination of research findings. Thus, this relationship places the researcher in the role of learner as he or she better understands the participants' experiences with respect to their disabling conditions and other relevant issues. For some researchers, such collaborations are viewed as a waste of time and energy. For others it is invited, appreciated, and used to develop a research process leading to outcomes that are of higher quality and relevance. Fawcett (1991) provides three suggestions to actively involve constituents in the research process: First, constituents should assess the social significance of the research goals (e.g., Is the research likely to lead to outcomes that will be beneficial to the constituent populations to whom it is targeted?); Second, constituents should validate the social appropriateness of the procedures (e.g., How effective or practical is this procedure or intervention for me?); Third, constituents should have opportunity to validate the social importance of the proximal, intermediate, and distal effects of the intervention (e.g., Is there an increased amount of function? Will it allow me to become more independent? Could I live alone?).

Many factors present potential challenges to developing the consumer's role in the project team. Plausible obstacles include the availability or willingness of constituents to participate in the research process, the lack of transportation to attend scheduled meetings, the education level of potential constituents, and the lack of funding to include constituents (and their personal assistants if needed) in the research process. Although these and other formidable obstacles may act as potential deterrents to research programs, rehabilitation and engineering researchers must be steadfast and proactive in involving their consumers in the research process.

CURRENT GOVERNMENTAL MECHANISMS

Many government agencies are designed to facilitate technology transfer. Some of the best opportunities for technology transfer occur either at entry and planning stages of a research project or at its conclusion. The former involves bringing participants from other research, academic, and industrial communities into the research and development program as partners who then have a stake in the research and who are free to commercialize or market the findings. The latter depends on disseminating the findings of research to the greater corporate, industrial, or health related communities. Implementation usually consists of conferences, publications, or other means of promulgating the results of the research. National Institutes of Health and the Veterans Administration provide two examples of how government research handles technology transfer.

NIH Mechanisms

As mentioned above, NIH has several means of transferring research results. The Office of Technology Transfer and the Community Clinical Oncology Programs are two mechanisms for this. Other offices that NIH has at its disposal are described below.

Office of Medical Applications of Research

The Office of Medical Applications of Research (OMAR) is another means of technology transfer for NIH as a whole, focusing on disseminating the results of research rather than developing partnerships for research. By linking the individual technology transfer sections of each institute, OMAR provides a coordinated effort in disseminating medical technologies and the applications of medical research, principally through the Consensus Development Program. Through this program NIH holds conferences on the most recent developments in medical research. The conferences bring together the scientific, governmental, industrial, and consumer communities and result in a NIH consensus statement, prepared by a nonadvocate, nonfederal panel of experts. The statement is based on (1) presentations during a 2-day public session by investigators working in areas relevant to the consensus questions, (2) questions and statements during open discussion periods from conference attendees that are part of the public session, and (3) closed deliberations by the panel. This statement is an independent report of the panel and is not a policy statement of NIH or the federal government. The conferences and consensus statements attract attention to new technologies and methods and corroborate the evidence with an independent, expert appraisal.

Other Technology Transfer Efforts

Most institutes maintain their own offices and programs for technology transfer. Some of these have goals and methods similar to those of NIH's Office of Technology Transfer, whereas others have different methods for encouraging dissemination. For example, some institutes, such as NCI, also offer a Technology Transfer Fellowship Program. This type of program provides an opportunity for professionals to receive specialized training in methods of technology transfer and become familiar with the issues and activities of technology transfer through 1- or 2-year fellowships. The program addresses strategies for dissemination, intellectual property development and management, mass communication, and market research, but it also personalizes each fellowship to meet the background and interests of the participants.

VA Mechanisms

Technology Transfer Section

The Rehabilitation Research and Development Service of VA includes a Technology Transfer (TT) Section that serves as its primary means of cooperation with and dissemination to industry. The TT Section initially brings in industry and other research partnerships at the beginning and planning stages of a project. Its goals are identifying potential products for development (the Product Recruitment Program, see Box 8-2), establishing criteria and processes for evaluating products, and commercializing government-developed products in the marketplace. The Rehabilitation Research and Development Service also works at the other end of the research process, distributing the findings through publications, holding conferences, and managing the interdisciplinary professional relations of the TT Section. By making developed products available to the market and making research findings accessible to clinicians and physicians, the Veterans Health Administration transfers and disseminates rehabilitation products to the private sector, where they can reach the most veterans with disabling conditions.

NIDRR Mechanisms

Although most governmental sponsored technology transfer activities focus on a specific product or piece of research, some programs exist exclusively for the purpose of disseminating extant technology. NIDRR has two such programs that focus on linking individuals with disabilities with organizations involved in research in assistive rehabilitation technology. These are the consumer assistive technology transfer network and ABLEDATA. A description of these two programs follow.

BOX 8-2
VA Product Recruitment Program

The goal of the VA Product Recruitment Program is to seek projects that have the potential to satisfy worthwhile ongoing clinical projects in the Neuromuscular Systems, Orthopedic Biomechanics, and Human Machine Integration sections of the Palo Alto Rehabilitation Research and Development Center and to seek projects with potential from clinical services in VA Medical Centers. The program conducts clinical needs assessments, solicits wish lists, holds focus groups, and contacts physicians and therapists to allow them to provide their input into this process.

Falls due to impaired balance present a serious health hazard to people who are elderly as well as to people who have just had surgery and people who are partially disabled but ambulatory. Balance, as well as hearing and vision, declines with age or injury. Each year one third of elderly people living at home will fall. Approximately 1 in 40 of these people will be hospitalized as a consequence of the fall. Impaired mobility due to balance deficits or a fear of falling can diminish a person's ability to perform activities of daily living, and often makes the difference between living independently at home or being supervised in a nursing home facility.

SOURCE: Sacks et al. (1994).

Consumer Assistive Technology Transfer Network

The Consumer Assistive Technology Transfer Network (CATN) is a 2-year project funded by NIDRR. The grant was awarded to the New Mexico Technology Assistance Program and is administered by Career Services for Persons with Disabilities, a consumer-driven organization in Albuquerque, New Mexico. Initiated in late spring 1996, CATN has established a network to link the primary stakeholders in the technology transfer process. It is anticipated that the network will eventually maintain itself.

CATN links consumers, family members, and service providers through the Rehabilitation Engineering Research Center for Technology Evaluation and Transfer that links federally funded research and development projects, manufacturers, and suppliers of assistive technology with the state technology projects and their companies. A National Board of Directors provides technical assistance. The Rehabilitation Engineering and Assistive Technology Society of North America's also provide support to link relevant activities within Tech Act programs.

CATN will provide the network through which advanced technology can be located to address disability-related issues and a means by which consumers may express unmet technology needs, researchers can obtain consumer and industry direction for the application of emerging technologies, and product developers can find commercialization assistance.

The use of the Internet is central to CATN, particularly because of the Internet's multimedia accessibility capabilities for people with disabilities. The CATN Internet's communication coordination facilitates and demonstrates the distribution and translation of assistive technology transfer requests or "cases" between consumers–providers and the engineers, researchers, and product developers.

ABLEDATA

The National Rehabilitation Information Center (NARIC) is an information service established by NIDRR in 1979. NARIC attempts to collect and disseminate publications and material pertinent to disability issues, as well as the results of federally funded research projects; NARIC acts as a library in that regard. Another information resource is ABLEDATA, is a national database that contains descriptions of some 22,000 commercially available assistive devices and new designs for accessibility. This provides the opportunity to link companies, universities, or individuals who have new rehabilitation equipment with others who need those products. Both ABLEDATA and NARIC provided information on disk and cassette, in large print, in braille, and over the Internet. Staff members of both projects can assist with a search if necessary. However, the utility of NARIC and similar approaches is largely unknown, and should be subjected to scientifically acceptable cost-benefit analyses.

CONCLUSIONS AND RECOMMENDATIONS

One of the major objectives of rehabilitation science and engineering research is to develop interventions that effectively limit disabling conditions and the environmental factors that contribute to the disabling process. Accomplishing this will require an effective dissemination of knowledge, both to consumers and to others who can develop products and services. Barriers to such dissemination include: (1) limited research, and (2) even more limited mechanisms for technology transfer. In contrast to other medically oriented technology transfer methods, rehabilitation science and engineering requires transfer mechanisms that go beyond physicians to include the spectrum of rehabilitation professionals, as well as people with disabling conditions and their families, architects, engineers, and policy makers (including elected officials, insurers, and administrators).

The following recommendations are presented to facilitate the development of technology transfer mechanisms that will improve the communication among relevant disciplines, bring consumers appropriately into the research process, and facilitate the translation of research from the bench to the consumer.

Recommendation 8.1 Mechanisms for the transfer of rehabilitation technology should be enhanced to ensure that consumers have access to the knowledge and technology generated with federally funded rehabilitation research. This includes developing models of technology transfer that involve local medical agents (including therapists, nurses, and physicians), particularly in underserved areas of the country.

Recommendation 8.2 Mechanisms should be developed to foster an evidence-based paradigm of rehabilitation practice, driven by scientifically based models that are tested or testable through clinical research. To assist in the development of this paradigm, a standardized database should be developed that allows for the characterization of the national variability in the provision of rehabilitation services. Characteristics of this paradigm would include:

- *effective intervention strategies that have been validated in outcomes and/or process-oriented research;*
- *reliable and responsive measures of impairments, functional limitations, disability, and quality of life that have predictive value for outcomes and which will promote standardization of rehabilitation services;*
- *patients and clients who are empowered with a greater ability to manage the long-term consequences of disabling conditions; and*
- *technology transfer mechanisms that provide incentives for practitioners to conform to best practice standards. At minimum, those health care programs that the federal government is currently in charge, including Medicare, Medicaid, VA, and CHAMPUS (Civilian Health and Medical Program of the Uniformed Services) should provide clear stipulations for practitioners to conform to best practice standards as they design and implement programs to meet the patients' or clients' needs.*

Recommendation 8.3 Consumers with potentially disabling conditions should be involved, whenever possible, throughout the process of research design, technology development, and dissemination to ensure that researchers understand the issues faced by consumers as they live their lives with disabilities.

Recommendation 8.4 More clinical research is needed to foster the development of rehabilitation science that can guide practice. This research must be equivalent in rigor, prestige, and funding to basic and other medical sciences. This includes but is not limited to more clinical outcomes studies. In particular, clinical research on functional limitations, disability, and the environment are needed to help guide clinical decisions.

Recommendation 8.5 The federal government should not allow payers to limit rehabilitation research conducted in the context of care. Such restrictions will impede the progress of medical research that is necessary to improve the health of the public and reduce the cost of care.

Recommendation 8.6 Clinical practice guidelines should be developed by the federal government that include not just diagnosis-related guidelines but also guidelines for rehabilitation of impairments, functional limitations, and disabilities.

Recommendation 8.7 University and federal researchers should seek partners in private industry to cooperate on the research and development of technologies that can ultimately benefit people with disabling conditions.

Recommendation 8.8 More rehabilitation-related research should be published in the peer-reviewed literature. Making material available on the Internet or directly to the public does not relieve rehabilitation scientists and engineers of their obligation to submit their work to peer-review.

9

Education and Training in Rehabilitation Science and Engineering

This chapter examines education and training as it prepares scientists and engineers to contribute to rehabilitation science and engineering and the status of current support and opportunities for such education and training. The chapter first outlines the committee's findings regarding the present status and need for the organization of a more widely recognized field of study, but not a new profession, of rehabilitation science and engineering. This is followed by a summary of the major sources of federal support for training in rehabilitation and opportunities in training and education among the practices and disciplines of rehabilitation. Finally, based on an analysis of the current status and needs, the committee presents several recommendations that are designed to encourage interdisciplinary education and training, and expanded capacity in the field.

THE FIELD OF REHABILITATION
SCIENCE AND ENGINEERING

As a part of its task, the committee considered the status and needs for education and training related to research in rehabilitation science and engineering,* and the potential need for a new discipline.

---

*As defined in Chapter 1, the committee uses the term *rehabilitation science and engineering* to emphasize the importance of both science and engineering in advancing rehabilitation efforts and addressing the needs of people with disabling conditions.

In doing this, the committee considered historical examples and rationale for the establishment and growth of other fields. It also considered the differences between academic and scientific fields of study and professional disciplines.

Assessing the Field

In analyzing the current state of knowledge and education related to rehabilitation science and engineering, the committee came to three initial observations. First, rehabilitation-related research is conducted within a variety of disciplines, and although this research is integral to each discipline, it is not dominant. Second, each of the separate existing disciplines has complementary and distinct perspectives on disability and rehabilitation, yet all address the enabling–disabling process as a fundamental concept. The third observation is that the research in the separate health, health professional, and engineering disciplines, although complementary, is not optimally interfaced or balanced. A distinct field of study—one that would contribute to other disciplines but that gives a conceptual structure across disciplines—could be beneficial if it enhances the current research, stimulates innovations, and coordinates the growth of knowledge. The following sections discuss each of these three findings.

Rehabilitation-Related Research in Existing Disciplines

The committee found that the existing health professional disciplines generate and use rehabilitation-related knowledge as the basis for preparing practitioners and delivering services. Many health professional disciplines participate in generating knowledge relevant to rehabilitation and the prevention of disability in the presence of disabling conditions. The most prolific and productive professional discipline in this regard is medicine and its subrealm of physical medicine and rehabilitation. Physical medicine and rehabilitation has also successfully coordinated with engineering in generating new knowledge and clinical therapeutic devices. Rehabilitation-related research is conducted from the perspectives of the disciplines of nursing (rehabilitation nursing), physical therapy, occupational therapy, and other health care professions. In each case, the professional disciplines all conduct research that contributes not only to their profession but also to the field of rehabilitation science and engineering. In each of these disciplines, however, rehabilitation-related research represents only a subset of knowledge and activity. Other areas of research are often more dominant in these disciplines, such as those related to acute illnesses, primary prevention of acute illnesses, health promotion, professional issues, or ethical issues related to health care. Thus, rehabilitation-related research, although integral to each discipline, is not dominant.

Multiple Perspectives on a Common Goal

The committee's second observation about the state of rehabilitation-related research was that each of the separate health professional, basic science, and engineering disciplines has complementary yet distinct perspectives on disability and rehabilitation reflecting the practical aims of the discipline. Medicine, for example, has pioneered the application of biological, medical, and engineering sciences in the elucidation of the pathological and pathophysiological bases of disabling conditions. The therapies developed by medicine are directed primarily toward preventing, treating, or ameliorating disease and the manifestations of disease that underlie disabling conditions. Medicine has developed innovative and effective therapies for reversing or compensating for losses in human functional capacity as a result of disabling conditions and disease. Medical therapies usually involve interventions directed toward the individual person. This success of medicine has been accomplished in part by the joining of forces of medical scientists with engineering scientists to develop assistive devices that replace body structures (e.g., artificial limbs), replace normal organ function (e.g., cardiac pacemaker), create changes in the physical environment to allow for independent living (e.g., smart environments), and prevent secondary conditions (e.g., pressure-controlled seats).

Engineering science has focused primarily on manipulation of the physical environment and development of assistive devices for use by medicine. Physical therapy emphasizes preservation and recovery of joint and muscle function for performing tasks related to independent living. Occupational therapy emphasizes a client-centered approach to help individuals gain skills and modify environments so that individuals with disabling conditions can perform the tasks and activities of self-maintenance and work. Nursing interventions are intended to promote health and optimize performance of activities of daily living, an independent and autonomous lifestyle, and achievement of overall comfort and well-being, despite the continued presence of disease and functional limitations.

Public health adds yet another perspective in developing the methods and knowledge to view disability and rehabilitation from a population perspective as opposed to the individual person- and person–environment-based foci of the preceding examples. Public health also offers knowledge for evaluating the cost-effectiveness of care and health promotion at the population level. Thus, the knowledge generated through public health research is important to changing the attitudinal and general societal views of disability and to changing health care policy. The other health-related disciplines (speech-language pathology, audiology, recreation, etc.) have similar distinct perspectives and research emphasis areas that are important to providing an understanding of disability and rehabilitation.

In each of these examples, it is evident that respective disciplines are investigating the same subject: the enabling-disabling process. The health professional disciplines and engineering are the primary sites for the integration of knowledge from the basic sciences (the physical, biological, social, and behavioral sciences) into conceptualizations that result in effective and innovative clinical interventions that constitute the basis of the enabling process. As explained in Chapter 3, this process encompasses (1) minimization of environmental barriers to independent functioning and (2) maximization of autonomous, independent functioning of the person in the face of a disabling condition(s). Because of this, the breadth of perspectives is essential in addressing the concerns of consumers and society. Some consumers request that disability be "demedicalized" by focusing on altering the social and physical environments for people with disabling conditions. Some consumers want to be cured. Society in general expresses a concern for the use of cost-effective strategies including prevention and reversal of functional limitations of people with disabling conditions. Each discipline, then, contributes to the process that addresses these multiple requests, concerns, and mandates. Although each discipline approaches the enabling–disabling process from its own area of expertise, ultimately they unite in the common goal of promoting health and preventing disease and disability in people with disabling conditions. This is the essence of rehabilitation science and engineering and a major reason that academic and scientific structure needs to organize the field of rehabilitation science and engineering.

Integrating the Multiple Perspectives

The third major finding of the committee is that the research in the separate health, health professional, and engineering disciplines, although complementary, is not optimally interfaced or balanced. This is especially noteworthy given that people with disabling conditions are demanding access to changes and interventions that range from reversal of the pathology (i.e., cure) to removal of all environmental constraints and barriers without altering the person with the disabling condition. There is a clear consumer mandate for options allowing personal choice and a provider mandate for cost-effective approaches. These mandates challenge the disciplines to build a balanced, coordinated, and broad scope of research. Research and core knowledge of this scope and balance are unlikely to emanate from the separate health, basic science, and engineering disciplines now conducting rehabilitation-related research without a mechanism to view each discipline's contribution within the context of an organizing situation, such as that offered by a field of study.

As mentioned above, a wide range of health care professionals is necessary to address the needs of people with disabling conditions and to prevent primary and secondary disabling conditions. Furthermore, changes in the health care delivery system show trends toward the greater use of primary care providers (including physicians, therapists, and nurse practitioners), multidisciplinary professional health care teams, and case management of clients by nonphysicians and diminished access to specialists. These forces do not call for a new type of rehabilitation clinician or practitioner; the roles and licensure of existing health care providers are established and complementary. There is, however, a growing need for better integration of the health care disciplines in the rehabilitative processes. This requires a common knowledge base upon which other disciplines can build. The committee sees an increased need for rehabilitation-related education in and across all existing health care professions so that knowledge pertaining to rehabilitation science and engineering can be integrated into the knowledge base of all general and primary care providers.

Assessing the Need for a New Discipline

The number and nature of disciplines have changed over time with the emergence of new disciplines, the merging of existing disciplines, and the loss of disciplines due to obsolescence of the knowledge (Flint, 1975). The committee explored the need for a new discipline of rehabilitation science and engineering with the understanding that new disciplines often are recognized as fields of study until their structure is well-established and organized. The process of organizing a new field of study usually stimulates the increased and coordinated generation of knowledge by scholars and researchers. This developmental perspective of the creation of new scientific disciplines guided the committee's evaluation, conclusions, and recommendations regarding the need for academic and scientific structure in the field of rehabilitation science and engineering.

The Nature of a Discipline

The nature of academic and scientific disciplines is to coordinate, emphasize the importance of, and stimulate research. By having a conceptual structure, disciplines provide an opportunity to coalesce the knowledge in a given field. Anthropology is an example from more than a century ago (Flint, 1975). A more contemporary example is the neurosciences, although this is more correctly considered to be an affinity group by most in the field. In both cases, however, the new science overlapped parts of the disciplinary matrix of existing disciplines; this did not necessitate removal of content or research from any existing disciplines.

Rehabilitation science and engineering is and should continue to be a part of the research in each of the contributing scientific, professional, and engineering disciplines. The existence of separate health professional and engineering disciplines represents an opportunity to generate and integrate knowledge for practice and to prepare the appropriate mix and numbers of health care team members knowledgeable in rehabilitation science and engineering for the emerging managed health care system. Still, it is necessary to understand the nature of the field as proposed here. Rehabilitation science and engineering is a scientific and academic field of study—but not a professional discipline—whose purpose is to generate new knowledge for use by professionals and consumers. Although rehabilitation science and engineering is not yet at a stage where it could call itself a discipline, the committee believes it to be an emerging field of study that could evolve into a discipline.

Scientific Disciplines Disciplinary syntax, that is, the methods and criteria for the acceptance of knowledge (Schwab, 1964), is the basis for distinguishing the sciences from the arts and humanities. Scientific disciplines use rigorous, objective methods and criteria to determine acceptable knowledge because they embody knowledge that is generalizable, predictable, and in the form of general laws describing the nature or behavior of events or phenomena. The sciences share a common assumption that some degree of predictability and order exists in the phenomena that make up the world and the universe (Flint, 1975). Empiricism, as a philosophy of science, uses the syntax of the rehabilitation-related scientific disciplines. Empiricism has evolved over time and was significantly changed into its modern form by Thomas Kuhn (1962). Kuhn characterized science as problem solving (Kuhn, 1979) rather than the means to absolute truth and emphasized the importance of prevailing paradigms, or world views, and revolutionary changes in paradigms (Kuhn, 1962). Contemporary empiricism requires deductive reasoning, objectivity, theoretical models, and substantiation of theoretical claims by observable or detectable and measurable phenomena (Cronbach and Snow, 1977; Serlin, 1987).

The committee considers rehabilitation science and engineering to be a field of study that fits well in the context of the existing scientific disciplines and within the context of contemporary empiricism.

Academic Versus Professional Disciplines Disciplines that are purely academic differ from those with a professional component (Donaldson and Crowley, 1978). Disciplines in both categories are sciences by virtue of their syntax. The distinction between academic and professional disciplines has to do with the intended use of the knowledge and the resultant requirements for the disciplinary theoretical matrix. The primary aim of an academic discipline is to elucidate and understand phenomena. *Basic research* in the academic disciplines is discovery for discovery's sake, and *applied research* is discovery of the applicability (i.e., real-world practicality) of the knowledge. In contrast, the professional disciplines (e.g., medicine, nursing, speech-language pathology, audiology, and occupational and physical therapy) have practical aims and generate knowledge to serve as the basis for service delivery. Professional disciplines discover how to use knowledge in the real world. The professional disciplines deal with the actual implementation of knowledge in a practical sense (Donaldson and Crowley, 1978). Prescriptive theories are thus the scientific basis for the clinical therapeutic interventions used by health care professionals.

Academic disciplines have educators and research scholars, whereas professional disciplines alone additionally have practitioners who use the knowledge to provide service and to influence the use of societal resources and implementation of policies addressing professional issues (Donaldson and Crowley, 1978). The academic versus professional disciplinary status of rehabilitation science and engineering was an important consideration for the committee. Ultimately, it was agreed that rehabilitation science and engineering should not be developed into a new professional discipline—neither is it an academic or scientific discipline. Rehabilitation science and engineering is, however, emerging as an organized, multidisciplinary field of study and as such makes unique contributions to the health, productivity, and quality of life of people with disabilities. Rehabilitation science and engineering also has the capacity to evolve into an academic and scientific discipline that will further enhance the growth (scope and balance) of knowledge and allow for a new perspective of rehabilitation, perhaps transcending and crosscutting the perspectives of the existing basic and applied sciences and professional disciplines.

Defining the Field of Rehabilitation Science and Engineering

The findings presented above led the committee to conclude that the organization of rehabilitation science and engineering as a field of study is key to stimulating innovations and coordinating the growth of knowledge emanating from rehabilitation-related research. The field is ripe for major advances through coordinated research efforts and the field's broad perspective of rehabilitation, engineering, and disabling conditions. Expanding research in the field is likely to provide the knowledge to respond to the needs of consumers with disabling conditions, health care providers, and policy makers. The developing field of rehabilitation science and engineering needs to be responsive to all of these mandates.

The Purpose of Rehabilitation Science and Engineering

Organizing rehabilitation science and engineering as a defined field of study that is more widely accepted as such should help generate new knowledge for use by professionals and consumers. As a science, rehabilitation science and engineering would crosscut and share with, rather than subsume or replace, research emphases in the existing health and engineering disciplines. This field would also identify and address gaps in knowledge and provide direction for multiperspective research and service unlikely to be accomplished within the separate, single-perspective health and engineering disciplines. Rehabilitation science and engineering could offer its own doctorate or provide a graduate minor curriculum for doctoral students in other programs.

The knowledge generated within the field of rehabilitation science and engineering can be used as a basis for practice by all health care professionals and can serve to train researchers in separate disciplines. Thus, a physician, nurse, physical therapist, occupational therapist, public health officer, basic scientist, or engineer might receive a part of his or her research training in rehabilitation science and engineering; this could be as a predoctoral or postdoctoral fellow. Rehabilitation science and engineering will create organizational units that can also serve as centers of excellence and training to expand the resources and services of the existing rehabilitation-related disciplines. The knowledge generated from the science should provide information to guide service delivery, support policy development, and propose strategies that will improve the lives of people with disabling conditions and their families.

Developing Paradigms in Rehabilitation Science and Engineering

As an emerging field of study, rehabilitation science and engineering operates under few accepted paradigms. Paradigms, defined as "universal achievements that for a time provide model problems and solutions to a community of practitioners," guide research and unite the ideas and terminology of a scientific field (Kuhn, 1962). The absence of paradigms in rehabilitation science and engineering should not be looked upon negatively; it is a state that all sciences pass through. When this is the case, however, agreement on the direction of action is difficult. Kuhn says, "In the absence of a paradigm or some candidate for paradigm, all of the facts that could possibly pertain to the development of a given science are likely to seem equally relevant" (Kuhn, 1962). Without paradigms, fact gathering tends to be random and to lack direction, and one practitioner's ideas are as valid as any other's. Kuhn suggests that when this is the case, practitioners write books to present their own views and that the material is often directed as much toward other schools of thought (or other practitioners) as toward the topic under consideration.

Is it practical to think that some aspects of rehabilitation can become a mature science? The process requires placing stronger emphasis on empirical knowledge through experimentation, case studies, and information gathering to learn how to best address the problems faced by people with disabling conditions. Ultimately, a global paradigm for rehabilitation science and engineering may never develop, but smaller areas, such as locomotion science, movement science, occupational science, nursing science, and others, may supplement developing or mature sciences that are already connected with the rehabilitation field (e.g., neurosciences, brain science, and medical science). In addition, the contributions made by the development of rehabilitation science and engineering will lead to more evidence-based practice in the clinical disciplines and which should result in more effective services for people with disabling conditions.

Summary

Rehabilitation science and engineering, defined in this report as encompassing basic and applied aspects of biology, medicine, and engineering as they relate to restoring human functional capacity and improving a person's interactions with the surrounding environment, is beginning to emerge as an organized, multidisciplinary field of study. As a field, rehabilitation science and engineering focuses on multidisciplinary research and provides a common knowledge base for individuals working on a rehabilitation team. Because the committee has determined that rehabilitation science and engineering is an evolving scientific and academic field of study, and that current professional fields will remain, the important issue in education and training becomes how to train researchers in an increasingly interdisciplinary field and how to educate professionals in the common knowledge of the many disciplines that make up the field of rehabilitation. Currently, many mechanisms exist for the purposes of providing training and education in rehabilitation science and engineering. The following section examines those mechanisms to illustrate the breadth of both the present opportunities and the needs in the field. The final section of this chapter outlines some general approaches that will encourage the development of the field of study rehabilitation science and engineering and the interdisciplinary use of new knowledge.

SUPPORT FOR EDUCATION AND RESEARCH TRAINING IN REHABILITATION SCIENCE AND ENGINEERING

Support for education specific to rehabilitation science and engineering is substantial in many respects. However, it is difficult to determine accurately the extent and nature of this support. Part of the difficulty is due to the various perceptions and definitions of rehabilitation and what actually constitutes rehabilitation research. In some instances it is evident that the activities supported by programs are within the mainstream of rehabilitation with respect to education, training, and research, but the relative priorities and commitments among these areas are not always evident.

National Institute on Disability and Rehabilitation Research

The National Institute on Disability and Rehabilitation Research (NIDRR) is part of the Office of Special Education and Rehabilitative Services of the U.S. Department of Education. NIDRR's mission is to contribute to the independence of people with disabling conditions. NIDRR accomplishes this mission by funding research, demonstration projects, training, and other related activities to maximize the full inclusion and integration of people with disabling conditions into society. Through grants, contracts, and cooperative agreements, NIDRR funds research designed to improve systems, products, and practices in the rehabilitation field. NIDRR is also charged with ensuring the widespread distribution of practical scientific and technological information in usable formats.

The research funded by NIDRR covers all aspects of disability, including brain injury, spinal cord injury, multiple sclerosis, and back pain, and broader areas, such as technology, accessibility, aging, service delivery, policy, ethics, recreation, and community integration. These programs are described in detail in Appendix B.

The exact nature of the education and training varies from project to project. In most instances project activities include the development of curricula and the presentation of training seminars. The target audiences are health and rehabilitation providers and people with disabling conditions. The educational and training activities carried out through these programs vary widely with respect to field, scope, content, audience, duration, medium, and other considerations. Education and training are targeted to health and rehabilitation professionals, individuals with disabling conditions and their families, students preparing for rehabilitation research careers, selected segments of the general public, and prospective employers of individuals with disabling conditions. The areas of training and education supported range from science and engineering design activities over an extensive range of applications to behavioral studies and social applications. The formulation and delivery of education and training to these audiences also vary considerably and include both informal and highly structured approaches and methods. The content areas supported by NIDRR projects reflect the widest spectrum that may be inferred in the scope of rehabilitation science and engineering. However, NIDRR supports two programs designed to train disability researchers.

Research Training Grants

The purpose of the NIDRR research training grants is to expand the capability in the field of rehabilitation research by supporting projects that provide advanced training in rehabilitation research. These projects provide research training and experience at an advanced level to individuals with doctoral or similar advanced degrees who have clinical or other relevant experience, including experience in the management of basic science research in fields pertinent to rehabilitation, to qualify those individuals to conduct independent research on problems related to disability and rehabilitation.

Fellowships

Fellowships, named for the late Mary E. Switzer, build future research capacity. NIDRR makes awards on two levels: Distinguished fellowships go to individuals of doctorate or comparable academic status who have had 7 or more years of experience relevant to rehabilitation research. Merit fellowships are given to people in earlier stages of their research careers.

National Center for Medical Rehabilitation Research

The National Center for Medical Rehabilitation Research (NCMRR) was established within the National Institutes of Health (NIH) by legislation passed in 1990. The center is a component of the National Institute of Child Health and Human Development. The mission of NCMRR is to foster development of the scientific knowledge needed to enhance the health, productivity, independence, and quality of life of people with disabling conditions. This is accomplished by supporting research on enhancing the rehabilitation and health care of people with disabling conditions and on assisting them with achieving the functional capabilities of relevance in their daily lives. A primary goal of the center is to bring the health-related problems of people with disabling conditions to the attention of the best scientists in the United States to capitalize on the advances occurring in the biological, behavioral, and engineering sciences.

The research initiatives and opportunities recommended in the *Research Plan for the National Center for Medical Rehabilitation Research* are discussed in terms of seven cross-cutting areas in which increased research effort is needed. Those areas are as follows:

- improving functional mobility;
- promoting behavioral adaptation to functional losses;
- assessing the efficacy and outcomes of medical rehabilitation therapies and practices;
- developing improved assistive technology;
- understanding responses of the whole body system to physical impairments and functional changes;
- developing more precise methods of measuring impairments, disabilities, and societal and functional limitations; and
- training research scientists in the field of rehabilitation.

Research grants make up the largest category of NCMRR research funding, but special grant categories are designed to train researchers in the field of rehabilitation.

The First Independent Research Support and Transition Award

The goal of the First Independent Research Support and Transition (FIRST) Award is to encourage new investigators (including those who have interrupted early promising research careers) in basic or clinical science disciplines to develop their research interests and capabilities in biomedical and behavioral research and to help bridge the transition from training status to established investigators.

To be eligible for a FIRST Award, the proposed principal investigator must be genuinely independent of a mentor, yet at the same time must be at the beginning stages of his or her research career, with no more than 5 years of research experience since completing postdoctoral research training or its equivalent. If the applicant is in the final stages of training, it is permissible to apply for the award, but no FIRST Award will be made to individuals in training. An important principle with regard to eligibility is that the more extensive the prior independent research experiences, regardless of funding sources, the greater likelihood for diminished enthusiasm among reviewers for the FIRST Award application.

FIRST Award applications must request 5 years of research support, and the principal investigator must commit to at least 50 percent of the research effort. The total direct costs requested must not exceed $350,000 for the 5-year period; no more than $100,000 may be requested in any 1 year. Funds for technical support, supplies, publication costs, travel, and equipment may be requested. The FIRST Award is not renewable, however, proposals to continue research originally supported by a FIRST award can be submitted as R01 Research Project Applications.

Mentored Clinical Scientist Development Award

The goal of the Mentored Clinical Scientist Development Award is to support the development of outstanding clinician-research scientists by providing specialized study for clinically trained professionals committed to a career in research. Individuals possessing a doctoral-level clinical degree and postgraduate clinical training are eligible for up to $50,000 per year plus $15,000 for other support.

Institutional Rehabilitation Medicine Scientist Development Program

The Institutional Rehabilitation Medicine Scientist Development Program provides physiatrists who recently completed their residency training with an opportunity to obtain intensive basic science experience with a highly qualified mentor. Participants' activities are divided into two phases. The first phase consists of a minimum of 2 years of training with an outstanding mentor in a basic science discipline. Thirty potential mentors in the fields of neuroscience, bioengineering, biomechanics, and orthopedics are identified by a 12-member steering committee. In the second phase, the individual joins a sponsoring department of physical medicine and rehabilitation at the junior faculty level for further research skill development. NIH provides support for the first 2-year period, and the sponsoring department supports the candidate for the last 3 years. The program provides $50,000 in salary for full-time research effort and $10,000 for other expenses.

Institutional National Research Service Award

The goal of the Institutional National Research Service Award is to enable institutions to make to individuals selected by them National Research Service Awards for predoctoral and postdoctoral research training in specified shortage areas. Grant funds may be used for personnel, equipment, supplies, trainee stipends (both pre- and postdoctoral), and related costs.

Postdoctoral Individual National Research Training Award

The Postdoctoral Individual National Research Training (NRTA) Award provides postdoctoral research training to individuals to broaden their scientific background and extend their potential for research in specified health-related areas. NRTA Awards provide stipends to postdoctoral researchers as a subsistence allowance to help defray living expenses during the research training experience and are based on the number of years of relevant postdoctoral experience at the time that the award is provided.

National Research Service Awards for Senior Fellows

The National Research Service Awards for Senior Fellows provide opportunities for experienced scientists to make major changes in the direction of their research careers, to broaden their scientific background, to acquire new research capabilities, to enlarge their command of an allied research field, or to take time from their regular professional responsibilities for the purpose of increasing their capabilities by engaging in health-related research. The award provides up to 2 years of support at up to $32,300 per year.

Research Supplement Awards for Underrepresented Minorities

Research Supplement Awards for Underrepresented Minorities are administrative supplements for ongoing research projects that provide funds to support and enhance the research capabilities of students and investigators belonging to a particular ethnic or racial group that has been determined by the grantee institution to be underrepresented in biomedical or behavioral research nationally. Support is provided throughout the continuum from high school to faculty level at grantee institutions.

Research Supplements to Promote the Recruitment of Individuals with Disabilities into Biomedical Research Careers

Research Supplements to Promote the Recruitment of Individuals with Disabilities into Biomedical Research Careers provide funds for ongoing research projects to support and enhance the research capabilities in biomedical research of individuals with disabling conditions. They promote the recruitment of individuals with disabling conditions who are interested in biomedical research along the continuum from high school to established investigator status, as well as established investigators who become disabled.

National Science Foundation

The National Science Foundation (NSF) is an independent federal agency created to promote and advance scientific progress in the United States. NSF is responsible for the overall health of science and engineering across all disciplines. In contrast, other federal agencies support research focused on specific missions, such as health or defense. NSF is also committed to ensuring the nation's supply of scientists, engineers, and science educators. NSF is led by a Presidentially appointed director and the National Science Board composed of 24 scientists, engineers, and educators from universities, colleges, industry, and other organizations involved in research and education.

All seven directorates in NSF support individual projects related to disabling conditions. These are typically investigator-initiated projects that are recommended for funding during regular competitive review cycles. NSF operates several programs dedicated specifically to research for people with disabling conditions.

Program for Persons with Disabilities

The Program for Persons with Disabilities in the Directorate for Education and Human Resources is dedicated to achieving full inclusion and participation of students with disabling conditions in science and math studies and in career development opportunities in science, engineering, mathematics, and technology. Many of the projects focus on developing instructional materials, media, and educational technologies that are usable by all students.

Experimental Projects for People with Disabling Conditions

Experimental projects for people with disabling conditions provide support for the development and demonstration of exemplary strategies for the recruitment, education, and retention of students with disabling conditions in science, engineering, and mathematics.

Model Projects for People with Disabling Conditions

Model projects for people with disabling conditions are designed to promote the development and dissemination of innovative intervention strategies to reduce the barriers that inhibit the interest, retention, and advancement of students with disabling conditions in science, engineering, and mathematics education and career tracks.

Facilitation Awards for Scientists and Engineers with Disabilities

Facilitation awards are an NSF-wide program that provides funding for students and faculty with disabling conditions to obtain special equipment and services needed to reduce or remove barriers so they can participate in the research and training activities supported by NSF.

Centers for Disease Control and Prevention

The mission of the Centers for Disease Control and Prevention (CDC) is to promote health and quality of life by preventing and controlling disease, disability, and injury. To accomplish this mission, CDC works with partners throughout the United States and the world to monitor health, detect and investigate health problems, conduct research to enhance prevention, develop and advocate sound public health policies, implement prevention strategies, promote healthy behaviors, foster safe and healthful environments, and provide leadership and training.

The Disabilities Prevention Program, located within the National Center for Environmental Health, has two major goals: (1) to reduce the incidence and severity of primary and secondary disabling conditions and (2) to promote the independence and productivity of people with disabling conditions and to further their integration into the community. Similarly, the National Center for Injury Prevention and Control (NCIPC) has as its goal the reduction of the incidence and severity of adverse outcomes (including secondary conditions) among injured individuals, with a special emphasis on traumatic brain injury and spinal cord injury. To accomplish this goal NCIPC: (a) establishes population-based injury surveillance systems, (b) develops population based outcomes surveillance systems, (c) identifies risk factors for adverse outcomes, and (d) develops community-based interventions to prevent adverse outcomes including secondary conditions.

CDC offers several opportunities for research, education, and training. The Epidemic Intelligence Service (EIS) is a 2-year program of training and service in applied epidemiology including infectious and chronic diseases, nutrition, reproductive health, injuries including those that occur as a result of violence, environmental health, and occupational health and safety. Each year 60 to 70 people are selected for the EIS program. The majority are physicians and include those in specialties such as preventive medicine and occupational medicine, but participation of professionals from other fields is increasing. EIS includes doctoral-level epidemiologists, statisticians, and nurses.

CDC also offers a Postdoctoral Research Associates Program, a Visiting Scientist Program, Visiting Associate Program, and a Guest Researcher Program.

U.S. Department of Veterans Affairs

Research and development in the U.S. Department of Veterans Affairs (VA) advances the diagnosis and treatment of health problems prevalent among patients who are veterans by applying findings of VA medical research studies throughout the hospital system. The scope of the VA-funded research portfolio extends from basic laboratory research on the cause, treatment, and cure of a variety of diseases and disorders to fundamental clinical research on patient care and management. There is emphasis on diseases and disorders affecting veterans, but the results are applicable to the health care of all Americans. VA is not a granting agency, but rather funds an intramural program for investigators at VA medical centers. The VA program encompasses three areas of research and development: medical research, health services research and development, and rehabilitation.

The VA rehabilitation research and development program integrates the multiple disciplines of science, engineering, and medicine to investigate and develop concepts, processes, and products that directly meet the special needs of veterans with disabling conditions. Scientific investigation is carried out in areas of physical orientation, mobility, and manual skills enhancement, spinal cord injury; prosthetics, amputation management, and orthotics, communication; cognition; auditory and visual sensory aids; vocational placement; and recreational opportunity. Priority emphasis is given to those investigator-initiated studies whose results benefit veterans with war-related injuries. Current special emphasis areas are

- orthopedics: prosthetics, orthotics, and amputation management;
- neurology: spinal cord injury, traumatic brain injury, and nerve injury;
- communications, cognition, and sensory aids: vision, audition, speech, and deglutition; and
- disabling conditions and conditions associated with aging: cardio-respiratory, metabolic, muscular, skeletal, and stability conditions.

VA investigators are guided by letters of information stating the current foci within these priority areas. Internal letters of information are developed through strategic planning workshops with the participation of rehabilitation clinicians and researchers, as well as users of rehabilitation technology.

VA currently operates four training and support programs, each targeting several different levels of investigators. Clinician investigators are trained either in the Medical Research Service or in the Health Services Research and Development Service Career Development Programs. Basic scientists are supported in Medical Research Service and Health Services Research Development Research Career Scientist Programs. VA recently completed a review of its research and training programs by the Research Realignment Advisory Committee (RRAC). This committee reviewed the restructuring of the VA system from a medical center-based system to a system based on integrated service networks, the current demographics of patients in VA medical centers, and the structure and function of the three VA research services (medical, health services, and rehabilitation), including the various training and career development programs associated with these research programs.

In a review draft released June 26, 1996, RRAC recommended that the Rehabilitation Research Service and Development Service consider a career development program similar in structure and funding to those in the Medical Research Service and Health Services Research and Development Service Career Development Programs. This career development program would include clinician-scientist career development consisting of three levels of awards: an entry level and two higher levels corresponding to an assistant professor and a more senior investigator. The Research Career Scientist Program would provide support for the recruitment and retention of basic science investigators. Career scientist awardees would be expected to seek extramural salary support and would be reviewed annually. Annual reviews should encourage excellence in at least two of the following three areas: VA service on committees, organized activities that contribute to clinical interest and the intellectual climate at the local VA medical center, and mentoring, including coauthorship of papers and grants.

PROFESSIONAL REHABILITATION EDUCATION AND TRAINING

Each profession within the scope of rehabilitation science and engineering maintains its own credentialing system for practitioners and an accrediting body for professional education. The following is a brief overview of current educational and certification requirements for rehabilitation practitioners.

Physical Medicine and Rehabilitation

Physical medicine and rehabilitation, also referred to as rehabilitation medicine or physiatry, is the primary medical specialty concerned with evaluating, diagnosing, and treating patients with disabling conditions that involve the musculoskeletal, neurological, cardiovascular, or other body systems. There are physicians in the fields orthopedic surgery and neurology who have received rehabilitation training. The primary focus of rehabilitation medicine is on maximal restoration of physical, psychological, social, and vocational function and on evaluation of pain. For diagnosis and evaluation, a physician may include the techniques of electromyography and electrodiagnosis as supplements to the standard history and physical, X-ray, and laboratory examinations. In addition to traditional treatment modes, specialists in rehabilitation medicine may use therapeutic exercise, prosthetics, orthotics, and mechanical and electrical devices. Physiatrists are certified by the American Board of Physical Medicine and Rehabilitation through the administration of written and oral examinations that assess candidate performance in basic sciences and clinical aspects of rehabilitation practice. Upon approval of the application and the candidate's successful completion of the examinations, the board grants a certificate to the candidate. The recipient of the certificate is known as a certificant or a diplomate of the American Board of Physical Medicine and Rehabilitation. In addition, an application and examination process are being developed for certification of special qualifications in spinal cord injury medicine.

The specialty of physical medicine and rehabilitation has 79 accredited residency programs. In 1994–1995 the training programs offered 1,313 residency positions, and 1,277 (97 percent) of these were filled. The board has given written and oral examinations annually since 1947 and has certified 4,940 physicians as diplomates; 2,562 of these have been certified in the past 10 years, with 298 certified in 1995.

Rehabilitation Engineering

Although the baccalaureate degree is most common in engineering practice, many engineers obtain master's degrees after they go into practice in order to specialize or to change career directions. Practicing biomedical engineers frequently have master's degrees. The doctorate has become more prevalent in engineering since the late 1950s and is still regarded as a research degree although that view has changed somewhat over the last few years as persons with doctoral degrees have become involved at decision-making levels related to development, implementation, or acquisition of new technologies. Engineering schools still emphasize practical application, uniting hand skills and intuitive knowledge with the precision of mathematics and the physical sciences. This blending of the practical and the theoretical was beneficial to good, practical engineering. Sometimes this creative kind of union of the practical and theoretical appears in individual persons, and sometimes it comes about mainly through design teams.

Future rehabilitation engineers who provide service to clients probably will need either education at least to the master's level in engineering, dual education in engineering and in a rehabilitation specialty (e.g., Physical Therapy, Occupational Therapy, Prosthetics or Orthotics, etc.), or specialized advanced degrees in rehabilitation science and engineering. Research in rehabilitation engineering will be led largely by engineering doctorates, doctorates dually educated in engineering and in rehabilitation (e.g., Physical Medicine and Rehabilitation or Occupational Therapy), or those with advanced degrees in rehabilitation science. Education programs will also need to have counterpart programs that foster the development of technical personnel in the rehabilitation field. Much of the practical day-to-day aspects of rehabilitation technology can be sustained by highly skilled people with appropriate technical backgrounds.

Rehabilitation Nursing

Professional schools of nursing prepare nurses for general practice in a variety of settings including the community. Graduates receive a baccalaureate degree from colleges or universities whose nursing program(s) is accredited by the National League for Nursing (NLN). Advanced practice nurses (clinical specialists, nurse practitioners) complete requirements for a master's degree in a given clinical area such as rehabilitation nursing (accredited by NLN). Doctoral nursing programs prepare nurses in theory and research to increase the body of nursing knowledge and practice.

In addition to the academic requirements for the levels of nursing practice, nurses may sit for a certification exam in rehabilitation. The Certified Rehabilitation Registered Nurse (CRRN) certification program was developed by the Association of Rehabilitation Nurses and is directed and implemented by the Rehabilitation Nursing Certification Board. The CRRN certification program has grown every year since its inception in 1984, and more than 12,400 rehabilitation nurses hold the CRRN credential. The goals of the CRRN program are to promote expertise in rehabilitation nursing, provide a standard for recognizing qualifications, and validate specialized knowledge to enhance the care of people affected by disabling conditions and chronic illness. Registered nurses with a minimum of 2 years of work experience as a registered professional nurse in rehabilitation nursing within the previous 5 years are eligible to take the examination. The certification is valid for 5 years. Renewal or certification may be obtained by reexamination or by achieving points of credit through a combination of continuing education, formal course work, professional publication, presentations, or submission of test items for the CRRN examination.

Assistive Technology

Rehabilitation Engineering and Assistive Technology of North America (RESNA) administers a credentialing program for rehabilitation professionals involved in assistive technology or rehabilitation engineering service delivery. Individuals with degrees in rehabilitation science who, in addition, have work experience related to assistive technology are eligible to take the credentialing examination. A rehabilitation science degree is defined as a degree in one of the following: occupational therapy, physical therapy, speech or language pathology, special education, medical doctor, nursing, rehabilitation counseling, orthotics, or prosthetics. RESNA offers two credentials: *assistive technology practitioner*, for service providers most frequently involved in a assessment of a consumer's need or training in the use of a particular device, and *assistive technology supplier*, for service providers most frequently involved in the sale and service of assistive technology devices. Requirements for credentialing are a combination of education, field of study, and work experience specific to client service in the area of assistive technology. RESNA's Rehabilitation Engineering Professional Specialty Group is in the process of developing the requirements for a rehabilitation engineer credential.

Rehabilitation Counseling

The Council on Rehabilitation Education (CORE) is a not-for-profit corporation that is the accrediting body for master's degree programs in rehabilitation counselor education. The purpose of CORE accreditation of rehabilitation counselor education programs is to promote the effective delivery of rehabilitation services to individuals with disabling conditions by promoting and fostering continuing review and improvement of master's degree-level rehabilitation counselor education programs. Another goal is to meet the personnel needs of both public and private rehabilitation agencies by providing graduates who have the skills, knowledge, and attitudes necessary to provide rehabilitation counselor services to individuals with physical, mental, or emotional needs. There are 84 accredited master's degree programs in rehabilitation counselor education.

Physical Therapy

Physical therapy exams, treats, and instructs individuals in methods to correct, alleviate, and limit physical disability. Physical therapy, which is the care and services provided by or under the direction of a physical therapist, includes the following activities:

1. Examining and evaluating individuals with impairment, functional limitation, and disability or other health-related conditions to determine a diagnosis, prognosis, and intervention. The tests and measures used may include assessment of functional capabilities in self-care and home management and in work, community, and leisure activities; balance and locomotion abilities; musculoskeletal, neuromuscular, cardiopulmonary, and integumentary systems; sensory and neurophysiologic functions (e.g., by electromyographic and motor nerve conduction testing); pain; need for and use of assistive, adaptive, orthotic, protective, supportive, or prosthetic devices; and environmental barriers.

2. Alleviating impairment, functional limitation, and disability by designating, implementing and modifying therapeutic interventions that may include patient-related instruction; therapeutic exercise; functional training in self-care and home management and in community, work,and leisure activities (including activities of daily living, instrumental activities of daily living, work hardening, and work conditioning); manual therapy techniques (including mobilization and manipulation); prescription, application, and, as appropriate, fabrication of assistive, adaptive, orthotic, protective, supportive, or prosthetic devices and equipment; airway clearance techniques; wound management; and electrotherapeutic, physical, and mechanical modalities;

3. Preventing injury, impairment, functional limitation, and disability, including the promotion and maintenance of fitness, health, and quality of life in all age populations.

4. Engaging in consultation, education, and research.

As of October 1996, the United States had 155 accredited physical therapy programs (48 at the bachelor's level, 102 at the master's level, 2 at the doctor of physical therapy level, and 195 accredited physical therapy assistant programs. The Commission on Accreditation in Physical Therapy Education of APTA determines the accreditation status of education programs for the physical therapist and physical therapist assistant. To meet the increasing need for qualified faculty, APTA recently initiated a program to support doctoral education for qualified physical therapists.

According to APTA, the United States has an estimated 97,000 licensed physical therapists. Of this number, 74 percent (71,780) practice full time, 19 percent (18,430) practice part time, and 7 percent (6,790) are not practicing or are retired. Thus, the current supply of physical therapists is estimated to be 90,210.

Occupational Therapy

Occupational therapy uses selected tasks and activities to restore, reinforce, and enhance performance in people with disabling conditions by facilitating learning of those skills and functions essential to help an individual adapt and achieve the capacity to perform with satisfaction to self and others those tasks and roles essential to productive living and to the mastery of self and the environment.

Occupational therapy serves a diverse population in a variety of settings such as hospitals and clinics, rehabilitation facilities, long-term care facilities, extended care facilities, industry sheltered workshops, schools and camps, private homes, and community agencies. Occupational therapists both receive from and make referrals to appropriate health, educational, or medical specialists.

The National Board for Certification in Occupational Therapy is the credentialing organization for occupational therapists. To become a registered occupational therapist, an individual must (1) be a graduate of an accredited occupational therapist education program and have successfully completed all therapist-level field work required by the education programs (but not less than 6 months) and (2) have successfully completed the certification examination for registered occupational therapist. There are currently 71,335 registered occupational therapists in the United States, and of these, the estimated workforce is 47,785 (Health Policy Alternatives, Inc. 1996).

The Accreditation Council for Occupational Therapy Education of the American Occupational Therapy Association accredits programs for occupational therapists. The council establishes, maintains, and promotes appropriate standards of quality for educational programs in occupational therapy and provides recognition for educational programs that meet or exceed the minimum standards. The standards are used for the development, evaluation, and self-analysis of baccalaureate and postbaccalaureate entry-level professional occupational therapy programs.

Orthotics and Prosthetics

An *orthotist* provides care to patients with congenital or traumatic disabling conditions of the musculoskeletal structure of the body by evaluating, designing, fabricating, fitting, and aligning braces knows an orthoses. A *prosthetist* provides care to patients with a partial or total absence of a limb by evaluating, designing, fabricating, fitting, and aligning those artificial limbs known as prostheses. There are currently 3,000 certified orthotists, prosthetists, and prosthetist-orthotists in the United States. Education programs are accredited by the National Commission on Orthotic and Prosthetic Education.

The American Board for Certification in Orthotics and Prosthetics, Inc. (ABC), is a credentialing body established by the orthotic and prosthetic professions to identify those practitioners who have satisfied the minimum qualifications to render public health services in these disciplines. ABC conducts examinations to test the competencies of those individuals engaged in or intending to be engaged in the practice of orthotics or prosthetics who voluntarily apply for the examination process. Three examinations are required: written, clinical patient management, and written simulation examinations. Examination content assesses performance in five domains: clinical assessment, patient management, technical implementation, practice management, and professional responsibility.

Audiology and Speech Pathology

The American Speech-Language-Hearing Association issues certificates of clinical competence to individuals who present evidence of their ability to provide independent clinical services to people who have disorders of communication. Individuals who meet the standards specified by the association's Council on Professional Standards may be awarded a certificate of clinical competence in speech-language pathology or a certificate of clinical competence in audiology. Individuals who meet the standards in both professional areas may be awarded both certificates.

The American Speech-Language-Hearing Association represents 87,060 members and nonmember certificate holders. There are currently 11,211 certified audiologists and 69,334 certified speech-language pathologists in the United States. Individuals holding dual certifications totaled 1,413 in 1996, which represents a decrease for the second consecutive year. More than one-third of audiologists are employed in a private practice setting, whereas 25 percent of speech-language pathologists are employed in such settings. More than 50 percent of speech-language pathologists are employed in a school setting and 39 percent are employed in a health care facility. Audiologists are generally employed in health care facilities (72 percent): 47 percent in nonresidential health care facilities such as physician or audiologist offices, 23 percent in hospitals, and 4 percent in residential health care facilities. The majority of speech-language pathologists (82 percent) and audiologists (80 percent) reported their primary employment function as clinical service provider.

ACADEMIC REHABILITATION EDUCATION PROGRAMS

The committee recommends interdisciplinary training in rehabilitation science and engineering and encourages the development of academic programs that promote research training for clinicians. Building a rehabilitation science requires highly trained professionals who can develop a knowledge base that can be disseminated to consumers of research and used to promote evidence-based rehabilitation practices. Foremost is the need for clinical trials of therapeutic interventions that rely less on clinical experience and more on systematic investigation by using standardized outcomes measures.

Support for rehabilitation science and engineering should be concentrated in environments that recognize and emphasize the interdependence of research, clinical service, education, and training. Education and training in rehabilitation science should also recognize and address the interdependence of professional disciplines serving the field of rehabilitation.

Examples of Existing Programs

Examples of such integrated academic programs include the master of arts in disability and rehabilitation currently offered at Washington University in St. Louis, Missouri. A doctoral program in rehabilitation science is planned to begin in the near future. An interdisciplinary doctorate program in rehabilitation science was initiated by the University of Pittsburgh with the admission of eight students in the fall of 1995. An additional 10 candidates were accepted to this program in the fall of 1996. This response reflects a significant demand for advanced research degree opportunities in rehabilitation science and engineering. The establishment of these programs reflects a trend in doctoral level study in rehabilitation science in the United States. Doctoral programs in rehabilitation science are also available in Canada (e.g., University of Alberta in Edmonton, University of Toronto, and McGill University) and in Australia (e.g., Curtin University in Perth). Although these programs have taken different approaches and vary with respect to their primary areas of emphasis, all embrace the concept of rehabilitation science as a contemporary academic discipline. The emergence of rehabilitation science and engineering education at this level seems quite consistent with the conclusions reached by the committee.

Such programs have been initiated because health professionals are now required to have an expanded set of skills and to work in interdisciplinary teams. The Pew Commission report *Healthy America: Practitioners for 2005* (1991) challenges faculty to give students a broad understanding of the determinants of health and to prepare them to be able to work with others to integrate a range of services that promote, protect, and improve the health of the public. Students must be trained to manage and use large volumes of scientific, technological, and patient information and to address issues spanning from basic mechanisms of cellular function to applied clinical science and policy. A rehabilitation science program is needed to guide rehabilitation practice and shape policies that will improve services and access for individuals with disabling conditions.

Programs in disability and rehabilitation provide students with advanced knowledge of the physiological, psychological, cognitive, social, and technological mechanisms that are related to and support the performance of individuals in everyday activities such as self-maintenance, school, work, leisure, and interaction with others. A rehabilitation science core curriculum of basic and advanced statistics and research design, measurement, and policy should link knowledge from the realms of pathophysiology, impairment, functional limitation, and disability to the performance of individuals with or at risk of developing disabling conditions. This would increase understanding of the mechanisms and issues that affect the lives of people with disabling conditions, including their specific health, work, cognitive, and social needs.

Rehabilitation science programs should be supported by an interdisciplinary faculty with diverse and complementary areas of expertise to build knowledge required to understand the factors that influence and improve the function of people with disabling conditions, and prevent unnecessary disabilities through the use of modified behaviors, technology, and environmental support.

RECOMMENDATIONS

All recommendations related to rehabilitation science and engineering are based on the presumption that research and training in this field will be consistent with the model of disability and rehabilitation presented in this report. In addition, it is assumed that many academic disciplines will be involved in these recommendations. This includes some that are not traditionally associated with rehabilitation, including health services research, public health, sociology, psychology, history, economics, and political science, among others.

Recommendation 9.1 Universities with extant programs in disciplines related to rehabilitation science and engineering should develop and offer doctoral and postdoctoral education in the field of rehabilitation science and engineering to help encourage the development of the field and respond to the expanding research needs.

Recommendation 9.2 The federal programs that support rehabilitation-related research and training should

- *tailor training grants to support professional education programs that integrate rehabilitation science and engineering into the knowledge base of primary care.*
- *encourage scientists from related fields to join in rehabilitation efforts to mentor rehabilitation scientists and engineering scientists in their formative years.*
- *develop new and improved mechanisms for enhancing multi-perspective transdisciplinary rehabilitation-related research representing the separate perspectives of the health professional and engineering disciplines.*
- *coordinate with and develop joint efforts with programs that support training and research in the separate health professional, engineering, and preclinical science disciplines, in order to facilitate the integration and translation of rehabilitation science and engineering knowledge into the full spectrum of issues related to the health and well-being of people with disabilities, from individual clinical care to health delivery systems to social policy reform.*

Recommendation 9.3 Researchers conducting rehabilitation-related research in the various existing disciplines should consider how their work fits into a broader concept of rehabilitation science and engineering described in this report.

Recommendation 9.4 Professional associations of rehabilitation-related disciplines (e.g., medicine, nursing, occupational therapy, physical therapy, speech-language pathology, prosthetics, orthotics, neuropsychology, and rehabilitation psychology) should collaborate in exploring opportunities to improve and enhance transdisciplinary activities among rehabilitation professionals.

10

Organization and Administration of Federal Research Programs

As described in Chapter 1, the U.S. government has a long tradition of establishing programs designed to aid Americans with disabling conditions. Today, more than 30 distinct federal programs exist to address either directly or indirectly the needs of people with disabling conditions. These needs have gained renewed national attention in recent years, partly in response to the Americans with Disabilities Act of 1990. One aspect of this renewed attention has been a focus on rehabilitation-related research.

As part of its charge from Congress, the committee reviewed and assessed the individual efforts of the major federal programs that support rehabilitation-related research, as well as the combined, overall federal effort. A series of options for improving the federal organization and administration of rehabilitation research was developed and is presented in this chapter as examples of what the committee considered in its deliberations. The chapter concludes with the committee's recommendations for improving the overall effort.

SCOPE OF FEDERAL RESEARCH EFFORTS

Federal expenditures in programs whose missions emphasize rehabilitation-related research are presented in Figure 10-1, showing that the National Institute on Disability and Rehabilitation Research (NIDRR) has the largest single program—accounting for 48 percent ($70 million) of the total ($147 million). Twenty-three percent ($32 million) of the funds are spent by the U.S. Department of Veteran Affairs (VA). The National Cen-

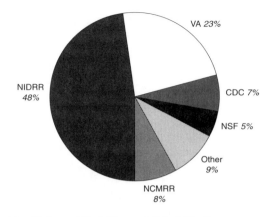

National Institute on Disability and Rehabilitation Research (NIDRR)	$69,625,000
U.S. Department of Veterans Affairs (VA)	32,398,000
National Center for Medical Rehabilitation Research (NCMRR)	11,707,000
Centers for Disease Control and Prevention (CDC)	9,500,000
National Science Foundation (NSF)	6,582,000
Other includes:	13,100,000
Architectural and Transportation Barriers Compliance Board	300,000
Office of Disability, Aging, and Long-Term Care Policy	5,000,000
Social Security Administration	5,000,000
U.S. Department of Housing and Urban Development, Office of Policy Development and Research	100,000
U.S. Department of Transportation	2,700,000

FIGURE 10-1 Traditional view of federal spending in rehabilitation-related research.

ter for Medical Rehabilitation Research (NCMRR) supports 8 percent ($12 million) of the federal spending on rehabilitation-related research. The Centers for Disease Control and Prevention (CDC) and the National Science Foundation (NSF) support 7 percent ($9.5 million) and 5 percent ($6.5 million), respectively. Five other federal agencies and programs with research activities focused specifically on rehabilitation spend the remaining nine percent of the federal government's rehabilitation-related research funds (the U.S. Department of Housing and Urban Development [HUD], the Office of Disability, Aging and Long Term Care of the U.S. Department of Health and Human Services [DHHS], the Social Security Administration [SSA], the U.S. Department of Transportation, and the Architectural and Transportation Barriers Compliance Board).

Other federal programs support and conduct research that is relevant to rehabilitation. Perhaps most notably is the NIH activity outside of NCMRR that is focused on a variety of areas, but that sometimes includes aspects of rehabilitation-related research (see NIH Research Priorities and Funding, below). In addition, but on a smaller scale, the National Aeronautics and Space Administration's work in engineering and space technology has had spin-offs in technology transfer to products for people with disabling conditions, although it does not directly fund rehabilitation research. The U.S. Department of Energy also supports projects (e.g., in hearing, visual modalities, and computer technology) with potential applications for people with disabling conditions. The net result is a highly diverse, but potentially complementary set of rehabilitation-related federal research activities that includes biomedical research, technological development, engineering, demonstration projects, outreach, and training.

In reviewing the scope of the federal programs, it is also important to consider congressional oversight of the programs. The numerous federal programs are authorized by various laws and are in the jurisdictions of different congressional committees. The largest rehabilitation-related federal research programs, however, i.e., NIH and the U.S. Department of Education, are both under the jurisdiction of the Labor, Health and Human Services and Education Subcommittee. Other programs have separate committees; for example, the VA Rehabilitation Research and Development Service is under the jurisdiction of the Veterans' Affairs Committee, and the Social Security Administration's efforts are under the jurisdiction of the Labor, Health and Human Services and Education Subcommittee. In the U.S. House of Representatives, the programs are similarly dispersed. All programs undergo separate authorization and appropriations processes conducted by different committees in both bodies.

In assessing the overall federal effort, the committee limited its review to the five largest programs that focus specifically on rehabilitation-related research (those with research budgets of more than $5 million, see Figure 10-1): NIDRR, VA, NCMRR, CDC, and NSF. Rehabilitation-related research at NIH, in addition to that which is supported by NCMRR, was also assessed. The following section provides a brief description and assessment of each of these.

MAJOR AGENCIES INVOLVED IN
REHABILITATION-RELATED RESEARCH

As mentioned above, numerous federal agencies have authority for and are conducting research in the field of rehabilitation science and engineering. To evaluate the major trends in federally funded research in rehabilitation science and engineering, the committee examined five agencies in greater detail. The following summary of the committee's findings includes a brief description of the each agency's mission, research priorities, and current funding level, and an assessment of the strengths and weaknesses of each agency. Appendix A details the actions that the committee took to collect information from the agencies (and other sources), and Appendix B contains a summary of relevant information for federal programs involved in rehabilitation-related research, as well as other programs that provide services, ensure compliance, or collect data.

National Institutes of Health

NIH is organized into 25 separate Institutes, Centers, and Divisions (ICDs), each with a specific focus on either a disease, an organ system, or a profession (e.g., cancer, musculoskeletal disorders, and nursing research, respectively). Disability and rehabilitation research is a part of many ICDs, but it is the central focus of only one, NCMRR, which is part of the National Institute of Child Health and Human Development (NICHD). The following sections discuss the overall effort of NIH (ICDs other than NCMRR) and NCMRR specifically.

Overall Effort of NIH

The goal of all NIH research is to acquire new knowledge to help prevent, detect, diagnose, and treat disease and disability, from the rarest genetic disorder to the common cold. NIH works toward that mission by conducting research in its own laboratories; supporting the research of nonfederal scientists in universities, medical schools, hospitals, and research institutions throughout the country and abroad; helping in the training of research investigators; and fostering communication of biomedical information.

Research Priorities and Funding To assess rehabilitation-related research at NIH, the committee collected abstracts from two sources: the Computer Retrieval of Information on Scientific Projects (CRISP) and the Institutes themselves (see Appendix A). As presented in Table 10-1, CRISP provided the committee with 764 abstracts (representing $114 million); the Institutes provided the committee with 973 abstracts (representing approximately $158 million). All 1,480 abstracts were reviewed to determine (1) relevance to rehabilitation, (2) state of the enabling–disabling process that was examined, and (3) type of experimental subject. An overlap of 17 percent (i.e., the percentage of total number of abstracts that were collected from both sources) was identified and duplicates were eliminated from the analysis, as were projects that were determined to be

TABLE 10-1 Medical Rehabilitation-Related Research at the National Institutes of Health ($thousands), 1995

Institute	Reported[a]	CRISP	Calculated[b]
National Cancer Institute	$23,512	$8,394	$20,050
National Heart, Lung, and Blood Institute	17,831	20,382	36,238
National Institute of Dental Research	9,559	930	8,193
National Institute of Diabetes and Digestive and Kidney Diseases	5,057	2,483	5,083
National Institute of Neurological Disorders and Stroke	17,742	19,089	30,337
National Institute of Child Health and Human Development (National Center for Medical Rehabilitation Research)	15,459	14,020	19,206
National Eye Institute	3,293	3,821	5,769
National Institute on Aging	20,790	25,715	22,650
National Institute of Arthritis and Musculoskeletal and Skin Diseases	13,670	6,897	17,095
National Institute of Deafness and Other Communication Disorders	19,941	9,429	27,466
National Center for Research Resources	9,504	212	7,041
National Institute of Nursing Research	1,680	2,619	4,130
National Institute of Allergy and Infectious Diseases		825	302
National Institute of General Medical Sciences		2,062	2,029
National Institute of Environmental Health Sciences		2,402	612
Total	158,038	113,991	206,201

[a]Values reported by Medical Rehabilitation Coordinating Committee August 29, 1996, in reponse to IOM committee request to NIH Director Harold Varmus.
[b]Values calculated by IOM committee according to review of individual abstracts.

non-rehabilitation related. Center grants were considered separately because rehabilitation was a minor component of their activities. The resulting total funding for individual rehabilitation-related research projects was $206 million. Although the committee's analysis (see Appendix A) indicated that NIH supported considerable research outside of NCMRR, that was determined to be relevant, the true focus of these activities lay elsewhere.

Although research priorities are established within individual ICDs, the analysis indicated the trends within NIH as a whole. Figure 10-2 shows that 12 percent (based on expenditures) of the abstracts were not related to rehabilitation science and engineering, 37 percent included a focus on rehabilitation science, another 39 percent focused on a single state of the enabling–disabling process (illustrated in Chapter 3), and 12

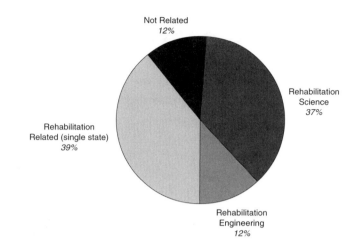

Not Related
12%

Rehabilitation
Science
37%

Rehabilitation
Related (single state)
39%

Rehabilitation
Engineering
12%

Relevance Category	Amount Funded	Number of Projects	Percent Funding
Rehabilitation science	$87,116,381	448	37
Rehabilitation engineering	$27,693,617	160	12
Rehabilitation related (single state)	$91,390,968	470	39
Not related	$29,091,590	184	12
Totals	$235,292,556	1,262	100

FIGURE 10-2 Percentage of research funding (not including center grants, which are summarized in Table 10-2) in four categories of relevance to rehabilitation research for the fiscal year 1995 program at the National Institutes of Health. Rehabilitation science: Projects that address movement among states in the enabling–disabling process. Rehabilitation engineering: Projects that address devices or technologies applicable to one of the rehabilitation states. Rehabilitation related (single state): Projects that address one rehabilitation state exclusively. Not related: Projects that do not clearly address any rehabilitation state. For additional information, see Appendix A.

percent involved rehabilitation engineering.[1] Within these categories of relevance, Figure 10-3 shows how many of the abstracts included a focus on the individual states of the enabling–disabling process. As expected, NIH research had a focus on pathology and impairment, as is appropriate with NIH's mission. A great majority of the single-state projects focused on pathology, and much of the identifiable rehabilitation-related research

---

[1]See Appendix A for details of the committee's analysis.

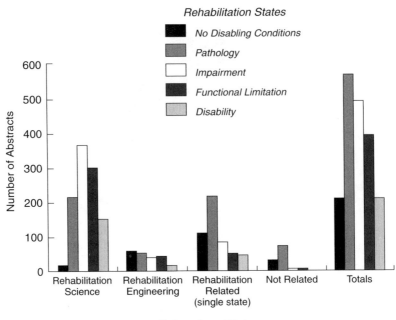

FIGURE 10-3 Number of abstracts within each category of relevance[a] that address the specific states of the enabling–disabling process[b] for Fiscal Year 1995. NOTE: Many abstracts address multiple states. For additional information, see Appendix A.

[a]Rehabilitation science: Projects that address movement among states in the enabling–disabling process. Rehabilitation engineering: Projects that address devices or technologies applicable to one of the rehabilitation states. Rehabilitation-related (single state): Projects that address one rehabilitation state exclusively. Not related: Projects that do not clearly address any rehabilitation state.

[b]No disabling conditions: Research that addresses the state of function or use of subjects with no disabling conditions to investigate mechanisms that are potentially relevant to assessing and treating disabling conditions. Pathology: Research that examines changes of molecules, cells, and tissues that may lead to impairment, functional limitation, or disability, distinguished from pathology by manifestation at organ or system level. Impairment: Research that analyzes changes in particular organs, systems, or parts of the body. Impairment is distinguished from functional limitation due to emphasis on organ and components instead of whole body. Functional limitation: Research that examines functional changes involving the entire subject, manifested by task performance. Disability: Research that focuses on the interaction of the subject with and in the larger context of the physical and social environment.

TABLE 10-2 National Institutes of Health Rehabilitation Funding Outside of Individual Research Projects

Activity	Amount Funded	Number of Projects
Center grants	$97,007,389	94
Community clinical oncology projects	$28,872,175	73
Total	$125,879,564	167

does not focus purposefully on rehabilitation. Approximately 17 percent of the NIH grants that the Institutes identified as being related to rehabilitation research involved materials, tissues, or subjects with no disabling conditions, as opposed to subjects in other rehabilitative states. In contrast, only one percent of the rehabilitation science projects dealt with subjects with no disabling conditions. In addition to individual research projects, broader-based center grants and community clinical oncology programs that also include rehabilitation-related activities receive funds amounting to $125 million dollars (see Table 10-2).

Strengths and Weaknesses There are many strengths in the rehabilitation-related research at NIH. As the center for biomedical research in the federal government, NIH maintains a high level of critical review that ensures high-quality research. In addition, the multiple perspectives of the many Institutes provide for significant potential synergy in addressing the array of rehabilitation-related issues. The drawback is that the overall effort is not well defined or coordinated, and rehabilitation per se is not a priority across all Institutes. Although a special emphasis panel on geriatrics and rehabilitation medicine was established in the Division of Research Grants to review rehabilitation-related research project applications, rehabilitation science still lacks a study section of its own.

NIH has a coordinating body for rehabilitation-related research in the Medical Rehabilitation Coordination Committee (MRCC) (see the NCMRR discussion below). The coordinating committee was established to facilitate communication among the Institutes engaging in rehabilitation-related research, but meaningful coordination seems to be lacking. The coordinating committee depends on the Institutes to conduct and report their efforts but has no effective mechanism for tracking these efforts independently or raising priorities within other Institutes. The result is a discordant effort in which even the definitions of rehabilitation-related research vary among the Institutes (see Appendix A).

Finally, although NIH now has a center for such research in NCMRR, rehabilitation-related research seems to receive relatively low priority

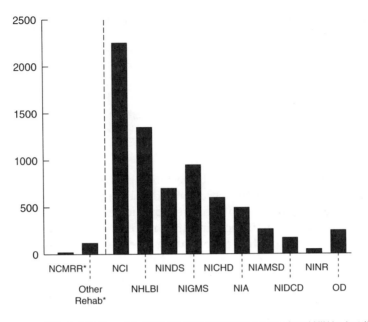

All rehabilitation related NIH research ($164M) is 1.54% of total NIH budget ($12 billion)

FIGURE 10-4 Funding levels within the National Institutes of Health: Comparison of funding for rehabilitation-related research with the total budgets for selected institutes, fiscal year 1996 estimates.

among the Institutes. Rehabilitation, although arguably one of the nation's most pressing needs, receives significantly less attention from NIH than other national health concerns (see Figure 10-4). Although NIH provides more than half of the gross federal effort in rehabilitation-related research, this seems to be more a result of the size of the aggregate budget than any special attention on the part of NIH.

National Center for Medical Rehabilitation Research

NCMRR was established within NIH by legislation passed in 1990 (Public Law 101-613). The mission of the Center, a component of NICHD, is to "conduct and support research and research training, the dissemination of health information, and other programs with respect to the rehabilitation of individuals with physical disabilities resulting from diseases or disorders of the neurological, musculoskeletal, cardiovascular, pulmonary, or any other physiological system" (Public Law 101-613). Beyond this, NCMRR strives to foster development of the scientific knowledge needed to enhance the health, productivity, independence, and quality of life of people with disabling conditions. A primary goal of the Center is to bring the health-related problems of people with disabling conditions to the attention of the best scientists in the United States in order to capitalize on the advances occurring in the biological, behavioral, and engineering sciences.

NCMRR also has responsibility as a federal coordinating body. Like the Interagency Committee on Disability Research (ICDR) of NIDRR, the MRCC, with the director of NCMRR as its chair, is authorized by legislation to "review and assess Federal research priorities, activities, and findings regarding medical rehabilitation research, and shall advise the Director of the Center and the Director of the Institute on the provisions of the Research plan" (Public Law 101-613). Its goals have actually been more modest in scope, choosing to work within NIH rather than across federal agencies. MRCC strives to foster communication among Institutes that have a significant interest in disability issues and rehabilitation research, but has met with limited success due to limitations in support and visibility.

Research Priorities and Funding NCMRR funded $15 million in research during fiscal year 1995. Between 17 and 23 percent of the NCMRR budgets between 1993 and 1996 were devoted to research training and career development. This level of support for research training is considerably higher than the norm for most components at NIH, but it is consistent with the emphasis on expanding research capacity that is called for in the NCMRR's research plan. The variety of funding mechanisms used by NICHD is used by NCMRR except for cooperative agreements, funding for clinical trials, and center grants. Centers tend to be expensive activities and have not been funded by NCMRR because overall budget restrictions have dictated that priority be given to less costly forms of research support. Supporting appropriately organized centers is a future priority of NCMRR, depending on the availability of funds.

As the focal point for rehabilitation-related research within NIH, NCMRR was of particular interest to the committee. NCMRR funded rehabilitation science to a slightly greater degree (43 percent of its research budget) than did NIH as a whole (37 percent), according to the committee's analysis. Likewise, rehabilitation engineering received 27 percent of NCMRR's budget as opposed to 12 percent from NIH. Many of the unrelated projects (22 percent) in NCMRR were training grants, and therefore not considered research in this definitional scheme. The emphasis of NCMRR's research tended to focus on pathologies and impairments (see Figures 10-5 and 10-6); 20 percent of the research awards address disability as defined in the committee's conceptual model (see Chapter 3).

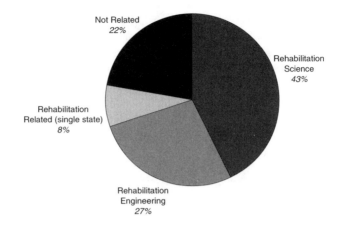

Relevance Category	Amount Funded	Number of Projects	Percent Funding
Rehabilitation science	$6,256,000	39	43
Rehabilitation engineering	$3,949,000	27	27
Rehabilitation related (single state)	$1,153,000	17	8
Not related	$3,266,000	27	22
Totals	$14,624,000	110	100

FIGURE 10-5 Percentage of research funding (not including center grants) in four categories of relevance to rehabilitation research for the fiscal year 1995 program at the National Center for Medical Rehabilitation Research. Rehabilitation science: Projects that address movement among states in the enabling–disabling process. Rehabilitation engineering: Projects that address devices or technologies applicable to one of the rehabilitation states. Rehabilitation related (single state): Projects that address one rehabilitation state exclusively. Not related: Training grants and projects that do not clearly address any rehabilitation state. For additional information, see Appendix A.

Strengths and Weaknesses As part of NIH, NCMRR is influenced by the predominant medical orientation of NIH. This is considered by some as a strength and by others as a potential weakness. The benefit is that NIH ensures rigorous review and a scientific basis for research findings. On the other hand, critics contend that the medical theory of disability is deterministic and frequently loses sight of the person. Although the *Research Plan for the National Center for Medical Rehabilitation Research* (NCMRR, 1993) focuses on the person with a disabling condition and on how that person's functional limitations are affected by interacting biological, personal, and societal forces, most emphasis seems to be on the biological underpinnings of

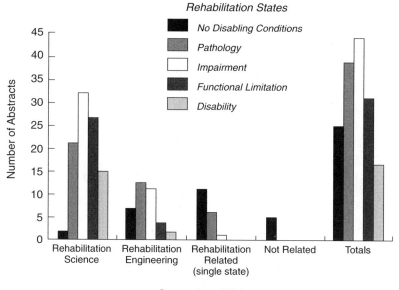

FIGURE 10-6 Number of abstracts within each category of relevance that address the specific states of the enabling–disabling process for the fiscal year 1995 program at the National Center for Medical Rehabilitation Research.

NOTE: Many abstracts address multiple states. Rehabilitation science: Projects that address movement among states in the enabling–disabling process. Rehabilitation engineering: Projects that address devices or technologies applicable to one of the rehabilitation states. Rehabilitation related (single state): Projects that address one rehabilitation state exclusively. Not related: Projects that do not clearly address any rehabilitation state. No disabling conditions: Research that addresses the state of function or use of subjects with no disabling conditions to investigate mechanisms that are potentially relevant to assessing and treating disabling conditions. Pathology: Research that examines changes of molecules, cells, and tissues that may lead to impairment, functional limitation, or disability, distinguished from pathology by manifestation at organ or system level. Impairment: Research that analyzes changes in particular organs, systems, or parts of the body. Impairment is distinguished from functional limitation due to emphasis on organ and components instead of whole body. Functional limitation: Research that examines functional changes involving the entire subject, manifested by task performance and can be readily distinguished from disability which involves interaction with the environment. Disability: Functional changes stemming from the interaction of the subject with and in the larger context of the physical and social environment. For additional information, see Appendix A.

conditions. The goals of NCMRR's research portfolio include methods of effecting greater and faster recovery from injury and disease and improving a person's ability to live independently.

MRCC, like ICDR, has problems with effective coordination of programs and research and also suffers from insufficient funds and staff. Rehabilitation-related research is not a general priority within NIH and helps to explain the limited success that MRCC has experienced in its effort to mold a coordinated and effective effort among the many NIH programs.

National Institute on Disability and Rehabilitation Research

The mission of NIDRR, a part of the Office of Special Education and Rehabilitative Services in the U.S. Department of Education, is "to contribute to the independence of persons of all ages who have disabilities by seeking improved systems, products, and practices in the rehabilitation process." NIDRR accomplishes this mission by funding research, demonstration projects, training, and other related activities to maximize the full inclusion and integration of this population into society. Through grants, contracts, and cooperative agreements, NIDRR funds research designed to improve systems, products, and practices in the rehabilitation field. NIDRR is also charged with ensuring the widespread distribution of practical scientific and technological information in usable formats.

Research Priorities and Funding

The research funded by NIDRR covers almost every aspect of disability including brain injury, spinal cord injury, multiple sclerosis, and back pain, as well as broader areas such as technology, accessibility, aging, service delivery, policy, ethics, recreation, and community integration. In fiscal year 1995, NIDRR funded approximately $57 million in rehabilitation-related research, which included individual research grants, center grants, and fellowships. NIDRR reported that $19 million of this went to medical rehabilitation, applied research that focuses on methods for improving function, and efforts aimed at reintegrating people with disabling conditions into the community (Seelman, 1996). A total of $13 million was directed toward engineering and technology development. In addition to supporting centers that include training in their activities, NIDRR also funded more than $2 million in individual research training grants and $200,000 in academic disability studies. Lastly, NIDRR funded approximately $2.5 million in dissemination and projects that pertained to ADA.

In addition to its operating budget of $70 million, NIDRR controls $39 million of State Technology Assistance under the Technology-Related

TABLE 10-3 National Institute on Disability and Rehabilitation Research Funding for Center Grants, Americans with Disability Act (ADA) Assistance, and Disability Studies in Fiscal Year 1995

Activity	Amount Funded	Number of Projects
Center Grants		
Rehabilitation Research and Training Centers	$24,536,852	47
Rehabilitation Engineering Research Centers	$10,844,615	16
Model Spinal Cord Injury Centers	$6,714,000	18
Total	$42,095,467	81
ADA assistance	$2,529,172	4
Disability studies	$198,787	8
Total	$44,823,426	174

Assistance for Individuals with Disabilities Act of 1988 (Public Law 100-407; the Tech Act). This program supports consumer-driven plans for the delivery of assistive technology. The purpose of these grants is to establish a program of statewide, comprehensive technology-related assistance for individuals of all ages with disabling conditions.

Using NIDRR's fiscal year 1995 Annual Program Directory to obtain abstracts for the projects NIDRR funded, the committee determined that approximately $10 to 13 million of NIDRR's $70 million operating budget went to training, ADA compliance support, and contracts, leaving approximately $57 million to fund research through various means such as individual research grants, center grants, small business cooperatives, and fellowships. A large portion of this ($44 million) supports centers—Rehabilitation Research and Training Centers, Rehabilitation Engineering Research Centers, and Model Spinal Cord Injury Centers (see Table 10-3).

Center grants compose the largest portion (78 percent) of NIDRR's $57 million research budget. Rehabilitation Research and Training Centers and Rehabilitation Engineering Research Centers conduct research targeted toward the production of new knowledge that will improve rehabilitation methodologies and service delivery systems, alleviate or stabilize disabling conditions, and promote maximum social and economic independence. They also institute related teaching and training programs that are used to disseminate and promote the use of research findings focusing on new engineering solutions to problems of disability.

NIDRR further supports projects for academic disability studies and issues pertaining to implementation of the ADA, leaving approximately $11 million to fund individual research projects into several areas of reha-

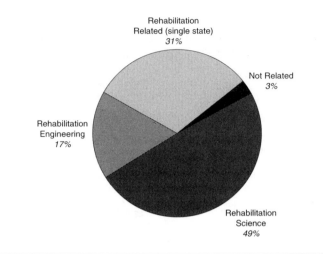

Relevance Category	Amount Funded	Number of Projects	Percent Funding
Rehabilitation science	$5,482,738	42	49
Rehabilitation engineering	$1,901,059	29	17
Rehabilitation related (single state)	$3,430,567	32	31
Not related	$374,618	3	3
Total	$11,188,982	106	100

FIGURE 10-7 Percentage of research funding (not including center grants, disability studies, or Americans with Disability Act-assistance projects; these are summarized in Table 10-3) in four categories of relevance to rehabilitation research for the fiscal year 1995 program at the National Institute on Disability and Rehabilitation Research. Rehabilitation science: Projects that address movement among states in the enabling–disabling process. Rehabilitation engineering: Projects that address devices or technologies applicable to one of the rehabilitation states. Rehabilitation related (single state): Projects that address one rehabilitation state exclusively. Not related: Projects that do not clearly address any rehabilitation state. For additional information, see Appendix A.

bilitation investigation. The committee's analysis[2] showed that 49 percent ($5.4 million) of the approximate $11 million went toward rehabilitation science in fiscal year 1995 (see Figure 10-7), 17 percent ($1.9 million) of the funding supported rehabilitation engineering, 31 percent ($3.4 million) was single-state research, and 3 percent ($0.4 million) funded research

[2] See Appendix A for details on the committee's analysis.

that was not related. Although NIDRR does fund some projects that address pathology and impairment, the bulk of its projects focus on functional limitation and disability (see Figure 10-8).

Strengths and Weaknesses

NIDRR is a valuable program with a unique mission that the committee believes should be preserved. The most important distinction that separates NIDRR from other agencies is its attention to consumers' needs and its emphasis on the interaction of the person and the environment. Most of the weaknesses seem to be derived from NIDRR's administrative placement within the U.S. Department of Education. The GAO (U.S. General Accounting Office, 1989) described NIDRR's poorly developed peer review process, its insufficient personnel, and its lack of authority over its own affairs as being due in large part to the policies and infrastructure of the U.S. Department of Education. Former NIDRR directors and others have expressed the view that—despite the efforts of NIDRR staff—the policies, procedures, and general interests of the U.S. Department of Education continually hinder the program. In addition, the core funding of center grants consumes a large portion of the agency's funds for 5-year periods, thereby reducing flexibility.

The weaknesses in the peer review process are manifold. The experience of past directors and staff indicates that the primary weaknesses of the process are that the panels are too small and there is no continuity between panels; these review panels are composed of only a few (3–5) reviewers who meet for just one review session rather than standing study sections or peer review panels that meet on a consistent basis. In addition, grant applications are occasionally not sent out prior to review meetings. Holding only one round of reviews per year for the field initiated research program is inadequate.

Reform of the peer review process would improve the quality of research, discipline the awards process, and attract quality scientists and personnel, but directors of NIDRR and secretaries of the U.S. Department of Education have been unable to implement the necessary changes. Another problem is the ineffectiveness of ICDR as a federal coordinating body. Congress and the executive branch established ICDR within NIDRR through the Rehabilitation Act of 1973, acknowledging the multiplicity of agencies engaged in rehabilitation-related research and the need to promote coordination and cooperation among those federal programs. Authorized by the Rehabilitation Act of 1973, the charge to the director of NIDRR, as the chair of ICDR, is "to identify, assess, and seek to coordinate all Federal programs, activities, and projects, and plans for such programs, activities, and projects with respect to the conduct of research

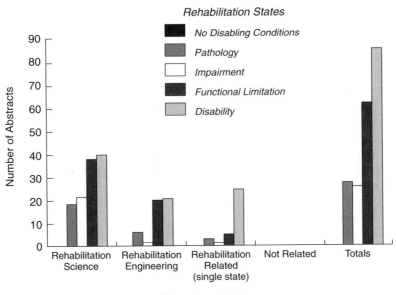

FIGURE 10-8 Number of abstracts within each category of relevance that address the specific states of the enabling–disabling process for the fiscal year 1995 program at the National Institute on Disability and Rehabilitation Research.

NOTE: Many abstracts address multiple states. Rehabilitation science: Projects that address movement among states in the enabling–disabling process. Rehabilitation engineering: Projects that address devices or technologies applicable to one of the rehabilitation states. Rehabilitation related (single state): Projects that address one rehabilitation state exclusively. Not related: Projects that do not clearly address any rehabilitation state. No disabling conditions: Research that addresses the state of function or use of subjects with no disabling conditions to investigate mechanisms that are potentially relevant to assessing and treating disabling conditions. Pathology: Research that examines changes of molecules, cells, and tissues that may lead to impairment, functional limitation, or disability, distinguished from pathology by manifestation at organ or system level. Impairment: Research that analyzes changes in particular organs, systems, or parts of the body. Impairment is distinguished from functional limitation due to emphasis on organ and components instead of whole body. Functional limitation: Research that examines functional changes involving the entire subject, manifested by task performance and can be readily distinguished from disability which involves interaction with the environment. Disability: Functional changes stemming from the interaction of the subject with and in the larger context of the physical and social environment. For additional information, see Appendix A.

related to rehabilitation of individuals with disabilities" (Public Law 93-112, as amended). The Rehabilitation Act did not, however, give ICDR the proper tools, that is, control of funding, to achieve this mission. Thus, it lacks the ability to entice cooperation or ensure compliance, which severely limits its effectiveness. Moreover, ICDR has no staff, budget, or real control, and thus does not have the ability to carry out its stated mission. In its present state it cannot exert the influence necessary to coordinate the overall federal efforts in rehabilitation-related research.

Perhaps because disability is not a priority of the U.S. Department of Education and because NIDRR does not have the budget to demand attention, NIDRR is neglected by the department and is not given adequate priority.

U.S. Department of Veterans Affairs

The VA program in rehabilitation-related research began shortly after the end of World War II as part of the effort to improve the quality of health care being provided to returning veterans with disabling conditions. VA medical research programs in general are meant to enhance the overall mission of the Veterans Health Administration (VHA), contribute new knowledge benefiting the nation as a whole, and provide training for future health care clinicians and researchers. The goals of VA's research program derive from its legislated mission as well as a continuously evolving shared vision of veterans' needs and VA's research potential. The VA Research and Development Office is divided into three services: the Medical Research Service, the Health Services Research and Development (HSR&D) Service, and the Rehabilitation Research and Development (Rehab R&D) Service.

Research that is relevant to rehabilitation can be found in almost all VA research activities. In addition to the services mentioned above, for example, the VA Geriatric Service maintains 16 Geriatric Research, Education, and Clinical Centers that include some rehabilitation-related research as it pertains to aging. The principal division for rehabilitation-related research within VA, however, is the Rehab R&D Service. Focusing most clearly on the needs of veterans with disabling conditions, the Rehab R&D Service:

- develops concepts, products, and processes that promote greater functional independence and improve the quality of life for "impaired and disabled veterans";
- supports a comprehensive program of investigator-initiated research, development, and evaluation of rehabilitation technology;
- provides for the immediate transfer of rehabilitation technology

and rapid dissemination of information into the VA health care delivery system; and
- contributes to the nation's knowledge about disease, disability, and rehabilitation.

Under the leadership of the Under Secretary for Health, VA effected a major reorganization of VHA at the beginning of Fiscal Year 1996. It is, as of this writing, not yet fully implemented. Incident to this reorganization and the associated staffing reduction for VA's Central Office, the Rehab R&D Service, having for some time been a separate office, was moved back under the Assistant Chief Medical Director for Medical Research and Development. Because of the overlapping areas of investigation, research that is relevant to patient rehabilitation can be found in the various VA research programs and services. VA leadership now believes this integrated organizational structure provides a linear model of interactions among the three categories (medical, rehabilitation, and health services) of research and encourages interservice coordination and support. Assurances has been given to this committee that the structural and functional integrity of the Rehab R&D Service will be maintained.

Research Priorities and Funding

The VA Rehab R&D Service received $26.7 million of the fiscal year 1995 VA budget, but unlike the VA Medical Research and HSR&D Services, which receive extramural support from other agencies, the Rehab R&D Service has no source of funding outside VA itself. In fiscal year 1995, the Rehab R&D Service supported 147 projects and about 150 principal investigators at VA medical centers. In addition, other departments in the Research Office fund rehabilitation projects amounting to approximately $6 million, itemized under the following categories:

Career Development	$234,000
Cooperative Studies	33,899
HSR&D Service	1,198,000
Biomedical	4,833,000.

Because of its legislative mandate and its appropriate historical role of supporting U.S. veterans, VA focuses a significant amount of its research efforts on rehabilitation. Research in VA's Rehab R&D Service is focused on prosthetics and orthotics, spinal cord dysfunction, aging, and cognitive and sensory impairments. The rehabilitation program is geared to improving functional independence and the quality of life of veterans with disabling conditions.

To assess rehabilitation-related research at VA, the committee reviewed abstracts that were provided by VA's Rehabilitation Research and Development program (funding amounts were not available for each project). Analysis[3] of the abstracts indicated that 33 percent were rehabilitation science (See Figure 10-9); rehabilitation engineering represented a full 46 percent of the studies funded in fiscal year 1995; 20 percent of the abstracts covered single-state research, and 1 percent were not related to rehabilitation. Within these categories of relevance, Figure 10-10 shows how many of the abstracts included a focus on the individual states in the enabling–disabling process. The distribution of VA research along the rehabilitative states reflected VA's mission, with most of the research concentrating on functional limitations.

Strengths and Weaknesses

VA research is a needs-based program, setting its priorities from the health care requirements of its veteran clientele. There is also a synergistic relationship between VA research and the veteran population that it serves. U.S. veterans display a proprietary interest in VA programs, are advocates for VA research, and are a unique test bed for VA clinical research and device studies. No other health care system, public or private, has a similar, unified research program with the breadth and depth of VA's.

Many of VA's research outcomes not only benefit veterans but serve national interests as well. Certain characteristics, however, make the VA research program unique. Research assignments commonly come to VA and DOD directly from Congress with legislative oversight of their progress and outcome. Not unlike VA's mandated clinical mission of combat contingency backup to the military medical services, VA's research department is DoD's primary designated agency for medical research support, as exemplified in VA's current multimillion dollar investment in Persian Gulf War veterans' illness.

Combat has many consequences. Most critical are the men and women with severe and permanent injuries. These veterans of war face complex issues throughout their lives. A VA program of Rehabilitation Research and Development gives flexibility to find solutions to these programs, whether they present themselves early on when as an injured soldier returns from Bosnia, or later, as disabled veterans of the Persian Gulf, Vietnam, Korea and World War II enter their fifties, sixties and seventies.

The comprehensive nature of the program is, in itself, unique. The VA Research and Development Office is organized in a way that reflects the

---

[3] See Appendix A for details of the committee's analysis.

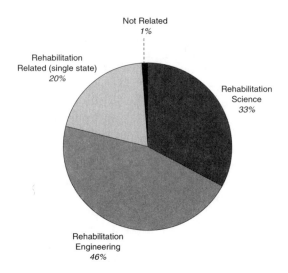

FIGURE 10-9 Percentage of research projects (not including center grants) in four categories of relevance to rehabilitation research for the fiscal year 1995 program at the Department of Veterans Affairs. Rehabilitation science: Projects that address movement among states in the enabling–disabling process. Rehabilitation engineering: Projects that address devices or technologies applicable to one of the rehabilitation states. Rehabilitation related (single state): Projects that address one rehabilitation state exclusively. Not related: Projects that do not clearly address any rehabilitation state. For additional information, see Appendix A.

Relevance Category	Amount Funded	Number of Projects	Percent of Projects
Rehabilitation science	NA	53	33
Rehabilitation engineering	NA	74	46
Rehabilitation related (single state)	NA	33	20
Not related	NA	2	1
Totals	$26,700,000	162	100

NA = Not available.

interrelated research questions that can be posed when a particular health outcome is desired. The acquisition of new knowledge spans the entire spectrum of research from basic to applied research to outcomes research, with each component of that spectrum being linked to the other. VA makes the strong claim that its intramural coordination of research, policy, and planning favors that linkage of interests.

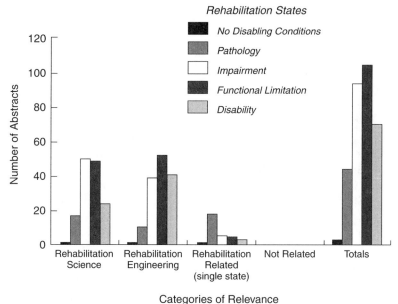

FIGURE 10-10 Number of abstracts within each category of relevance that address the specific states of the enabling–disabling process for the fiscal year 1995 program at the Department of Veterans Affairs.

NOTE: Many abstracts address multiple states. Rehabilitation science: Projects that address movement among states in the enabling–disabling process. Rehabilitation engineering: Projects that address devices or technologies applicable to one of the rehabilitation states. Rehabilitation related (single state): Projects that address one rehabilitation state exclusively. Not related: Projects that do not clearly address any rehabilitation state. No disabling conditions: Research that addresses the state of function or use of subjects with no disabling conditions to investigate mechanisms that are potentially relevant to assessing and treating disabling conditions. Pathology: Research that examines changes of molecules, cells, and tissues that may lead to impairment, functional limitation, or disability, distinguished from pathology by manifestation at organ or system level. Impairment: Research that analyzes changes in particular organs, systems, or parts of the body. Impairment is distinguished from functional limitation due to emphasis on organ and components instead of whole body. Functional limitation: Research that examines functional changes involving the entire subject, manifested by task performance and can be readily distinguished from disability which involves interaction with the environment. Disability: Functional changes stemming from the interaction of the subject with and in the larger context of the physical and social environment. For additional information, see Appendix A.

VA's research laboratories serve national interests as well. These VAMC based facilities, as a constituent element of the VA academic affiliation with 105 medical schools, provide an intimate coupling of advanced research activity with the nation's single largest source of graduate medical education. Today, more than 60 percent of doctors in the United States have received all or part of their training at VA medical centers.

Centers for Disease Control and Prevention

The mission of CDC is to promote health and quality of life by preventing and controlling disease, disability, and injury. To accomplish this mission, CDC works with state authorities and partners throughout the United States and the world to monitor health, detect and investigate health problems, conduct research to enhance prevention, develop and advocate sound public health policies, implement prevention strategies, promote healthy behaviors, foster safe and healthful environments, and provide leadership and training. Two of the centers have rehabilitation-related programs. The National Center for Environmental Health (NCEH) includes the Disabilities Prevention Program (DPP), and the National Center for Injury Prevention and Control (NCIPC) includes the Division of Acute Care, Rehabilitation Research, and Disability Prevention.

DPP, which funded $9 million in disability prevention research in fiscal year 1995, has two major goals: (1) to reduce the incidence and severity of primary and secondary disabling conditions and (2) to promote the independence and productivity of people with disabling conditions and further their integration into the community. To achieve these goals, DPP

- provides states with technical and financial assistance to build disability prevention capacity,
- establishes surveillance systems for disabling conditions,
- identifies risk factors for disabling conditions, and
- identifies and develops appropriate interventions to prevent secondary disabling conditions.

The goals of the Division of Acute Care, Rehabilitation Research, and Disability Prevention are to maximize the quality of life and productivity, minimize the health care costs of injured people, and reduce the impacts of injuries by improving acute care and rehabilitation services and systems. The division spends $500,000 to $600,000 annually on disability prevention, with a special interest in community-based injury and outcomes surveillance and research to prevent the occurrence of or reduce the severity of secondary conditions among people with traumatic brain and spinal cord injuries. Research includes identifying risk factors associated with adverse outcomes in the community setting, describing the natural history of the occurrence of adverse outcomes and secondary conditions, and evaluating interventions in the community setting.

Research Priorities and Funding

In fiscal year 1995, the two programs mentioned above supported a total of almost $10 million in rehabilitation-related research. Their grant-making process is modeled after that of NIH, but no training grants are available. Resources from both NCIPC and NCEH are used in a complementary fashion, occasionally within the same request for proposal, to cover a range of injury-related rehabilitation research that focuses on measuring the frequency and extent of disabling conditions caused by injury, measuring the secondary conditions, and developing and evaluating community-based interventions to prevent or reduce these disabling conditions. Secondary conditions are the clearest priority in CDC's disability and rehabilitation agenda, and the majority of CDC abstracts that the committee reviewed explicitly addressed this issue. Other abstracts described research involving prevention of disabling injury in the community.

The small number and uniform nature of the abstracts received from CDC made categorization through the abstract review process unnecessary. The projects funded by CDC consistently address prevention, specifically of secondary conditions among individuals with cerebral palsy, postpolio syndrome, spinal cord injury, or traumatic brain injury. All of the CDC abstracts were considered pertinent to rehabilitation research and a valuable contribution to the field.

Strengths and Weaknesses

The CDC program has several strengths including a community- or population-based approach to prevention and intervention, strong linkages with states, especially state health departments, and a history of effective surveillance activities. These links also help involve consumers in the process of setting research priorities.

CDC's focus on prevention as a means of reducing disabling conditions sets it apart from other federal programs and is an essential component of the overall federal effort. The CDC program makes a clear connection between prevention and rehabilitation, especially with its focus on preventing secondary conditions. Preventing secondary conditions as part of rehabilitation is an important area of research, especially from the perspective of aging with disabling conditions.

Monitoring events such as traumatic brain and spinal cord injuries, and the adverse outcomes associated with these injuries, also contributes to the goals of rehabilitation science and engineering. CDC's public health surveillance activities measure the incidence and prevalence of these injuries, and community-based intervention programs contribute to their prevention and control.

The weaknesses in the CDC program are the same as those seen in most other agency programs. For example, there is a need for more visibility within the agency and more involvement of other internal programs. Other centers (e.g., National Center for Chronic Disease Prevention and Health Promotion) should be more involved in the total effort. There is also a need to strengthen the links between CDC and other federal agencies to identify, validate, and adopt more uniform measurement strategies and terminologies in databases, as well as determining priorities and synergistic activities.

National Science Foundation

Established as an independent federal agency by the National Science Foundation Act of 1950, NSF is responsible for the overall health of science and engineering across all scientific disciplines and for promoting and advancing scientific progress in the United States. In contrast, other federal agencies support research focused on specific missions, such as health or defense. NSF is also committed to ensuring the nation's supply of scientists, engineers, and science educators.

All seven directorates in NSF support some projects related to rehabilitation, and in fiscal year 1995, NSF spent approximately $7 million on projects in this general area. The projects are typically investigator initiated and are recommended for funding during regular competitive review cycles. Most of the rehabilitation-related projects are supported through the Directorate for Engineering, which funds research pertinent to rehabilitation science and engineering through its Division of Bioengineering and Environmental Systems. The division operates two programs that support research for people with disabling conditions: the Biomedical Engineering Program and Research Aiding Persons with Disabilities (RAPD).

The Biomedical Engineering Program supports fundamental engineering research that has the potential to contribute to improved health care. The RAPD program is directed toward the characterization, restoration, and substitution of function in humans and tends to focus on basic science at the level of cells, tissues, organs, and organ systems. Emphasis is placed on the advancement of fundamental engineering knowledge, but many grants support product development. The program anticipates that the research will lead to the development of new technologies or the novel application of existing technologies by supporting research and training in basic science.

Research Priorities and Funding

One of NSF's goals is to expand the capacity for research, and therefore, the agency places importance on training. Approximately 20 percent of the abstracts that the committee reviewed for fiscal year 1995 involved training in research or product design. Although NSF does support faculty and graduate work, roughly three quarters of the training grants related to rehabilitation science and engineering went to undergraduate training.

Abstracts from NSF for fiscal year 1995 were retrieved from FastLane, the agency's on-line database, for the RAPD program. Figure 10-11 indicates that (on the basis of expenditures) 76 percent of the funding for rehabilitation-related research supported rehabilitation engineering activities. Single-state research represented 12 percent of the funding, and another 12 percent was not related to rehabilitation. None of the research was determined to be in the category of rehabilitation science. Within these categories of relevance, Figure 10-12 shows that most of the research tended to focus on functional limitation, disability, and impairment, in descending order.

The clearest priority is engineering. Not only did more than half of the abstracts that the committee reviewed pertain to rehabilitation engineering research, but the majority of the training grants funded rehabilitation engineering projects as well. The engineering grants tended to emphasize basic research, but many, including the training grants, were designed to advance product development. The accent on basic science continued in biomedical research as well, and the majority of all NSF research focused on impairment. NSF also sponsored grants that addressed health services, and all of these focused on cost reduction.

Strengths and Weaknesses

The strengths of NSF research emanate from its emphasis on basic science and rehabilitation engineering, a focus that is essential to the overall federal effort. NSF also addresses educational needs through the undergraduate design projects that recruit young engineers to the rehabilitation field. The relative size of the program, however, limits its ability to influence the overall field of rehabilitation science and engineering. NSF programs also experience a lack of coordination with other federal programs, thus limiting the potential synergy among the projects being supported by other agencies.

Additionally, none of the research projects emphasize rehabilitation

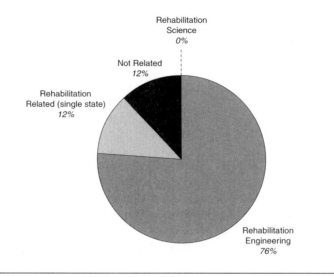

Relevance Category	Amount Funded	Number of Projects	Percent Funding
Rehabilitation science	$0	0	0
Rehabilitation engineering	$2,658,776	30	76
Rehabilitation related (single state)	$422,833	2	12
Not related	$420,314	4	12
Totals	$3,501,923	36	100

FIGURE 10-11 Percentage of research funding (not including center grants) in four categories of relevance to rehabilitation research for the fiscal year 1995 program at the National Science Foundation. Rehabilitation science: Projects that address movement among states in the enabling–disabling process. Rehabilitation engineering: Projects that address devices or technologies applicable to one of the rehabilitation states. Rehabilitation related (single state): Projects that address one rehabilitation state exclusively. Not related: Projects that do not clearly address any rehabilitation state. For additional information, see Appendix A.

science as defined by this committee, that is, concentration on the movement between the states in the enabling–disabling process (see Chapter 3). Although the research that NSF funds is an important component of the mix of interdisciplinary research in the field, the majority focuses on impairment without reference to other states. Thus, the focus of most NSF research is within each stage of the enabling–disabling process rather than the process itself. Only the grants aimed at products for individuals with disabling conditions offer the opportunity to provide an understanding of not only engineering principles but also effective rehabilitation and the interaction between the individual and the environment. Given ad-

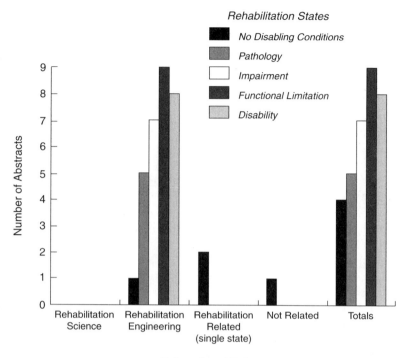

FIGURE 10-12 Number of abstracts within each category of relevance that address the specific states of the enabling–disabling process for the fiscal year 1995 program at the National. Science Foundation.

NOTE: Many abstracts address multiple states. Rehabilitation science: Projects that address movement among states in the enabling–disabling process. Rehabilitation engineering: Projects that address devices or technologies applicable to one of the rehabilitation states. Rehabilitation related (single state): Projects that address one rehabilitation state exclusively. Not related: Projects that do not clearly address any rehabilitation state. No disabling conditions: Research that addresses the state of function or use of subjects with no disabling conditions to investigate mechanisms that are potentially relevant to assessing and treating disabling conditions. Pathology: Research that examines changes of molecules, cells, and tissues that may lead to impairment, functional limitation, or disability, distinguished from pathology by manifestation at organ or system level. Impairment: Research that analyzes changes in particular organs, systems, or parts of the body. Impairment is distinguished from functional limitation due to emphasis on organ and components instead of whole body. Functional limitation: Research that examines functional changes involving the entire subject, manifested by task performance and can be readily distinguished from disability which involves interaction with the environment. Disability: Functional changes stemming from the interaction of the subject with and in the larger context of the physical and social environment. For additional information, see Appendix A.

equate funds, NSF should support clinical research efforts, perhaps in rehabilitation engineering centers, that involve a more comprehensive view of the enabling process.

Other Agencies

Several other federal agencies are also involved in rehabilitation science and engineering (see Appendix B). SSA for example, funded approximately $5 million in fiscal year 1995 in research for the purposes of developing intervention and service delivery models such as returning beneficiaries to work. SSA also recently initiated an Institute of Medicine (IOM) study for the purposes of reviewing its research plans for a revised process of determining whether a person has a disability.

In addition to the NIH and CDC programs described above, DHHS also administers a program in the Office of the Assistant Secretary for Planning and Evaluation (ASPE). This office is responsible for the development, coordination, research, and evaluation of DHHS policies and programs that support the independence, productivity, health, and security of children, working-age adults, and older people with disabling conditions. Within ASPE, the Office of Disability, Aging, and Long-Term Care Policy, along with other ASPE offices, provides staff support to the assistant secretary in carrying out these functions. One of this office's chief priorities concerns personal assistance services, which involve all forms of assistance, both human and technological, that enable people with disabling conditions to accomplish basic and instrumental daily living activities. In fiscal year 1995 ASPE funded $2.5 million in research that focused on the policy needs concerning personal assistance services and the delivery of those services.

Finally, it seems reasonable that the U.S. Department of Defense would be engaged in rehabilitation science and engineering research, but a survey conducted at the committee's request by the Assistant Secretary of Defense for Health Affairs revealed an insignificant volume of rehabilitation research being conducted within the military medical services. The U.S. Department of Defense does, however, subsidize, under contract, certain unspecified rehabilitation-related research. Various levels of clinical rehabilitation services are also provided in all military hospitals.

GENERAL ASSESSMENT OF FEDERAL REHABILITATION PROGRAMS

In addition to reviewing the individual federal programs that focus on rehabilitation-related research, the committee also reviewed the overall organization and administration of these programs for the purpose of assessing their combined adequacy in addressing the health needs of people with disabling conditions. In assessing a constellation of programs of this size and complexity with the overall mission of addressing health needs of such magnitude, it is not surprising to find some apparent problems. Foremost among these are the need for improved coordination among the various and numerous federal research programs and the need for additional research in rehabilitation science and engineering that will help to improve the health, quality of life, and productivity of the 49 million Americans with disabling conditions.

Further analysis of these programs—including the related efforts outside NCMRR at NIH—revealed certain trends in the overall federal research effort in rehabilitation science and engineering (see Figures 10-13 and 10-14). Given the current constraints and limitations of funding, these findings show a generally good balance of effort, but with most of the research focusing on pathology and impairment, and a relatively smaller proportion of research focusing on disability per se.

Adequacy of Current Efforts

The size of the combined federal research effort in the field of rehabilitation science and engineering is not adequate to address the health needs of people with disabling conditions. A clear disproportionality exists between the magnitude and significance of the health issues related to disability and rehabilitation and the amount of research that is currently supported to address them. This is not a new situation, as indicated by the NCMRR research plan from 1993, which states that one of the most important barriers "to improving rehabilitation research is inadequate funding. . . . Given the large numbers of Americans with disabilities, the social and economic impact of disability, and the opportunities for improvement of function through research, a significantly greater effort to fund medical rehabilitation research is clearly justified" (NCMRR, 1993, p. 48).

Chapter 2 of this report describes the significance of disabling conditions in various terms, including prevalence of conditions and the associated costs of health care and lost productivity. In 1996, for example, Trupin and colleagues used the National Medical Care Expenditures Survey to estimate that approximately 47 percent of the total medical care expenditures were for 17 percent of the population with an activity limitation. Expressed in 1994 terms, these medical care expenditures (direct costs) for people with disabling conditions would amount to $205.7 billion, or 3.1 percent of the gross domestic product (U.S. Bureau of the Census, 1995). Other studies, most notably Chirikos (1989), have estimated both direct and indirect costs. Expressed again in 1994 terms, the medical care expenditures (direct costs) would amount to $163.1 billion, and the indirect

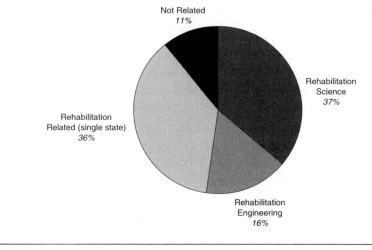

Relevance Category	Amount Funded	Number of Projects	Percent Funding
Rehabilitation science	$101,105,292	543	37
Rehabilitation engineering	$44,129,995	293	16
Rehabilitation related (single state)	$100,540,664	540	36
Not related	$30,207,510	193	11
Totals	$275,983,461	1,569	100

FIGURE 10-13 Percentage of research funding (not including center grants) in four categories of relevance to rehabilitation research for the fiscal year 1995 program for overall federal research. Rehabilitation science: Projects that address movement among states in the enabling–disabling process. Rehabilitation engineering: Projects that address devices or technologies applicable to one of the rehabilitation states. Rehabilitation related (single state): Projects that address one rehabilitation state exclusively. Not related: Projects that do not clearly address any rehabilitation state. For additional information, see Appendix A.

costs (lost productivity) would total $155 billion, for a grand total of more than $300 billion annually—more than 4 percent of the gross domestic product.

These cost estimates for disability and rehabilitation are in stark contrast to the relatively small amount of funding (approximately $245 million) that is directed toward research in rehabilitation science and engineering. Current expenditures amount to approximately $7 in research per year for each person with a disabling condition, whereas the costs of disability due to expenditures of health care and lost productivity, at about $7,500 per capita, are almost 1,000 times as great. Most importantly,

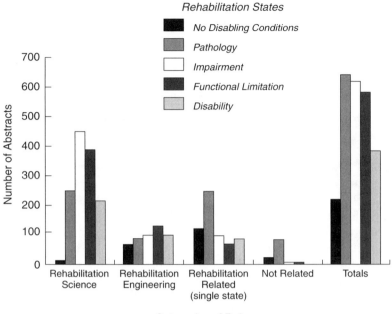

FIGURE 10-14 Number of abstracts within each category of relevance that address the specific states of the enabling–disabling process for the fiscal year 1995 program of overall federal research.

NOTE: Many abstracts address multiple states. Rehabilitation science: Projects that address movement among states in the enabling–disabling process. Rehabilitation engineering: Projects that address devices or technologies applicable to one of the rehabilitation states. Rehabilitation related (single state): Projects that address one rehabilitation state exclusively. Not related: Projects that do not clearly address any rehabilitation state. No disabling conditions: Research that addresses the state of function or use of subjects with no disabling conditions to investigate mechanisms that are potentially relevant to assessing and treating disabling conditions. Pathology: Research that examines changes of molecules, cells, and tissues that may lead to impairment, functional limitation, or disability, distinguished from pathology by manifestation at organ or system level. Impairment: Research that analyzes changes in particular organs, systems, or parts of the body. Impairment is distinguished from functional limitation due to emphasis on organ and components instead of whole body. Functional limitation: Research that examines functional changes involving the entire subject, manifested by task performance and can be readily distinguished from disability which involves interaction with the environment. Disability: Functional changes stemming from the interaction of the subject with and in the larger context of the physical and social environment. For additional information, see Appendix A.

however, significant savings in health care costs and reduced emotional costs may well be realized by enhancing research in rehabilitation science and engineering and improving the health, productivity, and quality of life of people with disabling conditions.

Coordination of Current Efforts

To be most effective, any set of research programs must be well coordinated. This is especially true for the set of federal research programs in rehabilitation science and engineering because of their distribution among so many different agencies and departments. Moreover, given the relatively limited amount of funding that is available for these research programs, good coordination is essential to maximize their combined productivity.

Despite a legislative mandate to NIDRR for coordination among the various and numerous federal agencies and programs there is a significant shortfall in achieving this important objective. Poor coordination and communication among programs severely limits their ability to develop and implement a cohesive vision for the overall federal effort or to establish well-defined research priorities that could complement one another. Territorial tension among the programs accentuates the problem and further limits possible interagency and multidisciplinary activities that are typically the hallmark of rehabilitation science and engineering.

Although some argue that there are benefits to the fact that responsibility for conducting and supporting current research in rehabilitation science and engineering is currently scattered among several agencies (e.g., multiple funding sources and replication of research), there are also drawbacks in terms of poor coordination and possible unnecessary duplication of effort. Inadequate monitoring of rehabilitation-related research activities among the various programs contributes to the potential problem of duplication of effort, and the different terminologies used by the various agencies complicate the issue even further, often making it nearly impossible to determine what is being done, and by whom. Moreover, although most programs have some means of cataloging and monitoring their respective research activities, each has its problems. For example, comparison of NIH research activities in rehabilitation and disability that are identifiable through the Computerized Retrieval of Information on Scientific Projects (CRISP) database with those activities identified by the NIH Institutes themselves shows only an 17 percent agreement (see Figure 10-15). In other words, most activities that were identified in CRISP as being rehabilitation-related research were not identified by the Institutes as such, and vice versa.

Even within agencies there are problems of coordination and communi-

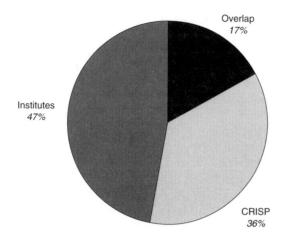

FIGURE 10-15 Sources of National Institutes of Health abstracts.

cation. The definition of rehabilitation-related research, for example, is not consistent among the Institutes at NIH (see Box A-2 in Appendix A). As described in Appendix A, this results in a variety of problems, including difficulty in even describing the current status of research. Moreover, with respect to NIH specifically, the lack of a study section to review rehabilitation-related research applications raises the question of whether there is a well-coordinated research effort in this field among the Institutes.

By law, the responsibility for coordinating federal disability research programs rests with ICDR, which is to be chaired by the director of NIDRR and whose membership includes 11 different agencies. The level of activity and relative success of ICDR, however, vary and are a function of both the energy and attention that ICDR receives from NIDRR and the goodwill, cooperation, and voluntary participation of its members.

Although ICDR has the potential (and the legislative mandate) to serve as a forum for agencies to discuss issues of mutual interest and concern and as a mechanism for them to identify research priorities and coordinate their research agendas, it has been relatively unsuccessful in these regards. This primarily seems to be a result of the fact that ICDR has no authority to ensure cooperation or even participation. It also has no full-time staff to manage and operate ICDR, nor any real means of providing incentives for member agencies to participate. Agency participation in ICDR meetings varies because the benefits of participation are not necessarily clear and the lack of participation has no observable negative effects on individual programs. Thus, the Holy Grail of effective coordination remains elusive, despite a clear need and the often valiant efforts on the part of NIDRR to compel and persuade the various agencies to participate.

One result of this disjointed effort is that potentially important areas of research in rehabilitation science and engineering may be either overlooked or underemphasized. For example, there seems to be inadequate attention to education and training of researchers in the field, especially nonmedical investigators, and health services research has largely been neglected. Perhaps the single greatest consequence of this disjointed effort, however, seems to be the lack of an appropriate emphasis on disability research per se, that is, the interaction of the person and the physical and social environments. NIDRR activities seem to address this particular area to a greater extent than the activities of other programs do, but the need still eclipses the effort. Far more studies are needed to address the environment as an independent variable and to identify and develop strategies for reducing and preventing disability and secondary conditions.

A well-coordinated federal effort in rehabilitation science and engineering with adequate funding and visibility is needed. This effort would address the following nine objectives:

• monitor the range of research activities in rehabilitation science and engineering among the various and numerous federal programs,
• ensure the highest-quality research (e.g., through peer review),
• identify and establish clear research priorities that would be complementary and mutually beneficial among the different federal programs,
• ensure interagency collaboration and joint research activities and reduce unnecessary duplication of effort,
• enhance the development of a cadre of rehabilitation scientists and engineers,
• develop effective technology transfer activities,
• help establish and maintain the use of consistent definitions and terminologies among agencies,
• optimize productivity through resource sharing and other cost-saving activities, and
• conduct clinical trials of therapeutic and environmental strategies to reduce and prevent disabling and secondary conditions.

The remainder of this chapter describes three of the many options that the committee developed and considered as means of addressing the problems and needs associated with inadequate support and coordination of federal programs in rehabilitation science and engineering. This is followed by recommendations for achieving enhanced coordination and visibility of the overall federal effort in rehabilitation science and engineering and for overarching areas of priority research.

SUMMARY OF POSSIBLE OPTIONS

The assessment of the current organization and administration of federal research in rehabilitation science and engineering described above reveals the deficiencies to be inadequate support, visibility, and coordination. Thus, any attempt to address these deficiencies must include strategies to increase support, enhance visibility, and improve coordination. More specifically, to improve the health, quality of life, and productivity of people with disabling conditions, the constellation of federal programs needs to address the nine objectives listed above.

In formulating its recommendations for the organization and administration of research in rehabilitation science and engineering by the federal government that address the needs and objectives articulated above, the committee considered several options. A summary of three of these is described below to characterize the spectrum of possibilities that the committee considered in developing the final recommendation.

Option 1: Improvement of NIDRR

All of the current programs that conduct and support research in rehabilitation science and engineering are important and make significant contributions to the overall need to improve the health of people with disabling conditions. If there is one program, however, that not only has possibly the largest potential for contributing to this effort but that is also the most limited by administrative and organizational constraints, it is NIDRR. The NIDRR mission and its constituency of people with disabling conditions are fundamentally important to the research agenda of rehabilitation science and engineering espoused by this committee. NIDRR has vigorously pursued this mission, but in the committee's estimation and as described above, it has been restricted in its ability to fully execute its mission primarily by virtue of its administrative position within the U.S. Department of Education, and the ICDR's lack of real authority.

Option 1 is designed to improve the overall constellation of federal programs by focusing on improving one of the most important components: NIDRR. In summary, this option would (1) improve peer review of grant applications at NIDRR and (2) move current medical research activities from NIDRR to NIH/NCMRR, limiting the focus in NIDRR to transportation, employment, independent living, parenting, and disability studies.

As discussed previously, the review of grant applications in NIDRR needs to be changed to improve its consistency and quality. To do this, review panels need to be established that would meet over a period of time rather than just once. In addition, although NIDRR is to be commended for its success in including consumers in the review of applications, there is a need to enhance the quality of the technical review.

One important aspect of the NIDRR program is its focus on person-environment interactions with an emphasis on the whole person. Implementing this option would refocus the NIDRR mission to emphasize the impacts of interventions and assistive technologies on improving the lives of people with disabling conditions in the following areas: employment, transportation, independent living, parenting, and disability studies. Thus, NIDRR would focus on programs that emphasize environment as an independent variable.

The advantages of keeping NIDRR in U.S. Department of Education include the following: constituencies remain intact, continuity of funding is ensured for Rehabilitation Research and Training Centers and Rehabilitation Engineering Research Centers, and costs of relocation are avoided. Because of its importance and particular focus of research activities, improving the NIDRR program would help to improve the present condition of the overall situation. However, these are minimal improvements that would improve only one important part of the constellation of activities and would not adequately address the need for a well-coordinated and well-supported overall federal effort.

Option 2: Consolidation of All Programs into a New Agency

Option 2 is at the opposite end of the spectrum of possible options for addressing the need for change in the organization and administration of research programs in rehabilitation science and engineering. This option would move all programs that currently support research in rehabilitation science and engineering into a single, newly created agency or department. The committee considered this option because the research issues related to the health of people with disabling conditions are significant enough, and large enough, to deserve such visibility and attention.

Many of the advantages and disadvantages of this option are readily apparent. With such consolidation of programs there would be economies of scale and potential savings in reduced bureaucratic waste. However, there would also be the costs associated with uprooting and displacing the many existing meritorious programs. Although the visibility of such a large, consolidated program would seem to be clearly justified, the hybrid vigor that results from various perspectives would be lost. In other words, consolidation would probably reduce the various agencies' broad range of approaches—and solutions—to the problems faced by people with disabling conditions. Finally, although the creation of a new agency or department with such a mandate is intriguing for many reasons, including the fact that it might facilitate the establishment of an integrated program with clear goals and vision, the fiscal and political realities of creating a new program of this size are probably unsurmountable at present.

Option 3: Move NIDRR to Create ADRR

The overall problems of coordination, visibility, support, and monitoring of federal programs are too large to be resolved by adjustments to the NIDRR program alone (Option 1). Consolidation into a single agency (Option 2) is similarly unacceptable, although for different reasons. A middle-ground approach is proposed as Option 3. This option would (1) move NIDRR to DHHS creating an Agency on Disability and Rehabilitation Research (ADRR) within DHHS that would coordinate the various federal programs, (2) establish a small set-aside fund from the agencies involved in rehabilitation research to support the coordination effort and help ensure participation, and (3) elevate other programs within their respective agencies to enhance visibility.

The committee believes that the unique mission of NIDRR needs to be preserved because it is fundamentally important to the research agenda of rehabilitation science and engineering espoused by this committee. NIDRR has vigorously pursued this mission as best as possible within the constraints of its administrative location. Moving NIDRR from U.S. Department of Education to DHHS, however, would facilitate, if not require, the implementation of a new system for grant application, review, and management—a major benefit to improving the quality of research.

There are three initial advantages and benefits to be gained from moving NIDRR to DHHS. First of all, the move would be an opportunity to review the program's mission and personnel, and make appropriate changes to the program's structure. Secondly, it would move NIDRR closer administratively to NIH and CDC, which should facilitate coordination among the agencies. Finally, it would allow NIDRR to amend its peer review process. In an environment more conducive to research, NIDRR could establish larger, more permanent peer review panels. These larger panels would allow review of a more heterogeneous mix of applications, and allow for broader representation (including people with disabling conditions) on the review panels. With increased investment in peer review, staff could make more site visits, making the peer review process more rigorous, attracting high quality scientists interested in rehabilitation-related research. Standing committees would have more time for reviewing and need less time getting to know the process.

After carefully considering all three options, the committee arrived at the conclusions and recommendations that follow.

CONCLUSIONS AND RECOMMENDATIONS

The current organization and administration of federal programs that support research in rehabilitation science and engineering are such that each program has a unique, worthwhile, and complementary mission. CDC investigates prevention and secondary conditions, NSF and NCMRR research basic engineering and medical rehabilitation, respectively, NIDRR focuses on disability and the whole person in the environment, and VA is able to tailor its research agenda to the needs of its constituents. This represents a sound spectrum of rehabilitation research. In general, weaknesses in the spectrum are not due to inappropriate priorities or other problems within the programs themselves, but rather to a general insufficiency in the magnitude of the overall program of research, its limited visibility, and lack of effective coordination of the overall constellation of programs. Thus, correcting this situation will require additional research activities, greater visibility within the administrative structure, and improved coordination. Any potential reorganization or restructuring of the rehabilitation science and engineering activities of the federal government should be designed to achieve these objectives and also pass the test of implementability, with an eye towards long term, effective function for the foreseeable future.

Due consideration was given to a spectrum of options for improving the current situation and achieving the objectives of expanded research, enhanced visibility, and improved coordination. Of the many options considered, three of which are described above, Option 3 was determined to be the most reasonable, appropriate, and effective one for addressing the identified needs for improved coordination and enhanced visibility for federal research in rehabilitation science and engineering. The committee therefore recommends that this option be implemented as a means of enhancing the overall federal effort in rehabilitation research and improving the health, quality of life, and productivity of people with disabling conditions (see Recommendation 10.1 below).

RECOMMENDATION 10.1 The committee recommends that the NIDRR program of activities and its annual appropriation of approximately $70 million should be moved from the U.S. Department of Education to HHS and serve as the foundation for the creation of a new Agency on Disability and Rehabilitation Research (ADRR). ADRR would assume the tasks that were formerly assigned to the Interagency Committee on Disability Research (ICDR) and be given enhanced authority through review of disability and rehabilitation research plans and control of funding for interagency collaboration. To further support and enhance the overall federal effort, all major *programs in disability and rehabilitation research should be elevated within their respective agencies or departments.*

There would be immediate benefits to the improvement of the quality and coordination of rehabilitation-related research from an administrative relocation of NIDDR to HHS. Expanding the overall research effort, however, will require additional funding. Table 10-4 shows what an expanded research effort such as this might cost.

Move NIDRR to Create ADRR

The major purposes of moving NIDRR are threefold: first, to explant it administratively to a more nurturing and supportive environment; secondly, to raise the visibility of disability and rehabilitation research as important health issues; and lastly to serve more effectively as the core of an interagency coordinating body. In serving as the basis for a new agency, the move would provide an opportunity to develop a better coordinated federal effort with enhanced visibility and well-defined, complementary goals for the overall effort. Moving NIDRR to DHHS and elevating it to an agency-level program (ADRR) would correct many of the deficiencies and problems that have been described above, and improve the overall productivity of federal research in rehabilitation science and engineering.

Moving NIDRR out of the Department of Education is an important component of the recommended changes to improve the overall federal effort. As indicated by the GAO in 1989, the U.S. Department of Education has not provided adequate resources to the development of NIDRR (GAO, 1989), and seems unlikely to do so in the future. Such things as the lack of consistent announcement dates for grant competitions and ad hoc review panels with only a few members prevent or at best interfere with high-quality reviews. The constant change in peer reviewers does not allow applicants to receive constructive criticism from the review process or the opportunity to respond to the same reviewers. Hence, investigators are discouraged from applying.

Administrative locations other than DHHS were considered by the committee, but the most reasonable choice seemed to be within DHHS, at the level of the Administration on Aging. There is also an historic precedent in that the origins of NIDRR reside in the former U.S. Department of Health, Education, and Welfare. But more importantly, and among other reasons, being located in DHHS would facilitate cross-fertilization with other relevant programs and activities, such as the Administration on Aging, the Bureau of Maternal and Child Health, the Administration on Developmental Disabilities. Moving to DHHS, as opposed to creating an independent agency, would

TABLE 10-4 Major Federal Programs in Disability and Rehabilitation-Related Research Showing the Organization of the Proposed New ADRR in DHHS and Two Levels of Funding to Enhance the Overall Federal Effort

Agency	Current Funds	$100 Million of Additional Funds		$200 Million of Additional Funds	
		New Funds	New Totals	New Funds	New Totals
U.S. DEPARTMENT OF HEALTH AND HUMAN SERVICES					
Administration on Disability and Rehabilitation Research (new agency)					
I. Coordination-Linkage Division	$70*	$52.5	$123	$105	$175
	0	25	25	35	35
a. Interagency committee and subcommittee					
b. Multiple agency projects					
c. Rehabilitation resource support centers					
II. Disability and Rehabilitation Research Division	39	15	54	39	78
a. Rehabilitation research, including centers and field-initiated research of issues such as employment, education, personal assistance services, parenting, policy, independent living.					
b. Disability studies					
III. Engineering and Environmental Research Division	22	7	29	22	44
a. Assistive technology and engineering, including centers and field-initiated research					
b. Universal design, including mass transportation and Americans with Disabilities Act compliance					
IV. Training and Career Development Division	3	2.5	5.5	3	6
a. Allied health and engineering					
b. Services training					
c. Recruitment of scientists with disabling conditions					

V. Information Integration and Dissemination Division
  a. Information integration
  b. Dissemination
	6	3	9	6	12

National Institutes of Health (NCMRR)	$15	$11.3	$26	$23	$38
Thematic program projects for six priority areas					
Develop clinical trials of new therapies (not cures) that improve health status and reduce secondary conditions, and coordinate with that of ADRR Centers program					
Centers for Disease Control and Prevention	$9	$6.8	$16	$14	$23
Current programs					
Establish population-based studies of people with disabling conditions, their needs for services and assistive technologies, and the effects of changing national, state, and local policies on participation by people with disabilities in major life activities, including their health costs and demographics					
Establish population-based surveillance systems for monitoring the incidence and impact of secondary conditions					
Develop and evaluate community-based interventions to reduce the incidence and impact of secondary conditions and promote the independence and productivity of people with disabling conditions.					
Fund longitudinal studies on disability (e.g., National Health Interview Survey-Disability Supplement expanded)					
Fund the development of a common terminology for the field					
U.S. DEPARTMENT OF VETERAN AFFAIRS	$32	$24	$56	$48	$80
NATIONAL SCIENCE FOUNDATION	$7	$5.3	$12	$11	$18
TOTAL	$133	$100	$233	$200	$333

*Current NIDRR funding.

also obviate the need to create a large workforce to handle the support functions of personnel, purchasing, and legal and public affairs, all of which would already be available in the department. Moreover, other agencies within DHHS (e.g., NIH and CDC) already perform the majority of disability and rehabilitation-related research.

To enhance its coordinating authority, ADRR would review plans for research in the following year submitted by all agencies with significant efforts in rehabilitation science and engineering. Such an evaluative function would allow ADRR to help ensure quality in each agency's research, eliminate duplication, identify priorities, and sustain a national agenda. ADRR would also maintain a database of projects and activities. Special efforts should be directed to the development of a common database for rehabilitation science and engineering that would facilitate monitoring, coordination, and priority-setting among the programs.

Part of ADRR's support could come from a set-aside fund (e.g., one percent) from each of the major programs that support research in rehabilitation science and engineering. These funds would be used to enhance coordination and interagency participation, as well as collaborative research activities.

ADRR should be provided with the authority to award research grants, contracts, cooperative agreements, and research and development with a rehabilitation science or engineering focus. Eligible entities would include universities, rehabilitation facilities, nonprofit organizations, and for-profit corporations. ADRR should also have the authority to award supplemental research funds. All award announcements should have proposal receipt dates that coincide with those of NIH, which will permit applicants to plan their research activities better.

This committee recognizes the strengths of center grant research and recommends continued support by ADRR. The committee further recommends, however, that ADRR enhance field-initiated research projects, environmental modifications training for people with disabling conditions and their families, and training for health and engineering personnel. Finally, ADRR staff should be grounded in relevant fields of rehabilitation science and engineering. Sufficient staffing, salary, equipment, and expenses must be provided to permit fulfillment of the defined missions.

Preferably, ADRR would be organized in a manner that reflects the major substantive activities of the program: coordination of federal research efforts, research, education, and dissemination. This would facilitate the implementation of a mission that focuses on substantive, multidisciplinary activities as opposed to those of the separate, individual disciplines.

The following section describes the committee's view on some of the details of the organization of the new agency.

Organization of ADRR

ADRR would have five divisions that would address the following areas: coordination and linkage; rehabilitation and disability research; engineering and environmental research; training for researchers and people with disabilities; and integration of rehabilitation-related research, practice and technology information. The sections that follow discuss each of these in detail.

Coordination and Linkage Division The coordination activities of this division would take on the responsibilities of ICDR currently assigned to NIDRR, but the division would have increased authority to fund colloborative activities. If NIDDR is moved to DHHS to create ADRR, but no additional funding is provided (e.g., one percent set-aside from other agencies), then support would need to be drawn from other internal programs for this purpose.

Interagency Committee The budget for these activities would need to cover staff salary, database management, conferences, cross-agency staff training and interagency committee meetings. The interagency committee would be composed of rehabilitation experts outside government, representatives of the major government funding agencies, major foundations funding rehabilitation-related research, leaders of organizations that provide services to people with disabling conditions, and people with potentially disabling conditions who represent major constituencies.

Multiple-Agency Projects A second branch of this division would support linkage projects that cross the boundaries of the missions of the various agencies. The projects would be on designated topics recommended by the interagency committee. Each participating agency would be required to dedicate some funds to the projects. Foundations and for-profit companies would be encouraged to cofund projects. Funding for these linkage activities would provide incentives for government agencies to cooperate in planning directed research activities, reduce costs of recruiting separate populations for studies of the same condition at different times in the course of the condition, and allow for more detailed cross-environmental studies of similarities and differences in societal level problem solving. The activities ideally funded at a level of approximately $1 million, would be supported through an interagency transfer of funds to a designated lead agency that would be responsible for managing the award.

Rehabilitation Resource Support Centers A second type of linkage program would be funded through a third branch of this division of ADRR and would provide funds to meet deficits in the study of the person–environment interaction. There is a need to support rehabilitation-related research projects that involve community sites that have not been traditionally funded through government agencies (e.g., in the cultural settings of minority groups, rural communities, inner cities, and home and at work). Moving from a laboratory-based approach to one based in communities will require new approaches that have little current research support. By using a variety of human assistance resources and physical environmental modifications, such studies will provide answers to questions regarding the participation by people with disabling conditions in major life activities. The idea would be to empower people with disabling conditions by using results based on scientific studies of what optimal conditions are best for each of life's major activities. The funds for these activities would provide support for community-based, longitudinal studies. The funds would be awarded through a peer reviewed, competitive process that would be managed by ADRR staff.

Rehabilitation and Disability Research Division The research on disability and rehabilitation currently funded by NIDRR would continue to be funded, but it would be funded by ADRR and would be managed by ADRR staff. Initially, no currently funded activities would be terminated and currently funded activities would continue through the existing award period. The program would be divided into two broad branches: rehabilitation science and disability studies.

Rehabilitation Science The rehabilitation science branch could be organized by topic areas rather than by the type of funding mechanism (i.e., via centers and field-initiated research). The mechanisms used to fund these activities could include special-emphasis projects, centers of excellence in areas of rehabilitation (such as Model Spinal Cord Injury Centers), research program grants, research and demonstration projects, new investigator awards, small grant awards, minority investigator awards, and awards to people with disabling conditions. The mechanisms would support work in topic areas by using a variety of funding mechanisms that could be awarded to sites at various locations. Thus, this branch could have several sections for programming and managing topics including but not limited to engineering, health and fitness, employment, transportation, housing, independent living, community integration, personal assistant services, and policy. The current effort in investigator-initiated research, currently funded at a level of approximately $39 million, is inadequate to meet the expansion to an inclusive approach to rehabilitation and disability recommended by this committee. It should be a priority to increase this effort.

Disability Studies A significant portion of the funding for this division of ADRR would be apportioned to support the field of disability studies. The committee encourages the development and support for the examination of people with disabling conditions and cultural response through a variety of lenses, including but not limited to economics, political science, religion, law, history, architecture, urban planning, literature, and fine arts.

Engineering and Environmental Research Division The activities of this committee revealed a significant weakness in the overall research activities related to rehabilitation engineering and environmental modification. Notably, the lives of people with disabling conditions can be enhanced through environmental strategies, including assistive technology and universal design, among others.

Assistive Technology and Engineering Few resources are allocated to studying the development, deployment, and use of assistive technologies. The coordination of these resources is minimal. The major source of current research effort, Rehabilitation Engineering Research Centers, which are currently funded through NIDRR, would continue to be funded for the existing award period. Again, the topics for funding would provide the organizational structure for the ADRR rather than the funding mechanism (e.g., Rehabilitation Engineering Research Centers). The topics in this branch of ADRR would include robotics, orthotics, prosthetics, wheelchairs, communication devices, visual aids, and others.

Universal Design A second branch in this division would fund those projects that are directed at modifying the built environment and assessing the natural environment for access. This branch would fund studies of universal design, special needs environments, mass transit vehicles (e.g., lightrail, passenger trains, airplane seating, and buses) and the structural and product engineering aspects of technologies. The branch would foster a Framingham-type study for several site examinations of the influence of changes in environmental access and accommodation mandated by the Americans with Disabilities Act of 1990 and how they change the participation of people with potentially disabling conditions in major life activities.

Training and Career Development Division This division would focus on three different areas of training. Not only would it include traditional career development awards to attract scientists and engineers to rehabilitation science and engineering but it would also provide training to caregivers and would bring scientists and engineers with disabling conditions into the field of rehabilitation-related research.

Allied Health and Engineering This branch would provide funding for training in sciences and engineering necessary for conducting research in rehabilitation-related topics that are not covered by NIH training programs. Support would be provided for early career development, midcareer transition and later career special summary projects. Several areas of research that have received little support for training personnel to conduct research would be funded by this branch (see Chapter 9).

Services Training A second branch within this division would provide training funds for professional development for those who provide service to people with disabling conditions. These professions include but are not limited to Occupational Therapy, Physical Therapy, Psychology, Physical Medicine and Rehabilitation, rehabilitation nursing, orthotics, and prosthetics. Additional efforts should be made to expand this program to train personal assistance providers, urban planners, architects, environmental specialists, lawyers, tax consultants, and other professionals who are beginning to develop programs for enhancing the lives of people with potentially disabling conditions.

Recruitment of Scientists with Potentially Disabling Conditions The third branch of this division would provide funding for training people with potentially disabling conditions and their families in the skills needed to understand, conduct, and participate in research. The funds would be provided as training supplements to existing grants, targeted fellowships, specialized career development grants, and small grants to advocacy organizations for short-term training in understanding and using research findings.

Information Integration and Dissemination Division *Information Integration* A one-time contract would be awarded to integrate the existing literature databases and to develop links to and from existing databases (e.g., NARIC, ERIC, and MEDLINE). The award would be in the range of $1 million to $2 million. The information division staff would then maintain the system.

Dissemination Information dissemination activities would be managed through this division. This would include making existing data accessible to the public, and the information would include publications and material pertinent to disability issues, as well as the results of federally funded research projects and clinical practice guidelines.

Elevate Other Existing Programs

The fact that focal points for most the rehabilitation research currently reside at the lower administrative levels—that is, programs, divisions, and centers as opposed to institutes and departments—indicates that rehabilitation is not yet the priority that it should be across the federal government.

The general levels of research activities within each program are the primary barrier to adequate attention to the pressing issues in rehabilitation research. The priorities within each program, although in need of coordination, seem appropriate within their respective missions. The problem lies not in the particular rehabilitation programs but in the constraints and limited visibility that they experience within their respective agencies or departments. Increasing the capacity of one program or directing another program to focus on a specific problem is not the solution to the general needs of rehabilitation-related research. The necessary programs exist, but they must be elevated and funded to more appropriate levels, increasing the resources, visibility, and importance of rehabilitation across the agencies.

The committee believes that NCMRR, for example, should at least be a separate Center at NIH. As a free-standing center, NCMRR could form one or more special emphasis review committees managed by the Division of Research Grants, NIH. This approach would follow the standard NIH operation of separating DRG study sections from Institutes and allowing the science of the projects to be reviewed for funding consideration by several institutes. The special emphasis panels would have scientists with experience in rehabilitation-related topics, giving these types of applications a more favorable chance for funding than currently exists at NIH. The net result would improve the science and encourage more applications in the area of medical rehabilitation. NCMRR should also be given the ability to support multidisciplinary research centers. This would allow NCMRR to fund thematic program projects in areas such as mobility, psychosocial, multiple organ systems, assessment and measurement, treatment effectiveness, and use of assistive technology (specifically prosthetics). Additionally, NCMRR would be able to fund clinical trials for effectiveness of old and new treatments, multiple organ system studies, cross condition comparisons, longitudinal studies of the natural course, primary health care for long-term illness and disabling conditions, and managed care.

Similarly, the DPP should be elevated within the CDC, perhaps to the

CDC Directors' office level. Like minority health and women's health, disability and rehabilitation-related research is a cross-cutting area that transcends definition at the Center level. Placement within the CDC Director's office would afford rehabilitation science and engineering the visibility that it deserves and help to ensure that these issues would be integrated into all programmatic activities.

Summary

By moving NIDRR to create ADRR, the federal government would take a very important step in enhancing the productivity, relevance, and coordination of the programs which support rehabilitation research. Each of the current programs provides vital information for various communities of people with disabling conditions, but heightened visibility of the individual programs would enhance their effectiveness. By augmenting the current research efforts, strengthening the efforts in coordination, and magnifying visibility, federal research efforts should become more productive and relevant. The following chapter describes the committee's overarching recommendations for improving the field of rehabilitation science and engineering.

11

Overarching Recommendations and Priorities

The previous chapters have illustrated the large potential for improving the health, productivity, and quality of life for the 49 million Americans with disabling conditions. Significant savings in health care costs, lost wages, and reduced emotional costs may well be realized by enhancing research in rehabilitation science and engineering. With this in mind, three fundamental needs emerged from the committee's assessment of the content, quality, and adequacy of the research and knowledge base in rehabilitation science and engineering. The first is a need to more widely recognize and accept rehabilitation science and engineering as an academic and scientific field of study, the continued development of which should result in significant contributions to the field, and ultimately to consumers. The second is a need to focus on a set of priorities for research that will advance the field of study and improve the health, productivity, and quality of life for people with disabling conditions. And perhaps most importantly, the third is a need to enhance the federal effort in rehabilitation science and engineering by expanding research, raising visibility, and improving coordination.

Each of these needs is important to improving research and enhancing knowledge. Enhanced education and training in rehabilitation science and engineering as a distinct multidisciplinary field of study will result in higher quality researchers and research. Setting research priorities will help focus the limited amount of energy and funding, and enhancing federal efforts should improve both the quantity and effectiveness of current federal efforts.

Three overarching recommendations are presented below to address these needs.

RECOGNIZE THE FIELD OF STUDY

Rehabilitation draws from a wide variety of disciplines—it is truly a multidisciplinary activity. Rehabilitation science and engineering is the body of knowledge that exists at the confluence of these disciplines—drawing from, and contributing to each. The continued development of a common knowledge base in rehabilitation science and engineering will be important to future research that can benefit people with disabling conditions.

At this point in the evolution of the science there is a sufficient knowledge base and level of research to justify the recognition of a new field of study. Such recognition would facilitate accelerations in multidisciplinary education, training, and research, all of which would combine to advance the field of rehabilitation science and engineering and more effectively address the needs of people with disabling conditions. For these reasons, the first overarching recommendation focuses on establishing rehabilitation science and engineering as a recognized field of study, as follows.

Overarching Recommendation 1.   Rehabilitation science and engineering should be more widely recognized and accepted as an academic and scientific field of study. As such, the field should receive greater financial support, serve as the basis for developing new opportunities in multidisciplinary research and education, and ultimately improve the health and quality of life of people with disabling conditions. This new field should be consistent with the model of the enabling–disabling process that is defined and described in this report.

EMPHASIZE PRIORITIES

Several chapters of this report provide specific recommendations for future research in rehabilitation science and engineering. In addition, Appendix A contains suggested research priorities from various professional associations.

Many topics and areas require investigation, and identifying priorities is not simple. The process cannot be based on prevalence alone or simply on cost. Moreover, the entire field has critical ecumenical needs such as creating a common terminology and taxonomy, agreeing on a model, and quantifying functional limitations and disability. Because of this, setting specific priority research topics may not be as important for this committee as setting general priorities for the field.

Acknowledging the limited ability of any assembly of individuals to identify research priorities with great acuity or detail, the committee chose instead to describe general priorities that should be fundamentally important to any rehabilitation-related research and to the advancement of rehabilitation science and engineering as a whole. Thus, the second overarching recommendation focuses on establishing general priorities for rehabilitation science and engineering.

Overarching Recommendation 2. As the field of rehabilitation science and engineering continues to evolve and gain recognition as an academic and scientific field of study, there are three general priorities that will and should be of fundamental importance to its growth and to the ultimate improvement of health, productivity, and quality of life for people with disabling conditions: strengthen the science, focus on the enabling–disabling process, and transfer the technology. (See Box 11-1.)

Within the context of these priorities, resource distribution should somewhat favor activities that address the states of functional limitation and disability. This would help to correct a current imbalance to the basic science end of the spectrum. These priorities are appropriate and relevant for all federal agency programs that were reviewed by this committee.

ENHANCE THE FEDERAL EFFORT

In general, weaknesses in the current spectrum of federal programs in disability and rehabilitation research are not due to inappropriate priorities or other problems within the programs themselves, but rather to a general insufficiency in the magnitude of the overall program of research, its limited visibility, and a lack of effective coordination of the overall constellation of programs. Thus, the constellation of federal research programs in rehabilitation science and engineering needs to be reorganized and administered in a fashion that will improve interagency coordination, enhance visibility, and expand research for the purposes of improving the health, independence, productivity, and quality of life for people with disabling conditions.

As the largest federal program with a focus on disability and rehabilitation research, NIDRR's program was of major interest to the committee. The NIDRR mission and its constituency of people with disabling conditions are fundamentally important to the research agenda of rehabilitation science and engineering espoused by this committee. The committee concluded, however, that despite vigorous pursuit of its mission, NIDRR has been restricted in its ability to fully execute its mission primarily by virtue of its administrative position within the U.S. Department of Educa-

BOX 11-1
General Priorities for Rehabilitation Science and Engineering

As the field of rehabilitation science and engineering continues to evolve and gain recognition as an academic and scientific field of study, there are three general priorities that will and should be of fundamental importance to its growth and to the ultimate improvement of health, productivity, and quality of life for people with disabling conditions.

1. **Strengthen the science.** Develop and validate accurate tools for measuring and predicting functional limitations, disability, and outcomes.

2. **Focus on the enabling–disabling process.** Investigate critical factors in the physical, social, and psychological environments that can affect transitions in the enabling–disabling process over the lifecourse.

3. **Transfer the technology.** Develop and implement effective linkages between research and practice that will involve consumers, assure quality, and enhance service delivery.

tion, and the Interagency Committee on Disability Research's lack of real authority. An important example of the former is the need for improved peer review processes that are unobtainable in the present administrative location.

For the purpose of improving the overall federal effort and addressing the priorities described in the second overarching recommendation, the committee restates Recommendation 10.1 as the third overarching recommendation since its implementation has such broad potential impact and significance.

Overarching Recommendation 3. The committee recommends that the NIDRR program of activities and its annual appropriation of approximately $70 million should be moved from the U.S. Department of Education to DHHS and serve as the foundation for the creation of a new Agency on Disability and Rehabilitation Research (ADRR). ADRR would assume the tasks that were formerly assigned to the Interagency Committee on Disability Research and be given enhanced authority through review of disability and rehabilitation research plans and control of funding for interagency collaboration. To further support and enhance the overall federal effort, all major programs in disability and rehabilitation research should be elevated within their respective agencies or departments. (Recommendation 10.1)

In keeping with the committee's task of making recommendations within differing levels of fiscal expenditure, Chapter 10 presents guidance on how funds could be distributed in a configuration of programs

TABLE 11-1 Overarching Recommendations and General Priorities for Rehabilitation Science and Engineering

Overarching Recommendation	Individual Chapter Recommendation	Government Agency Involved
1. Recognize the Field of Study. Rehabilitation science and engineering should be more widely recognized and accepted as an academic and scientific field of study. As such, the field should receive greater financial support, serve as the basis for developing new opportunities in multidisciplinary research and education, and ultimately improve the health and quality of life of people with disabling conditions. This new field should be consistent with the model of the enabling–disabling process that is defined and described in this report.	7.3, 9.1, 9.2, 9.3	U.S. Department of Health and Human Services (DHHS,) National Science Foundation (NSF), U.S. Department of Education, U.S. Department of Veteran Affairs (VA)
2. Emphasize General Priorities. As the field of rehabilitation science and engineering continues to evolve and gain recognition as an academic and scientific field of study, there are three general priorities that will be of fundamental importance to its growth and to the ultimate improvement of health, productivity, and quality of life for people with disabling conditions.	2.1, 2.2, 3.1, 3.2, 4.3, 5.1, 5.4, 6.4, 7.1 (Item 1), 7.2, 7.4, 8.3, 8.4	DHHS, NSF, U.S. Department of Education, VA DHHS, NSF, U.S. Department of Education, VA
General Priorities **1. Strengthen the science.** Develop and validate accurate tools for measuring and predicting functional limitations, disability, and outcomes.	4.1, 4.2, 5.2, 5.3, 5.5, 5.6, 5.7 6.1, 6.2, 6.3, 7.1 (Items 2 and 3), 9.4	
2. Focus on the enabling–disabling process. Investigate critical factors in the physical, social, and psychological environments that can affect transitions in the enabling–disabling process over the lifecourse.	8.1, 8.2, 8.5, 8.6, 8.7, 8.8 10.1	
3. Transfer the technology. Develop and implement effective linkages between research and practice that will involve consumers, ensure quality, and enhance service delivery.		

TABLE 11-1 continued

Overarching Recommendation	Individual Chapter Recommendation	Government Agency Involved
3. Enhance the Federal Effort. The NIDRR program of activities and its annual appropriation of approximately $70 million should be moved from the U.S. Department of Education to DHHS and serve as the foundation for the creation of a new Agency on Disability and Rehabilitation Research (ADRR). ADRR would assume the tasks that were formerly assigned to the Interagency Committee on Disability Research and be given enhanced authority through review of disability and rehabilitation research plans and control of funding for interagency collaboration. To further support and enhance the overall federal effort, all major programs in disability and rehabilitation-related research should be elevated within their respective agencies or departments.	10.1	DHHS, NSF, U.S. Department of Education, VA

consistent with this committee's recommendations. Table 10-4 in Chapter 10 shows the present funding levels and two options for expanded programs of research at a cost of $100 and $200 million.

Finally, Table 11-1 shows the relationship of the three overarching recommendations and general priorities to each of the individual recommendations in the preceding chapters.

References

Affleck, G., S. Urrows, H. Tennen, and P. Higgins. 1992. Daily coping with pain from rheumatoid arthritis, patterns and correlates. Pain 51:221–229.

Agency for Health Care Policy and Research. 1996. Managing Acute and Chronic Urinary Incontinence. Clinical Practice Guideline Update. Agency for Health Care Policy and Research Publication No. 96-0686, p. 1. Rockville, M.D. Public Health Service, U.S. Department of Health and Human Services.

Aguayo, A. J., S. David, and G. M. Bray. 1981. Influences of the glial environment on the elongation of axons after injury: Transplantation studies in adult rodents. J Exp Biol 95:231–240.

Aguayo, A. J., M. Benfey, and S. David. 1983. A potential for axonal regeneration in neurons of the adult mammalian nervous system. Birth Defects 19:327–340.

Aguayo, A. J., G. M. Bray, M. Rasminsky, T. Zwimpfer, D. Carter, and M. Vida-Sanz. 1990. Synaptic connections made by axons regenerating in the central nervous system of adult mammals. J Exp Biol 153:199–224.

Albrecht, G. 1992. The Disability Business. Newbury Park, Calif.: Sage Publications.

Allen, G. S., H. S. Ahn, T. J. Preziosi, R. Battye, S. C. Boone, S. N. Chou, D.L. Kelly, B. K. Weir, R. A. Crabbe, P. K. Lavik, S. B. Rosenbloom, F. C. Dorsey, C. R. Ingram, D. E. Mellits, L. A. Bertsch, D. P. Boisvert, M. B. Hundley, R. K. Johnson, J. A. Strom, and C. R. Transou. 1983. Cerebral arterial spasm—A controlled trial of nimodipine in patients with subarachnoid hemorrhage. N Engl J Med 308:619–624.

Allender, J., and A. W. Kaszniak. 1989. Processing of emotional cues in patients with dementia of the Alzheimer's type. Int Neurosci 146(3–4):147–155.

American Medical Association, Committee on Medical Rating of Physical Impairment.1958. A guide to the evaluation of permanent impairment of the extremities and back. J Am Med Assoc 166:3–109.

Aten, J. 1988. Spastic dysarthria: Revising understanding of the disorder and speech treatment procedures. Head Trauma Rehabil 3:63–73.

Baker, E. R., D. D. Cardenas, and T. J. Benedetti. 1992. Risks associated with pregnancy in spinal cord-injured women. Obstet Gynecol 80:425–428.

Baker, S. P., and A. H. Harvey. 1985. Fall injuries in the elderly. Clin Geriatr Med 1:501–512.

Balliet, R., K. B. Harbst, D. Kim, and R. V. Stewart. 1987. Retraining of functional gait through the reduction of upper extremity weight-bearing in chronic cerebellar ataxia. Int Rehabil Med 8(4):148–153.

Bandura, A. 1977. Social Learning Theory. Englewood Cliffs, N.J.: Prentice-Hall.

Bandura, A. 1986. Social Foundations of Thought and Action: A Social Cognitive Theory. Englewood Cliffs, N.J.: Prentice-Hall.

Baredes, S. 1988. Surgical management of swallowing disorders. Otolaryngol Clin North Am 21:711.

Basso, M., M. Beattie, J. Bresnahan, et al. In press. Multicenter analysis of open field test locomotory scores: Role of experience, teamwork, and field conditions on reliability. J Neurotrauma.

Batavia, A. I., and G. DeJong. 1990. Developing a comprehensive health services research capacity in physical disability and rehabilitation. Disabil Policy Studies 1:37–61.

Batavia, A. I., and G. S. Hammer. 1990. Toward the Development of Consumer-Based Criteria for the Evaluation of Assistive Devices. Journal of Rehabilitation Research and Development 27(4) 425–436.

Batavia, A. I., G. DeJong, J. Scheer, R. Brannon, M. Meehan, D. Wilkerson, and N. Naierman. 1991. Developing a Comprehensive Health Services Research Capacity in Physical Disability and Rehabilitation. National Institute of Disability and Rehabilitation Research. Washington, D.C.: National Rehabilitation Hospital.

Bauman, W. A., and A. M. Spungen. 1994. Disorders of carbohydrate and lipid metabolism in veterans with paraplegia or quadriplegia: A model of premature aging. Metabolism 43:749–756.

Bellaire, K., K. M. Yorkston, and D. R. Beukelman. 1986. Modification of breath patterning to increase naturalness of a mildly dysarthric speaker. J Commun Disorders 19:271–280.

Benfey, M., and A. J. Aguayo. 1982. Extensive elongation of axons from rat brain into peripheral nerve grafts. Nature 296:150–152.

Benjamin, K. 1995. Outcomes research and the allied health professional. J Allied Health 24:3–12.

Bergner, M., R. A. Bobitt, W. B. Carter, and B. S. Gilson. 1985. The SIP: Development and final revision of a health status measure. Med Care 19:787–805.

Bigos, S. J., M. C. Battie, D. M. Spengler, L. D. Fisher, W. E. Fordyce, T. Hansson, A. L. Nachemson, and J. Zeh. 1992. A longitudinal, prospective study of industrial back injury reporting. Clin Orthopaed Related Res 279(June):21–34.

Blaese, R. M., K. W. Culver, A. D. Miller, C. S. Carter, T. Fleisher, M. Clerici, G. Shearer, L. Chang, Y. Chiang, P. Tolstoshev, et al. 1995. T lymphocyte-directed gene therapy for ADA-SCID: Initial trial results after 4 years. Science 270:475–477.

Bloodstein, O. 1987. Treatment Efficacy Summary. A Handbook on Stuttering, 4th ed. Chicago: National Easter Seal Society.

Boult, C., M. Altmann, D. Gilbertson, C. Yu, and R. L. Kane. 1996. Decreasing disability in the 21st century: The future effects of controlling 6 fatal and non-fatal conditions. Am J Pub Health 86:1388–1393.

Bracken, M. B., M. J. Shepard, W. F. Collins, Jr., T. R. Holford, W. Young, D.S. Baskin, H. M. Eisenberg, E. Flamm, L. Leo-Summers, J. C. Maroon, et al. 1990. A randomized controlled trial of methylprednisolone or naloxone in the treatment of acute spinal-cord injury: Results of the Second National Acute Spinal Cord Injury Study. N Engl J Med 322:1405–1411.

Bracken, M. B., M. J. Shepard, W. F. Collins, Jr., T. R. Holford, D.S. Baskin, H. M. Eisenberg, E. Flamm, L. Leo-Summers, J. C. Maroon, L. F. Marshall, et al. 1992. Methylprednisolone or naloxone treatment after acute spinal cord injury: 1-year follow-up data. Results of the Second National Acute Spinal Cord Injury Study. J Neurosurg 76:23–31.

Braddom, R. L. 1996. Physical Medicine and Rehabilitation. Philadelphia: Saunders.

Brain Injury Association. 1995. Fact sheet on traumatic brain injury. Washington, DC.

Brandenburg, S., and G. Vanderheiden. 1987. Communication, control and computer access for disabled and elderly individuals: Communication aids. Austin, Tex.: ProEd.

Brandt, T., S. Krafczyk, and I. Mahbenden. 1981. Postural imbalance with head extension: Improvement by training as a model for ataxia therapy. Ann NY Acad Sci 636–649.

Bregman, B. S., E. Kunkel-Bagden, L. Schnell, H. N. Dai, D. Gao, and M. E. Schwab. 1995. Recovery from spinal cord injury mediated by antibodies to neurite growth inhibitors. Nature 378:498–501.

Brillhart, B. 1988. Family support for the disabled. Rehabil Nursing 13:216.

Brooks, C. A., J. Lindstrom, J. McCray, and G. G. Whiteneck. 1995. Cost of medical care for a population-based sample of persons surviving traumatic brain injury. J Head Trauma Rehabil 10:1–13.

Brown, R. T., K. J. Doepke, and N. J. Kaslow. 1993. Risk resistance adaptation model for pediatric chronic illness: Sickle cell syndrome as an example. Clin Psychol Rev 13(2):119–132.

Buchner, D. M., and B. J. deLateur. 1991. The importance of skeletal muscle strength to physical function in older adults. Ann Behav Med 13:91–97.

Buckner, R. L., M. Corberea, J. Schatz, M. E. Raichle, and S. E. Petersen. 1996. Preserved speech abilities and compensation following prefrontal damage. Proc Natl Acad Sci USA 93:1249–1253.

Burns, T. J., A. I. Batavia, Q. W. Smith, and G. DeJong. 1990. Primary Health Care Needs of Persons with Physical Disabilities: What are the research and service priorities? Arch Phys Med Rehabil 71:138–143.

Cameron, D.C., and D. Guy. 1990. The design of a light weight mobile chair for use with video fluoroscopy in the investigation of swallow disorders. Australas Radiol 34:272.

Cardenas, D. D. 1992. Neurogenic Bladder: Evaluation and Management. In: Physical Medicine Rehabilitation Clinic of North America, William E. Straas, Jr. (ed) 3:751–763.

Cardenas, D. D., and T. M. Hooton. 1995. Urinary tract infection in persons with spinal cord injury. Arch Physical Med Rehabil 76:272–280.

Cardenas, D. D., and M. E. Mayo. 1995. Lower urinary changes over time in suprasacral spinal cord injury. Paraplegia 33(6):326–329.

Carey, T. S., J. Garrett, J. Jackman, C. McLaughlin, J. Fryer, and D. R. Smucker. 1995. The outcomes and costs of care for acute low back pain among patients seen by primary care practitioners, chiropractors, and orthopedic surgeons. N Engl J Med 333:913–917.

Caroni, P., and M. E. Schwab. 1988a. Antibody against myelin-associated inhibitor of neurite growth neutralizes nonpermissive substrate properties of CNS white matter. Neuron 1:85–96.

Caroni, P., and M. E. Schwab. 1988b. Two membrane protein fractions from rat central myelin with inhibitory properties for neurite growth and fibroblast spreading. J Cell Biol 106:1281–1288.

Caroni, P., T. Savio, and M. E. Schwab. 1988. Central nervous system regeneration: Oligodendrocytes and myelin as non-permissive substrates for neurite growth. Prog Brain Res 78:363–370.

Center for the Evaluative Clinical Sciences, Dartmouth Medical School. 1996. Dartmouth Atlas of Health Care. 1996. Chicago: American Hospital Publishing.

Charlifue, S. W. 1993. Research into the aging process, pp. 9–12. In: Aging with Spinal Cord Injury, G. G. Whiteneck et al., eds. New York: Demos Publications.

Cheng, H., Y. Cao, and L. Olson. 1996. Spinal cord repair in adult paraplegic rats: Partial restoration of hind limb function. Science 273(5274):510–513.

Chirikos, T. N. 1989. Aggregate economic losses from disability in the United States: A preliminary assay. Milbank Q 67(2):59–91.

Choi, D. W. 1992. Excitotoxic cell death. J Neurobiol 23:1261–1276.

Clark, N. M., and W. Rakowski. 1983. Family caregivers of older adults: Improving helping skills. Gerontologist 23:627–642.

Conture, E. G. 1995. Treatment Efficacy Summary: Stuttering. Rockville, Md.: American Speech-Language-Hearing Association.

Conture, E., and B. Guitar. 1993. Evaluating efficacy of treatment of stuttering: School-age children. J Fluency Disorders 18:253–287.

Cope, D. N., and J. O'Lear. 1993. A clinical and economic perspective on head injury rehabilitation. J Head Trauma Rehab 8:1–14.

Corbet, B. 1990. A disabled person looks at aging, pp. 47–56. In: Aging and Rehabilitation II: The state of the practice, S. J. Brody and L. G. Pawlson, eds. New York: Springer.

Corcoran, M. A., and L. N. Gitlin. 1997. The role of the physical environment in occupational performance. In: Occupational Therapy: Enhancing Performance and Well-Being, C. Christiansen and C. Baum, eds. Thorofare, N.J.: Slack, Inc.

Cronbach, L., and R. Snow. 1977. Aptitudes and Instructional Methods. New York: Irvington.

Croog, S. H., A. Lipson, and A. Levine. 1989. Help patterns in severe illness: The roles of kin network, non-family resources, and institutions. J Marriage Fam (February):32–41.

Darley, F. L., A. E. Aronson, and J. E. Brown. 1969a. Differential diagnostic patterns of dysarthria. J Speech Hearing Res 12:246–269.

Darley, F. L., A. E. Aronson, and J. E. Brown. 1969b. Clusters of deviant speech dimensions in the dysarthrias. J Speech Hearing Res 12:462–496.

David, S., and A. J. Aguayo. 1981. Axonal elongation into peripheral nervous system "bridges" after central nervous system injury in adult rats. Science 214:931–933.

DeAngelis, G. C., I. Ohzawa, and R. D. Freeman. 1991. Depth is encoded in the visual cortex by a specialized receptive field structure. Nature 352:6331.

DeJong, G. 1979. Independent living: From social movement to analytic paradigm. Physical Med Rehabil 60:435–446.

DeJong, G., and J. P. Sutton. 1994. Rehab 2000: The evolution of medical rehabilitation in American health care. Washington, D.C.: National Rehabilitation Hospital.

DeJong, G., A. I. Batavia, Q. W. Smith, T. J. Burns, J. Scheer, R. Brannon, N. Naierman, and D. Butler. 1989. Meeting the Primary Health Care Needs of Persons with Physical Disabilities: Setting the Agenda. Washington, D.C.: National Rehabilitation Hospital.

DeJong, G., B. Wheatley, and J. Sutton. 1996. Perspective and analysis: Medical rehabilitation undergoing major shakeup in advanced managed care markets. Bureau of National Affairs Inc. 2:138–141.

DeLisa, J. A., G. M. Martin, and D. M. Currie. 1993. Rehabilitation medicine: Past, present, and future. In: Rehabilitation Medicine: Principles and Practice, J. A. DeLisa and B. Gans, eds. Philadelphia: J. B. Lippincott Co.

DePippo, K. L., M. A. Holas, and M. J. Reding. 1992. Validation of the 3-oz water swallow test for aspiration following stroke. Arch Neurol 49:1259.

Dietrich, W. D. 1992. The importance of brain temperature in cerebral injury. J Neurotrauma 2:S475–S485.

Dole, R. 1995. Senate Report 103-318. Washington D.C.: U.S. Senate.

Donaldson, S. K., and D. M. Crowley. 1978. The discipline of nursing. Nursing Outlook 26:113–120.

Duchek, J. 1991. Cognitive dimensions of performance, pp. 284–303. In: Occupational Therapy: Overcoming Human Performance Deficits, C. Christiansen and C. Baum, eds. Thorofare, N.J.: Slack, Inc.

Dunkel-Schetter C., L. G. Feinstein, S. E. Taylor, and R. L. Falke. 1992. Patterns of coping with cancer. Health Psychol 11(2):79–87.

Easton, D. F., D. T. Bishop, D. Ford, G. P. Crockford and the Breast Cancer Linkage Consortium. 1993. Genetic linage analysis in familial breast and ovarian cancer: Results from 214 families. Am J Human Genetics 52:678–701.

Eisenberg, M. G. 1995. Dictionary of Rehabilitation. New York: Springer.

Ellwood, P. M. 1988. Shattuck lecture. Outcomes management: A technology of patient experience. N Engl J Med 318(23):1549–1556.

Epstein, A. M. 1990. Sounding Board: The outcome movement—Will it get us where we want to go? N Engl J Med 323(4):266–270.

Eppley, Z. A., J. Kim, and B. Russell. 1993. A myogenic regulatory factor, $qmf1$, is expressed by adult myonuclei after injury. Am J Physiol:Cell 265:C397–C405.

Eslinger, P. J., and A. R. Damasio. 1986. Preserved motor learning in Alzheimer's disease: Implications for anatomy and behavior. Neuroscience 6(10):3006–3009.

Evans, R. L., R. D. Hendricks, R. T. Connis, J. K. Haselkorn, K. R. Ries, and T. E. Mennet. 1994. Quality of life after spinal cord injury: A literature critique and meta-analysis (1983–1992). J Am Parapleg Soc 17:60–66.

Fawcett, S. B. 1991. Social validity: A note on methodology. J Appl Behav Anal 24:235–239.

Fawcett, S. B., A. L. Paine, V. T. Francisco, and M. Vliet, M. 1993. Promoting health through community development, pp. 233–255. In: Promoting Health and Mental Health in Children, Youth, and Families, D. S. Glenwick and L. A. Jason, eds. New York: Springer.

Fawcett, S. B., G. W. White, F. E. Balcazar, Y. Suarez-Balcazar, R. M. Mathews, A. L. Paine, T. Seekins, and J. F. Smith. 1994. A contextual-behavioral model of empowerment: Case studies with people with disabilities. Am J Community Psychol 22:471–496.

Fiatarone, M.A., E. C. Marks, N. D. Ryan, C. N. Meredith, L. A. Lipsitz, and W. J. Evans. 1990. High intensity strength training in nonagenarians. J Am Med Assoc 263:3029–3034.

Flint, R. 1975. Philosophy as Scientia Scientarium and a History of the Classification of the Sciences. New York: Arno Press.

Fordyce, W. E. 1995. Back Pain in the Workplace: Management of Disability in Nonspecific Conditions. Seattle, Wash.: International Association for the Study of Pain Press.

Fougeyrollas, P. 1997. The social environment as external determinants of social participation of people with disabilities. In: Occupational Therapy: Enhancing Function and Well-Being, 2nd ed., C. Christiansen and C. Baum, eds. Thorofare, N.J.: Slack, Inc.

Fougeyrollas, P., and D. Gray. 1996. ICIDH, Handicap and Environmental Factors and Social Change: The Importance of Technology.

Foundation for Health Services Research. 1991. Conference Proceedings: Developing a Research Agenda for Outcomes and Effectiveness Research. Washington, D.C.: Foundation for Health Services.

Foundation for Physical Therapy. 1994. A Commitment to Research. Fairfax, Va.: Foundation for Physical Therapy Research.

Fowler, F. J., ed. 1989. Health Survey Research Methods: Conference Proceedings. DHHS Publication No. 89-3447. Rockville, Md.: National Center for Health Service Research.

Frith, C., and U. Frith. 1996. A biological marker for dyslexia. Nature 382:19–20.

Fuhrer, M. J. 1988. Rehabilitation Research in the 1980s. In: Advances in Clinical Rehabilitation, Vol. II, M. D. Eisenberg and R. C. Grzesiak, eds. New York: Springer.

Gates, G. A., W. Ryan, J. C. Cooper, et al. 1982. Current status of laryngectomy rehabilitation. I. Results of therapy. Am J Otolaryngol 3:1–7.

Gates, P. E. 1995. Think globally, act locally: An approach to implementation of clinical practice guidelines. J Qual Improve 21:71–85.

Geertz, C. 1973. The Interpretation of Cultures. New York: Basic Books, Inc.

Geertz, C. 1983. Local Knowledge: Further Essays in Interpretive Anthropology. New York: Basic Books, Inc.

Gehlsen, G. M., and M. H. Whaley. 1990. Falls in the elderly. Part II. Balance, strength, and flexibility. Arch Physical Med Rehabil 71:739–741.

Geirut, J. 1995. Treatment Efficacy Summary: Phonological Disorders in Children. Rockville, Md.: American Speech-Language-Hearing Association.

Gerhart, K. A., E. Bergstrom, S. W. Charlifue, R. R. Menter, and G. G. Whiteneck. 1993. Long-term spinal cord injury: Functional changes over time. Arch Physical Med Rehabil 74:1030–1034.

Gerratt, B. R., J. A. Till, J. C. Rosenbek, R. T. Wertz, and A. E. Boysen. 1991. Use and perceived value of perceptual and instrumental measures in dysarthria management, pp. 77–94. In: Dysarthria and Apraxis of Speech: Perspectives on Management. C. A. Moore, K. M. Yorkston, and D. R. Beukelman, eds. Baltimore, Md.: Paul H. Brookes.

Gleason, J. B., ed. 1985. The Development of Language, (2nd ed.) Columbus, Ohio: Merill Publishing.

Gonzalez, J., and A. Aronson. 1970. Palatal lift prosthesis for treatment of anatomic and neurologic palatopharyngeal insufficiency. Cleft Palate J 7:91–104.

Gordon, D. L., K. J. Sawin, and S. M. Basta. 1996. Developing research priorities for rehabilitation nursing. Rehabiliation Nursing Research 5(2):6–66.

Grady, M. L., ed. 1992. Medical Effectiveness Research Data Methods. AHCPR Publication No. 92-0056, Rockville, Md.: Agency for Health Care Policy and Research.

Graham, I. 1996. I believe therefore I practice (letter). Lancet 347:4–5.

Graitcer, P. L., and F. M. Maynard, eds. 1990. Preventing Secondary Disabilities Among People with Spinal Cord Injuries. Atlanta, Ga.: Centers for Disease Control.

Granger, C. V., G. L. Albrecht, and B. B. Hamilton. 1979. Outcome of comprehensive medical rehabilitation: Measurement by Pulses Profile and Barthel Index. Arch Phys Med Rehabil 60:145–154.

Gray, C., S. Sivaloganathan, and K. C. Simpkins. 1989. Aspiration of high-density barium contrast medium causing acute pulmonary inflamation—report of two fatal cases in elderly women with disordered swallowing. Clin Radiol 40:397.

Gray, D. 1996. Understanding spousal relations. Unpublished manuscript. Program in Occupational Therapy, Washington University, St. Louis, Mo.

Gresham, G. E., P. W. Duncan, W. B. Stason, et al. 1995. Post-Stroke Rehabilitation. Clinical Practice Guideline No. 16. AHCPR Publication 95-0662. Rockville, Md.: Agency for Health Care Policy and Research.

Griffiths, D. J., P. N. McCracken, G. M. Harrison, and K. N. Moore. 1996. Urge incontinence in elderly people: Factors predicting the severity of urine loss before and after pharmacological treatment. Neurorol-Urodyn 15(1):53–57.

Grisé, M. C. L., C. Gauthier-Gagnon, and C. G. Martineau. 1993. Prosthetic profile of people with lower extremity amputation: Conception and design of a follow-up questionnaire. Arch Phys Med Rehabil 74:862–870.

Groce, N. 1985. Everyone Here Spoke Sign Language: Hereditary Deafness on Martha's Vineyard. Cambridge, Mass.: Harvard University Press.

Gunsburg, A. P., D. W. Evans, R. Sekuler, and S. A. Harp. 1982. Contrast sensitivity predicts pilots' performance in aircraft simulators. Am J Optom Physiol Optics 59:105–108.

Guralick, J. M. 1994. Understanding the relationship between disease and disability. J Am Geriatr Soc 42:1128–1129.

Hadorn, D. C. 1992. The problem of discrimination in health care priority setting. J Am Med Assoc 268:1454–1459.

Hagen, K. B., K. Harms-Ringdahl, and J. Hallen. 1994. Influence of lifting technique on perceptual and cardiovascular responses to submaximal repetitive lifting. Eur J Appl Physiol 68:477–482.

Hahn, H. 1985. Disability policy and the problem of discrimination. American Behaviorial Scientist 28:293–318.

Hahn, H. 1988. Can disability be beautiful? Social Policy 18(Winter):26–32.

Haley, R. W., D. H. Culver, J. W. White, and W. M. Morgan. 1985. The nationwide nosocomial infection rate: A new need for vital statistics. Am Epidemiol 121:159–167.

Hall, J. M., M. K. Lee, B. Newman, J. E. Morrow, L. A. Anderson, B. Huey, and M. C. King. 1990. Linkage of early-onset familial breast cancer to chromosone 17q21. Science 250:1684–1689.

Hanson, S., S. P. Buckelew, J. Hewett, and G. O'Neal. 1993. The relationship between coping and adjustment after spinal cord injury: A 5-year follow-up study. Rehabil Psychol 38(1):41–52.

Harada, N., G. Kominski, and S. Sofaer. 1993. Development of a classification system for rehabilitation. Inquiry 30:54–63.

Harding, J. 1994. Cookbook medicine. Physician Executive 20:3–6.

Harvey, C., Wilson, S. E., Greene, C. G., Berkowitz, M., and Stripling, T. E. 1992. New estimates of the direct costs of traumatic spinal cord injuries: Results of a nationwide survey. Paraplegia 30:834–850.

Hayward, S. A., M. C. Wilson, S. R. Tunis, et al. 1995. Users' guides to the medical literature. VII. How to use clinical practice guidelines. A. Are the recommendations valid? J Am Med Assoc 274:570–574.

Health Policy Alternatives, Inc. 1996. Health care and market reform: Workforce implications for OT: Executive summary. OT Week 10(17):A2–A4.

Hegde, M. N. 1995. Introduction to Communicative Disorders. Austin, Tex.: Pro-Ed.

Heitmann, D. K., M. R. Gossman, S. A. Shaddeau, and J. R. Jackson. 1989. Balance performance and step width in noninstitutionalized, elderly, female fallers and nonfallers. Phys Ther 69:923–931.

Heinemann, A. W., J. M. Linacre, B. D. Wright, B. B. Hamilton, and C. Granger. 1994. Prediction of rehabilitation outcomes with disability measures. Arch Phys Med Rehabil 75:133–143.

Henneman, E., C. Somjjn, and D. Carpenter. 1965a. Functional significance of cell size in spinal motor neurons. J Neurophysiol 28:561–580.

Henneman, E., C. Somjjn, and D. Carpenter. 1965b. Excitability and inhibility of motor neurons of difference sizes. J Neurophysiol 28:599–620.

Hill, M. A. 1991. The economics of disability. Pp. 209–227 in S. Thompson-Hoffman and I. F. Storck, Eds., Disability in the United States: A portrait from national data. New York: Springer.

Hillel, A. D., R. M. Miller, K. M. Yorkston, E. McDonald, F. H. Norris, and N. Konikow. 1989. ALS severity scale. J Neuroepidemiol 88:142–150.

Holt, S., S. D. Miron, M. C. Diaz, et al. 1990 Scintigraphic measurement of oropharyngeal transit in man. Dig Dis Sci 35:1198.

Hopkins, H. 1988. An historical perspective on occupational therapy. In: Willard and Spackman's Occupational Therapy, H. L. Hopkins and H. D. Smith, eds. Philadelphia: J. B. Lippincott.

Hopp, J. F. 1993. Effects of age and resistance training on skeletal muscle: A review. Phys Ther 73:361–373.

Horner, J., E. W. Massey, and S. R. Brazer. 1990. Aspiration in bilateral stroke patients. Neurology 40:1686.

Hunt, L. A., A. A. Sadun, and C. J. Bassi. 1995. Review of the visual system in Parkinson's disease. Optom Vision Sci 72:92–99.

Institute of Medicine. 1990. Clinical Practice Guidelines. Washington, D.C.: National Academy Press.

Institute of Medicine. 1991. Disability in America: A National Agenda for Prevention. A. M. Pope and A.R. Tarlov, eds. Washington, D.C.: National Academy Press.

Institute of Medicine. 1993. Access to Health Care in America. M. Millman, ed. Washington, D.C.: National Academy Press.

Institute of Medicine. 1996. Primary Care: America's Health in a New Era. Washington, D.C.: National Academy Press.

Jackson, S., J. Donavan, S. Brookes, S. Eckford, L. Swithinbank, and P. Abrams. 1996. The Bristol Female Lower Urinary Tract Symptoms Questionnaire: Development and psychometric testing. Br J Urol 77(6):805–812.

Jarama, S. L. 1996. A model of psychosocial adjustment to disability among African Americans. Ph. D. dissertation. Department of Psychology, The George Washington University, Washington, D.C.

Jette, A. M. 1995. Outcomes research: Shifting the dominant research paradigm in physical therapy. Phys Ther 75:965–970.

Jette, A. M., A. R. Davies, P. D. Cleary, D. R. Calkins, L. V. Rubenstein, A. Fink, J. Kosecoff, R. T. Young, R. H. Brook, and T. L. Delbanco. 1986. The functional status questionnaire: Reliability and validity when used in primary care. J Gen Intern Med 1(3):143–149.

Johnson, E. R., S. W. McKenzie, C. J. Rosenquist, et al. 1992. Dysphagia following stroke: Quantitative evaluation of pharyngeal transit times. Arch Phys Med Rehabil 73:419.

Judge, J. O., C. Lindsey, M. Underwood, and D. Winsemius. 1993a. Balance improvements in older women: Effects of exercise training. Phys Ther 73:254–265.

Judge, J. O., M. Underwood, and T. Gennosa. 1993b. Exercise to improve gait velocity in older persons. Arch Phys Med Rehabil 74:400–406.

Kaluzny, A. D., T. R. Konrad, and C. P. McLaughlin. 1995. Organizational strategies for implementing clinical Guidelines. J Qual Improve 21:347–351.

Kaplan, R. M., J. B. Anderson, A. W. Wu, W. C. Mathers, F. Kozin, and D. Orenstein. 1989. The quality of well-being scale: Applications in AIDS, cystic fibrosis and arthritis. Medical Care 27(3):S27–S43.

Kasper, C.E. and L. Xun. 1996. Cytoplasm-to-myonucleus ratios in plantaris and soleus muscle fibers following hindlimb suspension. J Muscle Res and Cell Motility 17:1–8.

Kasper, C.E., T.P. White, and L.C. Maxwell. 1990. Running during recovery from hypodynamia induces transient muscle injury. J Appl Physiol 68(2):533–539.

Katz, J., ed. 1994. Handbook of Clinical Audiology, 4th ed. Baltimore, Md.: Williams & Wilkins.

Keith, R. A., C. V. Granger, B. B. Hamilton, and F. S. Sherwin. 1987. The functional independence measure: A new tool for rehabilitation, pp. 6–18 In: Advances in Clinical Rehabilitation, Volume I, M. G. Eisenberg, ed. New York: Springer.

Keith, A. R., D. B. Wilson, and P. Gutierrez. 1995. Acute and subacute rehabilitation for stroke: A comparison. Arch Phys Med Rehabil 78:495–500.

Keller, E., P. Vigneuz, and M. Lafamboise. 1991. Acoustic analysis of neurologically impaired speech. Br J Disord Commun 26:75–94.

Kelley, W. N., and M. A. Randolph. 1994. Careers in Clinical Research: Obstacles and Opportunities. Washington, D.C.: National Academy Press.

Kleinke, C. L. 1991. How chronic pain patients cope with depression: Relation to treatment outcome in a multidisciplinary pain clinic. Rehabil Psychol 36:669–685.

Klopsteg, P. E., and P. E. Wilson. 1954. Human Limbs and Their Substitutes. Washington, D.C.: National Research Council.

Knox, M., and T. R. Parmenter. 1993. Social networks and support mechanisms for people with mild intellectual disability in competitive employment. Int J Rehabil 16:1–12.

Koos, E. 1954. The Health of Regionville. New York: Columbia University Press.

Kottke. F. J., and M. E. Knapp. 1988. The development of physiatry before 1950. Arch Phys Med Rehabil 69:4–14.

Krause, J. S., and N. M. Crewe. 1991. Chronologic age, time since injury, and time of measurement: Effect on adjustment after spinal cord injury. Arch Phys Med Rehabil 72:91–100.

Krebs, D. E. 1982. Relationship of tourniquet time to postoperative quadriceps femoris muscle function. Phys Ther 62:670–672.

Krebs, D. E. 1989. Isokinetic, electrophysiologic and clinical function relationships following tourniquet-aided arthrotomy. Phys Ther 69:803–815.

Krebs, D. E. 1995. Interpretation standards in locomotor studies, pp. 334–354. In: Gait Analysis: Theory and Application, R. L. Craick and C. Oatis, eds. New York: C. V. Mosby.

Krebs, D. E., and S. Fishman. 1984. Characteristics of the child amputee population. J Pediatr Orthoped 4:89–95.

Krebs, D. E., and J. Lockert. 1995. Vestibulopathy and gait, pp. 93–116. In: Evaluation and Management of Gait Disorders, B. S. Spivack, ed. New York: Marcel Dekker.

Krebs, D. E., S. R. Harris, S. O. Herdman, and E. Michels. 1986. Theory in physical therapy (guest editorial). Phys Ther 66:661–662.

Krebs, D. E., D. K. Wong, D. S. Jevsevar, P. O. Riley, and W. A. Hodge. 1992. Trunk kinematics during locomotor activities. Phys Ther 72:505–514.

Kuhn, T. 1962. The Structure of Scientific Revolutions. Chicago: University of Chicago Press.

Kuhn, T. 1979. Metaphor in science, pp. 409–419. In: Metaphor and Thought, A. Ortony, ed. Cambridge, United Kingdom: Cambridge University Press.

Kunin, C. M. 1994. Urinary tract infections in females. Clin Infect Dis 18:1–12.

Lammertse, D. P., and G. M. Yarkony. 1991. Rehabilitation in spinal cord disorders. Outcomes and issues of aging after spinal cord injury. Arch Phys Med Rehabil 72:S309–S311.

Lancer, J. M., D. Syder, A. S. Jones, and A. Le Boutillier. 1988. The outcome of different management patterns for vocal cord nodules. J Laryngol Otol 102:423–427.

Landgraf, J. M., L. Abetz, and J. E. Ware. 1996. Child Health Questionnaire (CHQ): A user's manual. Boston, Mass.: The Health Institute, New England Medical Center.

Langmore, S. E., K. Schatz, N. Olson. 1991. Endoscopic and videofluoroscopic evaluations of swallowing and aspiration. Ann Otol Rhinol Laryngol 100:678.

LaPlante, M., and D. Carlson. 1995. Disability in the United States: Prevalence and Causes. 1992. Report of the Disability Statistics Rehabilitation Research and Training Center. National Institute on Disability and Rehabilitation Research. Washington, D.C.

LaPlante, M., and D. Carlson. 1996. Disability in the United States: Prevalence and causes, 1992. Disability Statistics Report (7). Washington, D.C.: National Institute on Disability and Rehabilitation Research, U.S. Department of Education.

Law, M., B. Cooper, S. Strong, D. Stewart, P. Rigby, and L. Letts. 1996. The person-environment-occupation model: A transactive approach to occupational performance. Can J Occup Ther 63:9–23.

Lazarus, R. S., and S. Folkman. 1984. Stress, Appraisal and Coping. New York: Springer.

Lehmkuhl, L. D., Hall, K. M., Mann, N., and Gordon, W. A. 1993. Factors that influence costs and length of stay of persons with traumatic brain injury in acute care and inpatient rehabilitation. J Head Trauma Rehabil 8:88–100.

Lewin-VHI, Inc. 1995. Subacute Care: Policy Synthesis and Market Area Analysis. Report to the Office of the Assistant Secretary for Planning and Evaluation. Washington, D.C.: U.S. Department of Health and Human Services.

Lindgren, S., and O. Ekberg. 1990. Cricopharyngeal myotomy in the treatment of dysphagia. Clin Otolaryngol 15:221.

Littell, E. 1989. Neurological training and retraining. In: Physical Therapy. R. M. Scully and M. R. Barnes, eds. New York: J. B. Lippincott Company.

Livingstone, M. S., and D. H. Hubel. 1987. Psychophysical evidence for separate channels for the perception of form, color, movement, and depth. J Neurosci 7:3416–3468.

Logemann, J. A. 1983. Evaluation and Treatment of Swallowing Disorders. San Diego: College Hill Press.

Logemann, J. 1995. Treatment Efficacy Summary: Oropharyngeal Dysphagia (Difficulty in Swallowing). Rockville, Md.: American Speech-Language-Hearing Association.

Lohr, K. N. 1995. Guidelines for clinical practice: What they are and why they count. J Law Med Ethics 23(1):49–56.

Lollar, D. J. 1994. Preventing Secondary Conditions Associated with Spina Bifida or Cerebral Palsy: Proceedings and Recommendations of a Symposium. Washington, D.C.: Spina Bifida Association of America.

Lord, S. R., G. A. Caplan, and J. A. Ward. 1993. Balance, reaction time, and muscle strength in exercising and nonexercising older women: A pilot study. Arch Phys Med Rehabil 74:837–839.

Lubeck, D., and E. Yelin. 1988. A Question of Value: Measuring the Impact of Chronic Disease. Milbank Quarterly 66(3):444–464.

Luepongsak, N., D. E. Krebs, E. Olsson, P. O. Riley, and R. W. Mann. In press. Hip stress during lifting with bent and straight knees. Scand J Rehabil Med.

MacKenzie, E. J., A. Damiano, T. Miller, and S. Luchter. 1996. The development of the Functional Capacity Index. Journal of Trauma 41(5):799–807.

Maddux, J. 1996. Self-Efficacy, Adaptation and Adjustment. New York: Plenum.

Mahoney, F. I., and D. W. Barthel. 1965. Functional Evaluation: The Barthel Index. Maryland State Med J 14:61–65.

Maklan, C. W., R. Greene, and M. A. Cummings. 1994. Methodological challenges and innovations in patient outcomes research. Medical Care 32(7):S13–S21.

Marge, M. 1988. Health promotion for persons with disabilities: Moving beyond rehabilitation. Am J Pub Health 2(4):29–35.

Martin, B. J., M. M. Corlew, H. Wood, et al. 1994. The association of swallowing dysfunction and aspiration pneumonia. Dysphagia 9:1.

Max, W., MacKenzie, E. J., and Rice, D. P. 1991. Head injuries: Costs and consequences. Journal of Head Trauma Rehabilitation 6:76–91.

Mayer, N. H., D. J. Keating, and D. Rapp. 1986. Skills, routines, and activity patterns of daily living: A functional nested approach, pp. 205–222. In: Clinical neuropsychology of intervention, B. Uzzell and Y. Gross, eds. Boston: Martinus Nijhoff.

Maynard, F. M. 1986. The Late Effects of Polio Create a Large Demand for Rehabilitation. Rehabilitation Report. Feb:2–3.

Maynard, F. M., M. Julius, N. Kirsch, R. Lampman, C. Peterson, D. Tate, W. Waring, and R. Werner. 1991. The Late Effects of Polio: A Model for Identification and Assessment of Preventable Secondary Disabilities: Final Report. Centers for Disease Control.

McDowell, B. J., S. J. Engberg, E. Rodriguez, and S. Sereika. 1996. Characteristics of urinary incontinence in homebound older adults. J Am Geriatr Soc 44(8):963–968.

McIntosh, T. K. 1992. Pharmacologic strategies in the treatment of experimental brain injury. J Neurotrauma 1:S201–S209.

McNeil, J. M. 1993. Americans with disabilities: 1991–1992. Current Population reports, Household Economic Studies P70-33. Washington, D.C.: U.S. Bureau of the Census.

Merzenich, M. M., C. Schreiner, W. Jenkins, and X. Wang. 1993. Neural mechanisms underlying temporal integration, segmentation, and input sequence representation: Some implications for the origin of learning disabilities. Ann NY Acad Sci 682:1–22.

Meyers, A. R., and R. Masters. 1989. Managed care for high risk populations. Journal of Aging and Social Policy. 1.

Miller, J. M., C. Kasper, and C. Sampselle. 1994. Review of muscle physiology with applications to pelvic muscle exercise. Urol Nurs 14:92–97.

Miller, R. M., M. E. Groher, K. M. Yorkston, and T. S. Rees. 1993. Speech, language, swallowing, and auditory rehabilitation. *In*: Rehabilitation Medicine: Principles and Practice, J. A. DeLisa and B. Gans, eds. Philadelphia, Pa.: J. B. Lippincott Co.

Moore, L. 1996. Job tests spell compo end for some. New Zealand Herald, p. A1.

Morey, M. C., P. A. Cowper, J. R. Feussner, R. C. DiPasquale, G. M. Crowley, D. W. Kitzman, and R. J. Sullivan, Jr. 1989. Evaluation of a supervised exercise program in a geriatric population. J Am Geriatr Soc 37:348–354.

Morgan, M. H. 1975. Ataxia and weights. Physiotherapy 61(11):332–334.

Morris, S. E. 1989. Development of oral-motor skills in the neurologically impaired child receiving non-oral feedings. Dysphagia 3:135.

Morton, R. E., R. Bonas, B. Fourie, et al. 1993. Videofluroscopy in the assessment of feeding disorders of children with neurological problems. Dev Med Child Neurol 35:388.

Nagi, S. 1976. An epidemiology of disability among adults in the United States. Milbank Memorial Fund Q 54:439–468.

Nagi, S. Z. 1965. Some conceptual issues in disability and rehabilitation. *In*: Sociology and Rehabilitation, M. B. Sussman, ed. Washington, D.C.: American Sociological Association.

National Center for Medical Rehabilitation Research. 1993. Research Plan for the National Center for Medical Rehabilitation Research. Washington, D.C.: National Institutes of Health.

National Council on Disability. 1993. A Disability Perspective on Access to Health Insurance and Health Related Services: A Report to the President and the Congress. Washington, D.C.: National Council on Disability.

National Spinal Cord Statistical Center. 1996. Spinal cord injury facts and figures. Birmingham, Ala.: Author.

Netsell, R., 1973. Speech physiology. *In*: F. D. Minifie, T. J. Hixon, and F. Williams, eds. Normal aspects of speech, hearing, and language. Englewood Cliffs, N.J.: Prentice-Hall.

Netsell, R., and B. Daniel. 1979. Dysarthria in adults: Physiologic approach to rehabilitation. Arch Phys Med Rehabil 60:502–508.

Netsell, R., and T. J. Hixon. 1978. A noninvasive method of clinically estimating subglottal air pressure. J Speech Hearing Dis 43:326–350.

Netsell, R., W. K. Lotz, and S. M. Barlow. 1989. A speech physiology examination for individuals with dysarthria, pp. 3–38. *In*: Recent Advances in Clinical Dysarthria, K. M. Yorkston and D. R. Beukelman, eds. Austin, Tex.: ProEd.

Newby, H. A., and G. R. Popelka. 1992. Audiology, (6th ed.) Englewood Cliffs, N.J.: Prentice-Hall.

Nockels, R., and W. Young. 1992. Pharmacologic strategies in the treatment of experimental spinal cord injury. J Neurotrauma 9(Suppl. 1):S211–S217.

Noll, S. F., C. E. Bender, and M. C. Nelson. 1996. Rehabilitation of patients with swallowing disorders, pp. 533–534. *In*: R. L. Braddom, ed. Physical Medicine and Rehabilitation. Philadelphia, Pa.: W.B. Saunders.

Norris, V. K., M. A. Stephens, and J. K. Kinney. 1990. The impact of family interactions on recovery from stroke: Help or hindrance? Gerontologist 30(4):535.

Northern, J. L., and M. P. Downs. 1991. Hearing in Children, 4th ed. Baltimore, Md.: Williams & Wilkins.

Nosek, M. A. 1993. Personal assistance: Its effect on the long-term health of a rehabilitation hospital population. Arch Phys Med Rehabil 74:127–132.

Ohry, A., Y. Shemesh, and R. Rozin. 1983. Are chronic spinal cord injured patients (SCIP) prone to premature aging? Med Hypoth 11:467–469.

Overstall, P. W., A. N. Exton-Smith, F. J. Imms, and A. L. Jonson. 1977. Falls in the elderly related to postural imbalance. Br Med J 1:261–264.

Parker, C. W. 1995. Practice guidelines and private insurers. J Law Med Ethics 23:57–61.

Patrick, D. L., and P. Erickson. 1993. Health Status and Health Policy: Quality of Life in Health Care Evaluation and Resource Allocation. Oxford, United Kingdom: Oxford University Press.

Patrick, D. L., M. Richardson, H. E. Satarks, and M. A. Rose. 1994. A framework for promoting the health of people with disabilities. In: Preventing Secondary Conditions Associated with Spina Bifida or Cerebral Palsy: Proceedings and Recommendations of a Symposium, D. J. Lollar, ed. Washington, D.C.: Spina Bifida Association of America.

Pentland, W. E., and L. T. Twomey. 1994. Upper limb function in persons with long term paraplegia and implications for independence. Part I. Paraplegia.

Pentland, B., P. Jones, C. Roy, and J. Miller. 1986. Head injury in the elderly. Age Aging 15:193–202.

Pew Commission. 1991. Healthy America: Practitioners for 2005. San Francisco: Pew Commission.

Pocock, S. O. 1987. Clinical Trials: A Practical Approach. New York: John Wiley & Sons.

Prigatano, G. P., and I. M. Altman. 1990. Impaired awareness of behavioral limitations after traumatic brain injury. Arch Phys Med Rehabil 71:1058–1064.

Rall, L.C., and R. Roubenoff. 1996. Body composition, metabolism and resistance exercise in patients with rheumatoid arthritis. Arthritis Care Res 9(2):151–156.

Ramig, L. 1992. The role of phonation in speech intelligibility: A review and preliminary data from patient with Parkinson's disease, pp. 119–156. In: Intelligibility in Speech Disorders: Theory, Measurement and Management, R. D. Kent, ed. Amsterdam, The Netherlands: John Benjamins.

Ramig, L. O. 1995. Treatment Efficacy Summary: Laryngeal-based Voice Disorders. Rockville, Md.: American Speech-Language-Hearing Association.

Rasley, A., J. A. Logemann, P. J. Kahrilas, et al. 1993. Prevention of barium aspiration during videofluoroscopic swallowing studies: Value of change in posture. Am J Roentgenol 160:1005.

Ratzka, A. 1986. Independent Living and Attendant Care in Sweden: A Consumer Perspective. New York: World Rehabilitation Fund, Inc., 75–78.

Relman, A. S. 1988. Assessment and accountability: The third revolution in medical care. N Engl J Med 319:1220–1222.

Resnick, B., D. Slocum, I. Ra, and P. Moffett. 1996. Geriatric rehabilitation: Nursing interventions and outcomes focusing on urinary function and knowledge of medications. Rehabil Nurs 21(3):142–147.

Revenson, T. A., and B. J. Felton. 1989. Disability and coping as predictors of psychological adjustment to rheumatoid arthritis. J Consult Clin Psychol 57:344–348.

Rice, D., and B. Cooper. 1967. The Economic Value of Human Life. Am J Pub Health 57:1954–1956.

Richardson, D. A., K. L. Miller, S. W. Siegel, M. M. Karram, N. B. Blackwood, and D. R. Staskin. 1996. Pelvic floor electircal stimulation: A comparison of daily and every-other-day therapy for genuine stress incontinence. Urology 48(1):110–118.

Rogers, E. M. 1983. Diffusion of Innovations, 3rd ed. The Free Press.

Rosenbek, J. C., and L. L. LaPoint. 1985. The dysarthrias: Description, diagnosis and treatment, pp. 97–152. In: Clinical Management of Neurogenic Communication Disorders, D. F. Johns, ed. Austin, Tex.: ProEd.

Rothstein, J. M. 1992. Who owns an idea? (editorial). Phys Ther 72:481–482.

Rubin, R. T. 1996. HMOs and AHCs—In defense of town and gown (editorial). Science 273:1153.

Russell, L. B., M. R. Gold, J. E. Siegel, N. Daniels, and M. C. Weinstein. 1996. The role of cost-effectiveness analysis in health and medicine. J Am Med Assoc 276(14):1172–1177.

Sacks, A. H., M. Le Blanc, and D. L. Jaffe. 1994. 1994 Rehabilitation R&D Center Progress Report. Palo Alto, Calif.: U.S. Department of Veterans Affairs.

Sage, G. H. 1984. Motor Learning and Control: A Neuropsychological Approach. Dubuque, Iowa: W. C. Brown.

Sauerbruch, F. 1916. An effective artificial hand. Literary Digest 53:452.

Schaefer, S. D., and D. F. Johns. 1982. Attaining functional esophageal speech. Arch Otolaryngol 108:647–649.

Scheier, M. F., K. A. Matthews, J. Owens, G. J. Magovern, Sr., R. C. Lefebvre, R. A. Abbott, and C. S. Carver. 1989. Dispositional optimism and recovery from coronary artery bypass surgery: The beneficial effects on physical and psychological well-being. J Personality Social Psychol 57:1024–1040.

Schima, W., G. Stacher, P. Pokieser, et al. 1992. Esphageal motor disorders: Videofluoroscopic and manometric evaluation—prospective study in 88 symptomatic patients. Radiology 185:487.

Schipplein, O. D., J. H. Trafimow, G. B. Andersson, and T. P. Andriacchi. 1990. Relationship between moments at the L5/S1 level, hip and knee joints when lifting. J Biomechanics 23(9):907–912.

Schulz, K. F., I. Chalmers, D. A. Grimes, and D. G. Altman. 1994. Assessing the quality randomization from reports of controlled trials published in obstetrics and gynecology journals. J Am Med Assoc 272:125–128.

Schulz, K. F., I. Chalmers, R. J. Hayes, and D. G. Altman. 1995. Empirical evidence of bias. Dimensions of methodological quality associated with estimates of treatment effects in controlled trials. J Am Med Assoc 273:408–412.

Schultz, R., and S. Decker. 1985. Long-term adjustment to physical disability: The role of social support, perceived control, and self-blame. J Personality Social Psychol 48:1162.

Schwab, J., ed. 1964. Structure of the disciplines: Meanings and significances. In: The Structure of Knowledge and Curriculum, G. W. Ford and L. Pugno, eds. Chicago: Rand McNally.

Schwab, M. E., and P. Caroni. 1988. Oligodendrocytes and CNS myelin are nonpermissive substrates for neurite growth and fibroblast spreading in vitro. J Neurosci 8:2381–2393.

Sechrest, L., E. Perrin, and J. Bunker, eds. 1990. Research Methodology: Strengthening Causal Interpretations of Nonexperimental Data. AHCPR Publication No. 90-3454. Rockville, Md.: Agency for Health Care Policy and Research.

Seelman, K. 1996. Presentation to IOM Committee on Assessing Rehabilitation Science and Engineering. February 1, Washington, D.C.

Selker, L. G. 1994. Clinical research in allied health. J Allied Health 23:201–228.

Serlin, R. 1987. Hypothesis testing, theory building, and philosophy of science. J Counseling Psychol 34:365–371.

Silagy, C., and T. Lancaster. 1995. The Cochrane collaboration in primary care: An international resource for evidence-based practice of family medicine. Fam Med 275:302–305.

Silver, K. H., D. Van Nostrand, K. V. Kuhlemeier, et al. 1991. Scintigraphy for the detection and quantification of subglottic aspiration: Preliminary observations. Arch Phys Med Rehabil 72:902.

Singer, M. I., and E. D. Blom. 1980. An endoscopic technique for restoration of voice after laryngectomy. Ann Otol Rhinol Laryngol 89:529–533.

Singer, M. I., E. D. Blom, and R. C. Hamaker. 1981. Further experience with voice restoration after total laryngectomy. Ann Otol Rhinol Laryngol 90:498–502.

Sitzmann, J. V. 1990. Nutritional support of the dysphagic patient: Methods, risks, and complications of therapy. J Parenteral Enteral Nutr 14:60.

Smitheran, J., and T. J. Hixon. 1981. A clinical method for estimating laryngeal airway resistance during vowel production. J Speech Hearing Dis 46:138–146.

Sommers, R. 1992. A review and critical analysis of treatment research related to articulation and phonological disorders. J Commun Disorders 25:3–22.

Splaingard, M. L., B. Hutchins, L. D. Sulton, et al. 1988. Aspiration in rehabilitation patients: Videofluoroscopy vs. Bedside clinical assessment. Arch Phys Med Rehabil 69:637.

Steinwachs, D. 1991. Health services research: Its scope and significance. Am J Pharm Ed 55:274–278.

Stewart, M. W., and R. G. Knight. 1991. Coping strategies and affect in rheumatoid and psoriatic arthritis: Relationship to pain and disability. Arthritis Care Res 4(3):116–122.

Stineman, M. G. 1995. Casemix measurement in medical rehabilitation. Arch Phys Med Rehabil 76(12):1163–1170.

Stineman, M. G., J. J. Escarce, J. E. Goin, B. B. Hamilton, C. V. Granger, and S. V. Williams. 1994. A case-mix classification system for medical rehabilitation. Medical Care 32(4): 366–379.

Stuss, D. T. 1992. Biological and psychological development of executive functions. Brain Cognition 20:8–23.

Sudarsky, L. 1990. Geriatrics: Gait disorders in the elderly. N Engl J Med 322:1441–1446.

Sullivan, E. V., H. J. Sagar, J. D. Gabrieli, S. Corkin, and J. H. Growdon. 1989. Different cognitive profiles on standard behavioral tests in Parkinson's disease and Alzheimer's disease. J Clin Exp Neuropsychol 11:799–820.

Talbot, L. A., and M. Cox. 1995. Differences in coping strategies among community-residing older adults with functional urinary continence, dysfunctional urinary continence and actual urinary incontinence. Ostomy-Wound-Manage 41(10):30–32, 34–37.

Taubes, G. 1996. Looking for the evidence in medicine: News and comment. Science 272:22–24.

Taylor, S. E., V. S. Helgeson, G. M. Reed, and L. A. Skokan. 1991. Self-generated feelings of control and adjustment to physical illness. J Soc Issues 47(4):91–109.

Teasell, R. W., H. M. Finston, and L. Greene-Finestone L. 1993. Dysphagia and nutrition following stroke. Phys Med Rehabil 7:89.

Thompson, M. 1984. Feasibility of Willingness-to-pay Measurement In Chronic Arthritis. Medical Decision Making 4:195–215.

Thompson, M., J. Read, and M. Liang. 1982. Willingness-to-pay Concepts for Societal Decisions in Health. In: Values and Long-term Care. R. Kane and R. Kane, eds. Lexington, Mass.: D.C. Heath.

Thompson, R. F., D. M. Crist, M. Marsh, and M. Rosenthal. 1988. Effects of physical exercise for elderly patients with physical impairments. J Am Geriatr Soc 36:130–135.

Tinetti, M. E., and S. F. Ginter. 1988. Identifying mobility dysfunctions in elderly patients: Standard examination or direct assessment? J Am Med Assoc 259:1190–1193.

Toal, S. B., R. L. Burt, and E. C. Tomlinson, eds. 1993. Proceedings of the National Conference on the Prevention of Primary and Secondary Disabilities. Centers for Disease Control and Prevention, U.S. Department of Health and Human Services. Atlanta, Ga.: Centers for Disease Control and Prevention.

Troup, J. D. G. 1965. Relation of lumbar spine disorders to heavy manual work and lifting. Lancet 1:857–861.

Trupin, L., and D. P. Rice. 1996. Health Status, Medical Care Use, and Number of Disabling Conditions in the United States. Disability Statistics Abstract 9:1–4.

Trupin, L., D. Rice, and W. Max. 1996. Medical Expenditures for People with Disabilities in the United States, 1987. Disability Statistics Report 5, National Institute on Disability and Rehabilitation Research.

Turk, M. A., R. J. Weber, M. Pavin, C. A. Geremski, and C. Brown. 1995. Medical secondary conditions among adults with cerebral palsy. Arch Phys Med Rehabil 76:1055.

Turk, M. A., R. J. Weber, C. A. Geremski, C. Brown, and S. Segore. 1996. Pain complaints in adults with cerebral palsy. Arch Phys Med Rehabil 77:940.

Umlauf, M. G., S. Goode, and K. L. Burgio. 1996. Psychological issues in geriatric urology: Problems in treatment and treatment seeking. Urol Clin North Am 23(1):127:136.

Urbscheit, N. L. 1990. Cerebellar dysfunction, pp. 597–618. In: Neurological Rehabilitation, 2nd ed. D. A. Umphred, ed. St. Louis, Mo.: C. V. Mosby.

U.S. Bureau of the Census. 1995. Statistical Abstract of the United States: 1995 (115th edition). Washington D.C.: U.S. Bureau of the Census.

U.S. Bureau of the Census. 1989. Labor force status and other characteristics of persons with a work disability: 1981 to 1988. Current Population Reports, Series P-23, No. 160. Washington, D.C.: U.S. Department of Commerce.

U.S. Department of Health and Human Services. 1995. Managed Care for People with Disabilities: Developing a Research Agenda. Washington, D.C.: U.S. Department of Health and Human Services.

U.S. General Accounting Office. 1989. Department of Education: Management of Office of Special Education and Rehabilitative Services. Washington, D.C.: U.S. Government Printing Office.

U.S. Preventive Task Force. 1989. Guide to Clinical Preventive Services: An Assessment of the Effectiveness of 169 Interventions. Baltimore, Md.: Williams & Wilkins.

Vasudevan, S. V. 1992. Impairment, disability and functional capacity assessment. In: Handbook of Pain Assessment, D. C. Turk and R. Melzack, eds. New York: Guilford Press.

Verbrugge, L. M. 1994. The disability supplement to the 1994–95 National Health Interview Survey (NHIS-Disability). (Available from the Division of Health Interview Statistics, National Center for Health Statistics, Hyattsville, MD 20782).

Wagner, T. H., D. L. Patrick, T. G. Bavendam, M. L. Martin, and D. P. Buesching. 1996. Quality of life of persons with urinary incontinence: Development of a new measure. Urology 47(1):67–71.

Wallerstein, N. 1992. Powerlessness, empowerment, and health: Implications for health promotion programs. Am J Health Promotion 6(3):197–205.

Ware, J. E. 1995. The status of health assessment 1994. Annu Rev Public Health 16:327–354.

Ware, J. E., and C. D. Sherbourne. 1992. The MOS 36-Item Short-Form Health Survey (SF-36). Med Care 30:473–483.

Ware, J. E., M. S. Bayliss, W. H. Rogers, M. Kosinski, and A. R. Tarlov. 1996. Differences in 4-year health outcomes for elderly and poor, chronically ill patients treated in HMO and fee-for-service systems. J Am Med Assoc 276:1039–1047.

Weiner, J. P., and G. de Lissovoy. 1993. Razing a Tower of Babel: A taxonomy for managed care and health insurance plans. Journal of Health Politics, Policy, and Law 18(1):75–103.

Wenger, B. L., H. S. Kaye, and M. LaPlante. 1996. Disability Among Children. Disability Statistics Abstract 15:23.

Wetmore, S. J., K. Krueger, K. Wesson, and M. L. Blessing. 1985. Long-term results of the Blom-Singer speech rehabilitation procedure. Arch Otolaryngol 111:106–109.

White, G. W., A. L. Paine-Andrews, R. M. Mathews, and S. B. Fawcett. 1995. Home access modifications: Their effects on community visits of people with physical disabilities. J Appl Behav Anal 28:457–463.

White, G. W., T. Seekins, and R. T. Gutierrez. 1996. Preventing and managing secondary conditions: A proposed role for independent living centers. J Rehabil July, August, September, 14–21.

Whiteneck, G. G., S. W. Charlifue, K. A. Gerhart, D. P. Lammertse, S. Manley, R. R. Menter, and K. R. Seedroff. 1993. Aging with Spinal Cord Injury. New York: Demos.

Whiteneck, G. G., M. A. Charlifue, M. B. Frankel, M. H. Fraser, B. P. Gardner, K. A. Gerhart, D. Krishnan, R. Menter, I. Nuseibeh, D. J. Short, and J. R. Silver. 1992. Mortality, morbidity, and psychosocial outcomes of persons spinal cord injured more than 20 years ago. Paraplegia 30:617–630.

Whyte, W. F., ed. 1991. Participatory Action Research. Newbury Park, Calif.: Sage Publications.

Wiechers, D. O. 1985. Acute and latent effects of poliomyelitis on the motor unit as revealed by electromyography. Orthopedics 8:870–872.

Wilkerson, D. L., A. I. Batavia, and G. DeJong. 1992. Use of functional status measures for payment of medical rehabilitation services. Arch Phys Med Rehabil 73:111–120.

Williams, R. 1994. Increasing Access to Personal Assistance: Americans with Disabilities' insurance policy for staying healthy, well and productive. In: Preventing Secondary Conditions Associated with Spina Bifida or Cerebral Palsy: Proceedings and Recommendations of a Symposium, D. J. Lollar, ed. Washington, D.C.: Spina Bifida Association of America.

Wilson, I. B., and P. D. Cleary. 1995. Linking clinical variables with health-related quality of life: A conceptual model of patient outcomes. J Am Med Assoc 273(1):59–65.

Winstein, C. J. 1983. Neurogenic dysphagia: Frequency, progression and outcome in adults following head injury. Phys Ther 63:1992.

Winter, D. A., A. E. Patla, J. S. Frank, and S. E. Walt. 1990. Biomechanical walking pattern changes in the fit and healthy elderly. Phys Ther 70:340–347.

Wolk, S., and T. Blair. 1994. Trends in medical rehabilitation. Reston, Va.: American Rehabilitation Association.

Woolf, S. H. 1990. Practice guidelines: A new reality in medicine. I. Recent developments. Arch Intern Med 150:1811–1818.

Woolf, S. H. 1993. Practice Guidelines: A new reality in medicine. III. Impact on patient care. Arch Intern Med 153:2646–2655.

World Health Organization. 1980. International Classification of Impairments, Disabilities, and Handicaps: A Manual of Classification Relating to the Consequences of Disease. Geneva, Switzerland: World Health Organization.

Yelin, E. 1989. The social context of the work-disability problem. Milbank Q 67:114.

Yelin, E. 1992. Disability and the Displaced Worker. National Institute of Child Health and Human Development. New Brunswick, N.J.: Rutgers University Press.

Yelin, E., and P. Katz. 1994. Making work more central to work disability policy. Milbank Q 72(4):593–619.

Yorkston, K. M. 1995. Treatment Efficacy Summary: Dysarthria (Neurological Motor Speech Impairment). Rockville, Md.: American Speech-Language-Hearing Association.

Yorkston, K. M., and D. R. Beukelman. 1981. Assessment of Intelligibility of Dysarthric Speech. Tigard, Oreg.: C. C. Publications.

Yorkston, K. M., and D. R. Beukelman. 1991. Motor speech disorders, pp. 251–316. In: Communication Disorders Following Traumatic Brain Injury: Management of Cognitive, Language, and Motor Impairment, D. R. Beukelman and K. M. Yorkston, eds. Austin, Tex.: ProEd.

Yorkston, K. M., D. R. Beukelman, and C. D. Traynor. 1984. Computerized Assessment of Intelligibility of Dysarthric Speech. Tigard, Oreg.: C. C. Publications.

Yorkston, K. M., V. L. Hammen, D. R. Beukelman, and C. D. Traynor. 1990. The effect of rate control on the intelligibility and naturalness of dysarthric speech. J Speech Hearing Dis 55:550–561.

Young, L. D. 1992. Psychological factors in rheumatoid arthritis. J Consult Clin Psychol 60:619–627.

Zautra, A. J., and S. L. Manne. 1992. Coping with rheumatoid arthritis: A review of a decade of research. Ann Behav Med 14:31–39.

Zborowski, M. 1952. Cultural Components in Responses to Pain. J Social Issues 8(4):16–30.

Zea, M. C., F. Z. Belgrave, T. Townsend, S. L. Jarama, and S. P. Barks. In press. The influence of social support and active coping on depression among African Americans and Latinos with disabilities. Rehab Psychol.

Zeki, S. 1993. A Vision of the Brain. Oxford, United Kingdom: Blackwell Scientific Publications.

Zola, I. 1966. Culture and symptoms—An analysis of patients presenting complaints. Am Sociol Rev 31:615–630.

Appendixes

A

Data Collection and Analysis

In an effort to be comprehensive in addressing the committee's overarching task of assessing the current status of rehabilitation science and engineering and developing recommendations for future needs in the field, the committee pursued several avenues of data collection and analysis. In addition to what might be the obvious, that is, reviewing federally funded research in the field, the committee also explored many other sources in a concerted attempt to cast a broad net for the collection and assessment of information. These sources included discussions with federal agency representatives, a variety of presentations at committee meetings, focus groups with consumers and professional associations, surveys of private and public organizations, and commissioned papers. A summary description of these follows.

REVIEW OF REHABILITATION RESEARCH ABSTRACTS

As part of the charge to this committee to assess and evaluate federal rehabilitation research programs and make recommendations for future research, the committee collected, reviewed, and analyzed research abstracts from the major agency programs in rehabilitation research. The general purposes were to (1) assess the current status of research, (2) identify research needs and gaps, and (3) provide an objective basis for the committee's consideration in the development of recommendations for future research. More specifically, the committee was interested in the following questions (among others):

1. How much research is clearly related to rehabilitation according to the committee's definition of rehabilitation as the "process" of movement in the enabling/disabling process?

2. How much rehabilitation-related research is being done in the various categories of pathology, impairment, functional limitation, and disability?

3. What are the common study designs and experimental subjects?

4. What are the major areas of research emphasis for each federal agency? Do the areas of research emphasis complement each other?

5. How much rehabilitation-related research focuses on factors such as: environmental factors, policy issues, developing assistive technology, secondary conditions, quality of life, and health outcomes.

The remainder of this section describes the process that the committee used in collecting, reviewing, and analyzing the abstracts, a summary of the results of the analysis, and a discussion of some of the problems encountered as part of the process.

Sources and Numbers of Abstracts

Abstracts of rehabilitation-related research activities were obtained for fiscal year 1995 from the following agencies for review (numbers in parentheses indicate how many abstracts were received):

- Centers for Disease Control and Prevention (CDC) (17)
- National Institutes of Health (NIH) (1,480)
- Agency on Health Care Policy and Research (AHCPR) (12)
- National Science Foundation (NSF) (124)
- National Institute for Disability and Rehabilitation Research (NIDRR) (288)
- U.S. Department of Veterans Affairs (VA) (176)

Of the 17 abstracts provided by CDC, 12 were from the Disability Prevention Program 2 were from National Center for Injury Prevention and Control, and 3 were from the National Institute on Occupational Safety and Health. The 124 abstracts from NSF were from its Bioengineering and Environmental Systems Division. The 288 NIDRR abstracts were obtained from its Annual Program Directory for fiscal year 1995. All of the VA abstracts were from the Rehabilitation Research and Development Program—although other rehabilitation-related research is apparently conducted by VA, abstracts were not obtainable for review. The 1,894 NIH abstracts were obtained from two different sources. The first set (973 abstracts) was provided in response to a committee request to the director

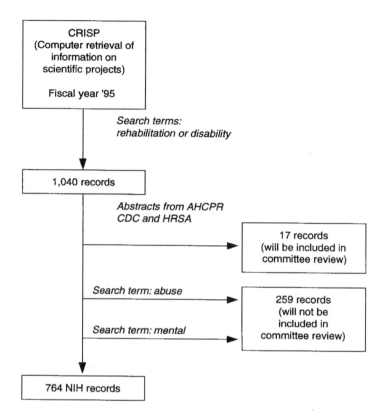

FIGURE A-1 PHS research in rehabilitation: process for identifying, retrieving, and reviewing rehabilitation related abstracts.

of NIH.[1] The second set (764 abstracts, 257 of which corresponded with abstracts identified by the Institutes) was retrieved from the Computer Retrieval of Information on Scientific Projects (CRISP) database on CD ROM for fiscal year 1995. The CRISP database is an online computer-based system that contains information on funded extramural and intramural research in the Public Health Service. CRISP was also the source for the abstracts from AHCPR that were reviewed. Finally, the committee received one abstract from the Health Resources and Services Administration and three abstracts from the Office of Disability, Aging, and Long Term Care within the Office of the Assistant Secretary for Planning and Evaluation. Figure A-1 describes the process that the committee followed in identifying and retrieving abstracts from CRISP.

---

[1]NIH was asked to provide the committee with abstracts from each of the institutes at NIH, along with their respective definitions of rehabilitation-related research.

In general, the keywords "rehabilitation" and "disability" were used and the keywords "mental health" and "substance abuse" were excluded. Through the Medical Rehabilitation Coordinating Committee, the various NIH institutes submitted their definitions of rehabilitation research and a listing of all the rehabilitation or rehabilitation-related research that was funded in fiscal year 1995.

Review and Analysis of Abstracts

The committee performed a pilot examination of the abstracts using a form that it created to assess whether certain types of information would be available for review and analysis. The form included six major sections (see Box A-1), each with a subset of several variables for evaluation. The results of the pilot study indicated that the varied quality and limited amount of information in the abstracts were inadequate to address many of the committee's questions and the review needed to be reduced in scope.

Following the pilot review and in accord with the limited amount of information available in the abstracts, the abstract review process was scaled back to address only the first three sections (see Box A-1). All abstracts from the federal agencies were then reviewed by a subcommittee and staff, and classified according to rehabilitation relevance, rehabilitation state addressed, and experimental subject.

The intent of these three categories is to provide a succinct summary of the rehabilitation science and engineering research that is funded by the federal government, the extent to which the research projects identified by the agencies fulfill this committee's definition of rehabilitation science, and whether the work involved human subjects, animals, tissue culture, synthetic materials, or computer models. In this way, the committee could assess the current range, trends, and general priorities in the field of federally funded research in rehabilitation science and engineering. The operational definitions for the different categorizations are described below.

BOX A-1
Major Sections of the Abstract Review Form

1. Relevance to rehabilitation science and engineering
2. Rehabilitation states
3. Experimental subjects
4. Targeted population and condition
5. Study design
6. Other descriptors

TABLE A-1 Rehabilitation Relevance Classification

Category	Description of Research
Rehabilitation science	Research that addresses the transition between states of the enabling–disabling process (i.e., pathology, impairment, functional limitation, and disability)
Rehabilitation engineering	Research that emphasizes the development of devices or other technology applicable to the enabling–disabling model states
Drug or alcohol abuse and mental health	Research that addresses rehabilitation of drug and alcohol abuse; mental health studies were also classified here
Rehabilitation related (single state)	Research that is related to rehabilitation but not emphasizing transition among rehabilitative states and that can include studies of materials, tissues, or subjects with no disabling conditions
Not related	Research that is not clearly relevant to rehabilitation

Rehabilitation Relevance

This classification had five mutually exclusive categories (see Table A-1). "Rehabilitation science" includes research projects that address two or more rehabilitative states (defined in the following section), and in some cases can span all of the rehabilitative states from pathology to disability. Because these are exclusive categories, any project that cut across rehabilitation states, and therefore met the definition of rehabilitation science, but that was predominantly an engineering modality, was categorized as "rehabilitation engineering." The "rehabilitation-related/ single state" category includes projects that are relevant to rehabilitation but that focus on only one state in the enabling–disabling process (not transitions among the states). Research involving drug or alcohol abuse and mental health research were specifically excluded from this committee's charge. Finally, the category "not related" described projects that did not have a research component or that were not clearly relevant to rehabilitation research. Among such abstracts were grants to purchase equipment for research, training with no research component, and seminars that did not produce a report.

Rehabilitative States

Under this classification the project abstracts were categorized ac-

TABLE A-2 Rehabilitative States Classification

Category	Description of Research
No disabling conditions	Research that addresses the state of function or use of subjects with no disabling conditions to investigate mechanisms that are potentially relevant to assessing and treating disabling conditions
Pathology	Research that examines changes of molecules, cells, and tissues that may lead to impairment, functional limitation, or disability, distinguished from pathology by manifestation at organ or organ system level
Impairment	Research that analyzes changes in particular organs, systems, or parts of the body; impairment is distinguished from functional limitation due to emphasis on organ and body components instead of the whole body
Functional limitation	Research that examines functional changes involving the entire subject, manifested by task performance
Disability	Research that focuses on the interaction of the subject with and in the larger context of the physical and social environments

cording to the states described in the enabling–disabling process developed by this committee (see Table A-2; for more detailed discussion, see Chapter 3). The four basic states of pathology, impairment, functional limitation, and disability are those that were initially described by Nagi and more recently elaborated by the Institute of Medicine (1991).

A category called "no disabling conditions" was added to accommodate research that dealt with nonpathological materials. Note that this category is intended for studies that focus exclusively on materials or subjects with no disabling conditions (excluding those that only have control subjects with no disabling conditions). This category includes research that addresses technology or mechanisms contributing to disability without directly studying pathology, impairment, functional limitation, or disability.

Experimental Subjects

A third categorization of the projects is summarized in Table A-3. Note that this categorization distinguishes between "human" and nonhu-

TABLE A-3 Subject Classification

Category	Description of Research
Human	Clinical studies involving human subjects, including noncultured human tissues such as brain slices, tissues, and blood samples, and cadaver materials
Animal	In vivo studies involving nonhuman animal subjects, including noncultured animal tissues such as brain slices
Cultures	In vitro studies involving animal tissue cultures; this includes cell lines, as well as primary cell cultures
Synthetic	Studies of synthetic materials, both organic and inorganic; this includes electrodes, plastics, biopolymers, and inorganic materials
Computer	Computer and other models, including mathematical models

man "animal" preparations and that these two categories include both cadaver and living tissues from these two sources. "Cultures" are different in that they involve living cells that are cultured from either human or animal sources. The "synthetic" category includes both organic and inorganic materials that are used, particularly for prostheses and other devices. Finally, a category of "computer" and other modelling is included. These are not exclusive categories; many studies involve studies of multiple subjects, ranging from human to computer modelling.

Results

As mentioned previously, the committee was limited in their efforts to assess the current status of research by the quality of the abstracts. The abstracts often did not contain enough detail to ascertain study designs, for example, or whether the projects adequately addressed environment, policy, secondary conditions, quality of life, or outcomes measures, among other concerns. Furthermore, because the data were culled from the abstracts, some of which were quite brief, it is likely that our results do not reflect every experiment that was supported by the larger grants. Additionally, the abstract analysis was dependent on the efforts of a small subcommittee and IOM staff. No formal evaluation of internal validity was performed, e.g., inter-rater reliability evaluation. The committee does have confidence, however, these results provide a reasonable indication of the general trends that currently exist in rehabilitation-related research in the federal government.

The committee's specific results which describe each program and its research priorities can be found in Chapter 10.

General Conclusions

Table A-4 summarizes the federal spending on rehabilitation-related research, according to the committee's findings. The committee segregated the programs into two groups. Those with budgets greater than $5,000,000 were analyzed individually and are listed first; those with budgets less than $5,000,000 were not examined and are listed on the bottom of the table. The first column enumerates the funding levels reported by the programs themselves. The second column then lists the amount of the funding associated with the total number of research abstracts that were reviewed for each program. NIDRR, for example, has a budget of $70,000,000, but much of this supports such items as centers and training—activities that were assessed separately from the examination of research activities. The third column lists the amount of funding that the committee classified as not related to rehabilitation-related research. The following three columns then delineate the amounts of the programs' budgets that support rehabilitation-related research, through individual research projects, center grants, and other spending, respectively. The final column provides the committee's best approximation of the amount of each program's budget that supports rehabilitation-related research.

The evaluation process itself led to several important conclusions. First, the task of identifying and collecting the abstracts illuminated the need for centralized administrative control of rehabilitation research. Agencies seemed unsure of their own rehabilitation efforts, much less those of other agencies. NIH's lack of a unified definition for rehabilitation research (see Box A-2), for example, and the lack of correlation between NIH and the CRISP system of projects identified as being rehabilitation related indicates a discordant effort inside NIH and reflects the lack of true coordination throughout the federal government.

The committee also drew conclusions from the size of the research effort. The relatively small size of the research funding pool suggests that there are several gaps in the overall research efforts, but this is not meant to fault any particular agency for ignoring a specific issue. The fiscal limitation on rehabilitation research limits investigation to a narrow level of effort in each field. Of the rehabilitation states described above, pathology and impairment receive the most attention, primarily because it is within the mission of NIH to address these and NIH has the largest budget. NIDRR, among others, does focus on functional limitation and disability, but it only has approximately $12 million to support field-initiated or other investigative research efforts, as opposed to center grants or State Technology Assistance, for example.

Rehabilitation has yet to become a high priority for NIH and other agencies for which rehabilitation is not the primary goal. The current level of research activity for NIDRR and other agencies is not sufficient to address the many pressing issues in rehabilitation today. A coordinating body equipped with the tools required to organize the federal agencies would not only bring much needed attention to the field would, but also increase the quality and efficiency of the present research efforts. The current status of research in the field of rehabilitation science and engineering is that it is small and could benefit greatly from additional funds, greater attention, and better overall administrative control.

A majority of the grants regarded by federal agencies to be for rehabilitation research involved studies of humans or human materials. Many studied both animals and human subjects. Rehabilitation research that involve human subjects and studies of functional limitation and disability were substantially more costly than grants that dealt with animals, tissue cultures, or subjects with no disabling conditions. For example, although only 58 percent of the grants at NIH involved human subjects, those grants took up a lion's share of the funds (80 percent). Within rehabilitation science research specifically, human studies dominated and outnumbered studies involving animal, tissue culture, synthetic, and computer models by a 2:1 ratio. A small minority of studies used tissue cultures. Use of computer models was relatively rare.

Finally, the committee analyzed the research projects of each agency in terms of the agency's mission. (The committee used a series of interviews and questionnaires to investigate the agencies' missions, the method for which is described below, and a more detailed discussion of the mission and research analysis is available in Chapter 10.) In summary, each of the primary agencies involved in funding research in rehabilitation science and engineering has a unique mission and identity, and they do fund projects whose topics are related to the mission of the agency. The committee found no programs that need to be eliminated or consolidated, but it did feel that the efforts could be better coordinated. In all, the committee reviewed many promising projects and quality research which have the potential to influence the lives of people with potentially disabling conditions. There is still a pressing need for more research, and a better coordinated federal effort.

AGENCY QUESTIONNAIRES AND INTERVIEWS

In order to obtain a better understanding of the federal agencies involved in funding research related to Rehabilitation science and engineering, the committee developed two questionnaires: one designed to characterize the general mission and composition of each agency (see Box A-3, the second to characterize training activities (see Box A-4). The committee also interviewed federal agency representatives in person.

TABLE A-4 Summary of Federal Funding in Support of Rehabilitation-Related Research

	Reported Federal Funding	Calculated Federal Funding				Other Spending	Best Approximation
		Total Project Abstracts Reviewed[a]	Not Related[b]	Research	Center Grants[c]		
NIH[d]	$142,579,000	$220,668,556[e]	$25,825,590	$194,842,966	$125,530,564		$320,024,530
NCMRR	15,459,000	14,624,000	3,266,000	11,358,000	349,000		11,707,000
NIDRR	70,000,000	11,188,982[f]	374,618	10,814,364	44,823,426	13,987,592[g]	69,625,382
VA	32,700,000	25,006,009[h]	320,988	24,685,021	993,991	6,700,000[i]	32,379,012
CDC	9,500,000	993,991[j]	0	993,991	8,506,009		9,500,000
NSF	7,000,000	3,501,923[k]	420,314	3,081,609	0	3,500,000[l]	6,581,609
Subtotal	$277,238,000	$275,983,461	$30,207,510	$245,775,951	$179,853,990	$24,187,592	$449,817,533
Subtotal (excluding Institutes)[m]	$134,659,000	$55,314,905	$4,381,920	$50,932,985	$54,627,426	$24,187,592	$129,793,003
ODALTCP		5,000,000					
SSA		5,000,000					
DOT		2,700,000					
ATBCB		300,000					
HUD		100,000					
Subtotal		$13,100,000					$13,100,000
Total	$290,338,000						$462,917,533

[a]Project abstracts reviewed excluded center grants and abstracts that pertained to Mental Health or Drug/Alcohol Abuse.

[b]Abstracts that were not related included funding for seminars with no research component, equipment purchases, and research that did not clearly pertain to any stage of the enabling–disabling process.

[c]Center Grants were segregated because the abstracts did not provide enough detail to categorize them as the individual research projects were.

[d]This excludes NCMRR figures, listed in the line below.

[e](Estimate) Sum of abstracts provided by CRISP and Institutes, minus a 17 percent overlap.

[f](Actual) Abstracts provided by FY95 Program Directory. This excludes funding for training, and center grants, ADA compliance, academic disability studies, and miscellaneous contracts.

[g]Other spending includes training, ADA compliance, academic disability studies, and miscellaneous contracts.

[h](Estimate) Abstracts provided by VA only for projects funded through VA Rehab R&D Service. Because individual funding levels were unavailable, they are approximated here using trends from abstract analysis. $25 million excludes $1 million for center grants funding. No abstracts from other R&D programs were provided.

[i]$6.7 million from other R&D programs within VA included in final approximation.

[j](Actual) Abstracts provided by CDC and CRISP. CDC abstracts described center grants and had no individual funding levels. CRISP-identified individual research projects totaled $993,991.

[k](Actual) Abstracts for all projects funded through RAPD program at BES were obtained from FastLane database. Other Directorates also fund rehabilitation research but do not have programs directed at disability or rehabilitation, and those abstracts were not obtained.

[l]$3.5 million from other Directorates within NSF included in final approximation.

[m]Subtotal excludes NIH funding outside of NCMRR.

BOX A-2
Examples of Definitions Used by Various Institutes Within NIH

National Institute of Arthritis and Musculoskeletal and Skin Diseases and National Institute of Neurological Disorders and Stroke

Rehabilitation is the study of physical disability in a group of diseases, including neurological, musculoskeletal, cardiovascular, and system disorders in which impairment, disability, and handicap are defined by quantified physiologic, physical, behavioral, and functional parameters. It is also the study of the reduction of residual disability, prevention and reduction of secondary complications, the restoration of physical function, communicative ability, and physiological, social, and vocational adaptation by interventions which include, but are not limited to, physical agents and exercises, bioengineering applications, and their mode of delivery. Finally, it is the study of maintenance of function in chronic disorders during the course of the disorder.

National Institute of Nursing Research

Research is restoring or bringing to a condition of health or useful and constructive activity, usually involving learning new ways to do functions that have been lost. Nursing research addresses many aspects of rehabilitation to restore lost function and improve quality of life. Examples include such scientific areas as muscle restoration and urinary incontinence and areas that involve patient and family adaptation to chronic illness and disability. Nursing research represents a blending of both the physiological and psychological aspects of rehabilitation.

National Institute of Deafness and Other Communication Disorders

Medical rehabilitation-related research is directed toward acquiring knowledge on functional restoration, improvement, or stabilization of performance and independence. It includes any research—basic, clinical, or applied—that may lead to the development of improved or new treatment or techniques.

The following agencies responded to the questionnaire:

National Center for Injury Prevention and Control, Centers for Disease Control and Prevention

Disabilities Prevention Program, Centers for Disease Control and Prevention

National Institute for Disability and Rehabilitation Research

Clinical Center, Rehabilitation Medicine Department, National Institutes of Health

National Center for Medical Rehabilitation Research, National Institutes of Health

National Science Foundation

Social Security Administration

U.S. Department of Veterans Affairs

BOX A-3
Questions for Federal Agencies

GENERAL DESCRIPTION
1. How is your agency unique (in terms of its mission, context, and research priorities?
2. Who works at your agency (in terms of number of personnel, average education, years of service)?
3. Where are the results of the research published?

FUNDING REHABILITATION RESEARCH AND TRAINING
4. Regarding specific research funding awards, describe profiles of principal investigators, duration of funding, and areas of emphasis.
5. What percentage of the budget is driven by agency announcements targeting research areas versus field or investigator-initiated research?
6. What percentage of funding is targeted for training?

INTERAGENCY ACTIVITY
7. How well do you communicate with other agencies with similar missions?
8. Discuss interagency overlap in missions, applications, funded grants, and requests for grants or proposals.

U.S. Department of Defense/Army
Rehabilitation Services Administration

PROFESSIONAL ASSOCIATIONS

Over the course of the study, the committee requested and received presentations and papers from organizations and associations representing many of the different professional fields involved in rehabilitation science and engineering. This enabled the committee members to discuss current issues with representatives with different perspectives and to develop a more complete understanding of the trends and topics within the rehabilitation field as a whole.

Presentations and Papers

The committee invited a variety of organizations to participate in the public sessions of each meeting. Committee members heard presentations and asked questions so that they could become familiar with the particular issues of the constituency that each organization represented. A listing of the organizations that addressed the committee and some of the issues that they presented follows.

BOX A-4
Current Training Opportunities in the Rehabilitation Sciences

1. Does your agency fund training?
   a. What occupations does the training target?
   b. Where is the training emphasis?
   c. What is considered a success in training?
   d. What programs does your agency have for training people with disabling conditions, women, and minorities?
2. What is the nature of your agency's training program?
   a. What types of research methods are most emphasized in the training programs?
   b. What are the predominant approaches used in the training programs?
   c. What is the pedagogical balance used in the training program?
   d. What disciplines are involved in your training programs?
   e. Are your training programs multidisciplinary?
   f. Do your training programs focus on multiple disabling conditions?
   g. How many trainees do your training programs graduate each year?
3. Who are the mentors of the trainees supported by your agency's training programs?
4. What is setting for the training program?
   a. Laboratory
   b. Hospital
   c. University clinic
   d. Freestanding rehabilitation facility
   e. Community health care facility
   f. Community advocacy-based facility
   g. Home
5. How long is the training experience?
   a. Undergraduate
   b. Predoctoral training
   c. Postdoctoral training
   d. Career development
   e. Continuing education
6. To what extent are the people being studied involved in the training program?
7. Does your program sponsor training in any of the following areas?
   a. Effective and efficient community provision of service
   b. Influence of ILCs and, in general, self-help or advocacy groups for a wider span than rights and political change
   c. Environmental mapping for barriers and facilitators of social participation by people with disabling conditions
   d. Measurements (psychometric, clinometric and communometric) that measure phenomena valued by people with disabling conditions and that have scientific rigor
   e. Social policy influences on resource availability
   f. Natural histories and longitudinal studies of the unexpected minorities (those living with conditions from which they would have died in earlier days)
   g. Engineering and assistive technology development, commercialization and use factors.
   h. Academic research training sites for prosthetists and orthotists.
   i. Economic analyses (e.g., employment and disability and the health care costs of disability
8. Who reviews the training grant applications made to your agency?

American Academy of Physical Medicine and Rehabilitation, American Congress of Rehabilitation Medicine, Association of Academic Physiatrists (jointly)

• New models of research centers (multidisciplinary and with clinical research capacity enhancement) need to be developed and implemented.

• A governmentwide oversight body is needed to ensure proper direction and coordination of the various individual agencies involved.

• The multiplicity of funding agencies is an advantage for promoting and conducting rehabilitation research, especially if greater coordination at the top can occur.

• New rehabilitation research disciplines are not needed; however, the creation of collaborative multidisciplinary research teams and environments is needed.

• Much greater financial support ($300 million) is mandatory to support a truly effective rehabilitation research agenda.

American Physical Therapy Association

• Rehabilitation practice must shift to an evidence-based paradigm.

• The training of a cadre of rehabilitation clinicians to become clinical investigators must be supported.

• Priorities for research in rehabilitation must be established and focused research programs must be developed to accomplish these priorities.

• Fewer academic programs and more academically qualified faculty are needed.

• Rehabilitation clinicians must open their doors and develop more collaborative relationships between disciplines.

American Speech-Language-Hearing Association

The general area of communication sciences and disorders covers a broad spectrum of subdisciplines many of which are involved with rehabilitation science and engineering. Priorities for research in these areas are:

• Augmentative communication, especially devices such as language boards or computerized synthetic speech instruments

• Prosthetic laryngeal devices, especially the surgical implantation of electrolaryngies to be used for sound generation

• Assistive listening devices including, but not limited to, wearable hearing aids

• Cochlear implants which are being surgically implanted to link the current capability of implanted devices to finer auditory discrimination involved in speech perception.

• Static structures (i.e., prostheses) for craniofacial anomalies, especially cleft palate, and the sequelae of the removal of structures surgically from the orifacial region (cheeks, tongue, palate, pharynx, etc.) as a result of cancer.

• Interventions for childhood and adult neurogenic disorders (e.g., cerebral palsy in children and head injuries in both children and adults), such as behavior therapy and augmentative and prosthetic devices.

Medlantic Research Institute

• Consumer-driven markets best aid rehabilitation research, making it more creative, dynamic, and ultimately, more responsive.

• Market-based health care systems are only effective if there are organized, informed consumer groups and competition on price and on quality and outcomes.

• A consumer-driven system will empower the consumer to make choices and enable the provider to compete on a level playing field.

Sandia National Laboratories

• There exists a need in rehabilitation science and engineering for central integrating projects to draw together existing funded research.

• Private industry is efficient in molding and proliferating useful research as products.

• University and federal researchers must be encouraged to seek private partners to cooperate with each other to share technologies.

• Government agencies should be encouraged to cooperate with each other to share technologies.

• A legitimate role of government is to promote partnerships with private industry, and agencies should be allowed and encouraged to actively establish such partnerships.

Rehabilitation Nurses Foundation/Association of Rehabilitation Nurses

Top 10 clinical rehabilitation nursing research priorities:

1. Interventions to support health-promoting behaviors in people with disabling conditions
2. Effects of bladder management techniques on urinary tract infections, quality of life, and cost of care in individuals with neurogenic bladder
3. Educational strategies to optimize patient and family learning in rehabilitation
4. Therapeutics that enhance and maintain independence and self-care

5. Effect of caregiving on family members who care for individuals with chronic illness/disabilities or disabling conditions in the home

6. Interventions to prevent physiological complications and secondary disabilities

7. Family characteristics that contribute to successful functional outcomes in rehabilitation

8. Efficiency/effectiveness of specific bowel protocols on patient outcomes

9. Interventions to assess and improve quality of life in people with disabling conditions

10. Impact of a violence-induced disabling conditions on the rehabilitation trajectory

Top 10 contextual rehabilitation nursing research priorities:

1. Relationship of functional outcomes to type, intensity, and length of rehabilitation services

2. The effect of changing health care priorities on the practice of rehabilitation nurses

3. Cost and contributions of rehabilitation nurses as a component of the rehabilitation process

4. Influence of the rehabilitation nursing staff mix on patient outcomes

5. Impact of case management in the community on patient outcomes

6. Effects of advanced-practice nursing in ambulatory care on patient outcomes

7. Relationship between patient acuity, functional index measures, and patient care staffing

8. Comparisons between comprehensive community-based and facility-based rehabilitation program outcomes

9. Effect of levels of nursing competence on patient outcomes

10. Issues of transferring newly learned skills to the home environment

Paralyzed Veterans of America

• Rehabilitation outcomes measures are the clearest priority.

• Rehabilitation research is woefully misdefined because the line between basic scientific research and rehabilitation research is increasingly unclear.

• Rehabilitation program development must increase greatly its focus toward more immediately affecting the functional limitations of people with disabling conditions.

• The level of training has fallen increasingly so that the gap between the rehabilitation clinician and the rehabilitation scientist has widened.

Submitted Papers

Several of the organizations continued their contribution to the committee's efforts by preparing background and position papers. The committee received the following papers:

• Comments to the Committee Assessing Rehabilitation Science and Engineering, Pamela Duncan, American Physical Therapy Association
• Comments Regarding the Assessment of Rehabilitation Science and Engineering—Research Priorities, John Melvin, Research Priorities Task Force—Physical Medicine and Rehabilitation
• Statement of the Paralyzed Veterans on America Before the Committee Assessing Rehabilitation Science and Engineering, Frank Morrone, Paralyzed Veterans of America
• Research Priorities for Rehabilitation Nursing: A Summary, Dorothy Gordon, Rehabilitation Nursing Foundation

Educational Standards

To investigate the current state of education, specifically interdisciplinary exposure and training in different specialties, the committee contacted several organizations that certify individuals or accredit institutions. The following boards and associations provided information about the educational standards in their respective fields:

• American Board for Certification in Orthotics and Prosthetics
• American Board on Physical Medicine and Rehabilitation
• American Occupational Therapy Association
• American Occupational Therapy Certification Board
• American Physical Therapy Association
• American Speech-Language-Hearing Association
• Council on Rehabilitation Education
• Rehabilitation Engineering and Assistive Technology of North America
• Rehabilitation Nursing Certification Board

Education and Research Training Survey

To understand the research and training requirements and opportunities within certain academic disciplines better, the committee designed a short questionnaire inquiring into the levels of research experience of educators and graduates in certain rehabilitation-related fields. In addition to the boards and associations contacted for educational standards (listed above), the committee contacted the following organizations: American Academy of Pediatrics, American Nurses Association, and the Institute of Electrical and Electronics Engineers-Engineering in Medicine and Biology Society.

FOCUS GROUPS

In conjunction with the meetings and conferences, committee members held a series of small focus group meetings with the following professional and consumer groups:

- American Academy of Physiatry
- American Occupational Therapy Association
- American Physical Therapy Association
- American Speech-Language-Hearing Association
- American Spinal Injury Association
- First International Conference on Aging and Cerebral Palsy
- National Association of Rehabilitation Research and Training Centers
- National Council on Independent Living
- Society for Disability Studies

Purpose and Method

The focus group sessions were convened to assist the committee in casting a broad net for the collection of information about the current state of rehabilitation science and engineering and to help ensure the inclusion of the unique perspectives of the specific professional or consumer groups (see Box A-5). In this way, the committee was able to hear firsthand the concerns and desires of the people at the heart of rehabilitation and the people best able to form new directions for the field.

Response and Analysis

The focus groups represented a wide spectrum of individuals in-

---

BOX A-5
Forum and Focus Group Questions

Question 1: Regarding the various and numerous federal research programs in rehabilitation, what is good? What is bad? What is missing?

Question 2: What are the important unmet needs in rehabilitation?
Do some of these require new approaches from science and engineering?
Do some of these require new approaches from social and behavioral sciences?

Question 3: What types of research are needed?

Question 4: What are the problems that could interfere with developing and improving rehabilitation science?

Question 5: What would be the best strategies for achieving the necessary level of research and professional expertise?

---

volved in rehabilitation—professionals from different disciplines, researchers, trainers, and consumer groups. Although there was very little overlap in the responses from the different groups, some themes did appear. These included the following:

- a desire to see increased funding of research projects, primarily from the federal government,
- the importance of increased communication between different disciplines involved in rehabilitation and the emphasis on the interdisciplinary nature of the science as the science grows, and
- the two most common research priorities were identified to be secondary conditions and aging with disabling conditions.

The following is a summary of the focus groups' responses to the questionnaire.

Summary of Responses to Focus Group Questions

In response to the first question, focus group participants identified several recent government initiatives as good developments for the field of rehabilitation. NCMRR's new funding mechanisms and NIDRR's application emphasis were mentioned as improvements in federal administration. The NIDRR Spinal Cord Injury Model System is a valuable example of how investments in centers of excellence can have an enormous impact on improving clinical care. Finally, the availability of training programs from NCMRR and the recent gathering of all the NCMRR trainees indicates growing cohesion in the field.

Some problems with federal programs were also recognized. In general, it was felt that not enough programs are funded to handle clinical studies, due to expense. Furthermore, the lack of a definition of rehabilitation research within the federal programs does not facilitate the integration of rehabilitation scientists in their studies, and hinders transfer of findings into applications that can be tested in applied studies. Grant review committees were also identified as lacking strength and experience in dealing with applied research as opposed to pathophysiology and impairment level strategies.

There was also concern about health care delivery. Some felt that insurance companies currently dictate the standards of patient care, relying on nonprofessionals and economics rather than the expertise of health care professionals. A solution for this is to have health care professionals set the standards of care, which would provide patients with an appropriate quality of life. The dilemma of how decisions will be made about those disabling conditions that affect only small number of individuals also caused some concern. The major issue pertains to researching the condition with so few subjects available. A possible solution might be to sponsor consensus conferences (1) to discuss the state of the art, (2) to determine whether consensus can be reached, and (3) determine where to concentrate resources. Clinical practice guidelines and consumer information might also be developed.

Some felt that the current system lacks real opportunity for research within rehabilitation science. A limited mentoring system, scarce career opportunities, and a paucity of funding all restrict the amount of research. There is little research focusing on (1) the environment as a determinant of disabling conditions. Some also felt that (2) prevention does not receive the attention it deserves. Presently there are no means for identification, screening and public education of at-risk groups, for example, the elderly for falls. Additionally, primary prevention or prerehabilitation is not reimbursable despite the need to identify medical conditions before they cause a problem.

The second question addressed unmet needs, and participants identified education as one such need. Education at the onset of disability should not take place in so short a period of time, but instead, it should imitate physician training: A long-term model for learning that involves simultaneous instruction and experience. Many barriers to independent living do not develop from a want of services, but from a lack of knowledge about available resources in the community.

There also needs to be a better interface between rehabilitation and education. The primary and secondary school systems are dealing with problems which had been handled by pathologists, and therapies designed for laboratory or office situations are being transferred to school settings and conducted by people with training in special education.

Rehabilitation needs evaluation of *efficacy* and *cost effectiveness* of surgical and behavioral treatments. Especially in regard to assistive technology, treatment efficacy must research both the efficacy of the device itself and the process of teaching the person to use the device. Industry needs inducements to bring down the costs of technological equipment for those with disabilities. Often, technology does not reach the consumer because of the costs associated with possible liability, or because only a limited number of devices are needed to serve those with a specific disability.

Some of these needs require new approaches from science and engineering. Current rehabilitation models tend to see rehabilitation as the process encompassing only recovery from acute injury. Re-rehabilitation, as defined by Frederick Maynard, envelopes rehabilitation as a dynamic process, with an understanding that people with a disability are at heightened risk of secondary conditions. Implementing feedback loops from the consumer to the rehabilitation professionals regarding quality of care, and training directed towards replacing the current medical model with the "Independent Living/Consumer Empowerment" model would improve current services vastly, bridging the gap between medical professionals and their patients with disabilities who view the quality of life very differently. End-users of technology and programs should be involved in the earliest part of the design process, especially in regard to rehabilitation engineering.

Some of these needs require new approaches from social and behavioral sciences. There is a need for measurement studies that capture the issues beyond impairment. The Functional Independence Measure is a start, but does not look at the factors that support community integration. Some felt that part of the problem is that Behavioral Medicine is largely missing from current research activities. Psychosocial issues are very important, and individual outcomes measures should be closely tailored to the individual's psychology. There is a real need for Behavioral Medicine to be integrated into medical education and rehabilitation training, and for long-term care to take psychosocial needs into account.

The third question addressed current needs in research. Many felt that secondary conditions themselves need to be better defined and understood, especially the risk factors involved, the timing of the onset of certain secondary conditions, and the interventions necessary to prevent or treat these efficiently. Research of secondary conditions should not be limited to the frequency and time frame of the occurrence, but should include subgroups, in order to get a better understanding of how the disabilities affect specific sets of people. Rehabilitation Science needs longitudinal studies that determine the impact of conditions over time, and studies that bridge the levels of pathophysiology to disability. These studies should also focus on the time in life at which disability occurs, as it impacts outcome. This could also involve aging with a disability, specifically the simultaneous declines in cognitive, auditory, and visual functioning which may accompany aging.

Rehabilitation also needs research into the environment. The effects of different kinds of family support and health care delivery patterns were identified as worthy subjects of research. Scientists should also investigate how capacities can be *developed* instead of *restored*, making progress toward higher levels of functioning that may not have existed prior to impairment. Finally, one of the largest unmet research needs is how to measure unmet needs of individuals with disabilities, especially the "unserved" population.

The fourth question dealt with problems that could interfere with developing and improving rehabilitation science. The lack of training and experience of rehabilitation researchers to compete successfully for NIH funding and the increasing burden of clinical care responsibilities faced by physicians who care for people with disabilities severely limit advances to the field were both mentioned as impediments to the development of rehabilitation science. Another major obstacle is the perceived lack of value for the applied sciences. In academe, rehabilitation is "applied" science and often has "second class citizen" status. This perception about rehabilitation needs to be changed. In addition, a poorly understood taxonomy for rehabilitation and poor communication among disciplines and the disability community contribute to the slow development within rehabilitation.

Dissemination of rehabilitation-related information was also cited as a major deterrent to better rehabilitation. First of all, general dissemination is not adequate to reach the grass roots level. Compounding this is the fact that critical information comes too quickly to the individual and the family at the initial onset of the disabling condition; they simply cannot retain and therefore utilize the material. "Survivors' Councils" may be one solution to this, but frequently, the information needed to identify patients and their families is not available, which is another barrier to community development and education. Another solution is to disseminate information better via a variety of sources, for example, the Internet. Independent Living Centers (ILCs) could also serve as a valuable tool for informing consumers, but they are largely isolated from other resources. Frequently, contacts in housing accessibility associations are not known, and often ILCs, Community Wellness Centers, and Rehabilitation Centers need a go-between. Whether the problem is a lack of services or a lack of coordination and dissemination, it was felt that most settings can only currently offer fragmented resources to uninformed consumers. Community development should be a major goal of rehabilitation science so that the community itself becomes a tool for each individual's long-term rehabilitation.

The final question asked participants to identify the best strategies for achieving the necessary level of research and professional expertise. Some mentioned infusions of federal research dollars: A large investment in rehabilitation research would change the academic and clinical institutions according to need. In education and training, long-term care and prevention should be the focal points of a new paradigm. Also, a decrease in the teaching loads of rehabilitation faculty would allow more time for research. The teaching loads are too high and need to be decreased if research productivity is to increase. This could occur if more grant funding was available.

Dissemination was also identified as a means of developing research. Fostering the sharing of research results in interdisciplinary journals and scientific conferences, rather than limiting publication to strictly professional publications, would aid communication. A rehabilitation world wide web site that links scientists from different disciplines to the issues, questions, resources, and needs of persons and communities for knowledge to guide practice and design to limit disability, and that facilitates career mentorship for faculty, researchers, and scientists. Some felt that the promotion of community awareness and building community networks of services and education is key to establishing a coordinated system of care for the people with disabilities. Independent Learning Centers need to make themselves available to Vocational Rehabilitation Counseling students of all disciplines, because ILCs do what VR should be doing: faster, better, cheaper, and from a consumer-driven perspective.

Finally, some called for a "War on Disability" similar to the "War on Cancer" in the 1960s, establishing a National Institute for Rehabilitation Research with appropriate accompanying study sections.

PRIVATE ORGANIZATIONS

The committee felt that it was important to get as much feedback as possible from individual consumers and small consumer groups. Because focus groups could not be held with each constituency, the committee designed a questionnaire to send to identifiable organizations that might have interest in rehabilitation science and engineering.

Method

Questionnaires were mailed to approximately 500 private organizations. The National Rehabilitation Information Center provided a list of disability-related organizations with a national constituency. The questionnaires were sent along with a one-page description of the study, the committee roster, and a cover letter explaining the committee's purpose for the information.

The questionnaire consisted of 33 questions designed by the committee on issues raised in the initial focus group sessions (see Box A-6). The form identified unique issues or aspects of rehabilitation and asked the individual to rate the importance of each as a research, educational, or governmental priority in the current state of rehabilitation as a whole. The scale ranged from 1 to 7, with 7 being the most important or the most pressing need. Finally, the questionnaire contained several lines for the respondents to identify issues not addressed by the questionnaire.

Response and Analysis

The response rate was low: a total of 43 of 488 (less than 10 percent) of the questionnaires sent. Twenty-seven additional questionnaires were returned due to invalid addresses. Of those that did respond, there was little deviation from an average score of 5, with the maximum and minimum average scores very seldom fluctuating beyond ±0.7. To enhance the minor differences, the staff created a relative scale from 0 to 10 in which the lowest average score rated a 0 and the highest average score rated a 10. The other scores were then given proportional scores within this new scale. Figure A-2 illustrates this in a graph displaying the relative scores as a bar chart.

Highest and Lowest Priorities

Acknowledging some overanalysis and enhancement of the findings, the following is a list of the highest and lowest priorities identified in the survey of private organizations.

Highest Priority Concerns or Needs

1. Determine what quality means to people who have and who are restricted in social participation (Question 5; Score: 5.85)

2. Involve consumers in advisory committees to understand the needs and potential contribution of science to improving social participation of people with disabling conditions (Question 23; Score: 5.76)

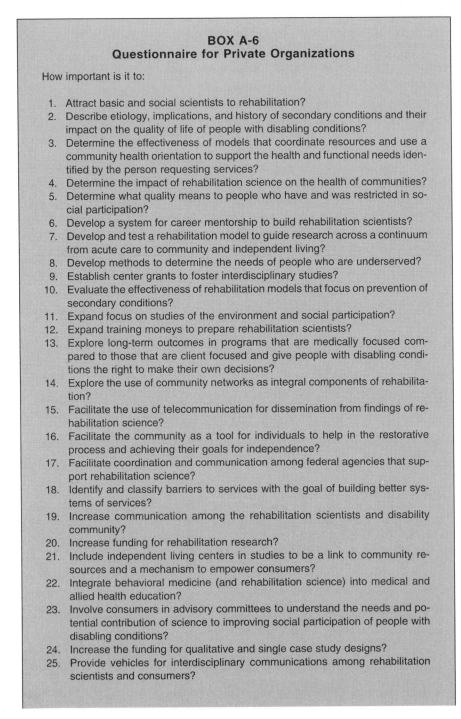

BOX A-6
Questionnaire for Private Organizations

How important is it to:

1. Attract basic and social scientists to rehabilitation?
2. Describe etiology, implications, and history of secondary conditions and their impact on the quality of life of people with disabling conditions?
3. Determine the effectiveness of models that coordinate resources and use a community health orientation to support the health and functional needs identified by the person requesting services?
4. Determine the impact of rehabilitation science on the health of communities?
5. Determine what quality means to people who have and was restricted in social participation?
6. Develop a system for career mentorship to build rehabilitation scientists?
7. Develop and test a rehabilitation model to guide research across a continuum from acute care to community and independent living?
8. Develop methods to determine the needs of people who are underserved?
9. Establish center grants to foster interdisciplinary studies?
10. Evaluate the effectiveness of rehabilitation models that focus on prevention of secondary conditions?
11. Expand focus on studies of the environment and social participation?
12. Expand training moneys to prepare rehabilitation scientists?
13. Explore long-term outcomes in programs that are medically focused compared to those that are client focused and give people with disabling conditions the right to make their own decisions?
14. Explore the use of community networks as integral components of rehabilitation?
15. Facilitate the use of telecommunication for dissemination from findings of rehabilitation science?
16. Facilitate the community as a tool for individuals to help in the restorative process and achieving their goals for independence?
17. Facilitate coordination and communication among federal agencies that support rehabilitation science?
18. Identify and classify barriers to services with the goal of building better systems of services?
19. Increase communication among the rehabilitation scientists and disability community?
20. Increase funding for rehabilitation research?
21. Include independent living centers in studies to be a link to community resources and a mechanism to empower consumers?
22. Integrate behavioral medicine (and rehabilitation science) into medical and allied health education?
23. Involve consumers in advisory committees to understand the needs and potential contribution of science to improving social participation of people with disabling conditions?
24. Increase the funding for qualitative and single case study designs?
25. Provide vehicles for interdisciplinary communications among rehabilitation scientists and consumers?

**BOX A-6
continued**

How important is it to:

26. Put more emphasis on transfer of information?
27. Establish means of supporting measurement studies across the continuum of rehabilitative services, including those provided in the community?
28. Conduct longitudinal studies to determine implications of conditions over time?
29. Conduct clinical trials of applied technology?
30. Establish grant review committees that are oriented to the continuum of science, from pathology to disability?
31. Develop mechanisms to fund studies that address questions at the functional limitation, disability, and environmental levels?
32. Study issues of care givers to determine the needs and issues that relate to their quality of life as well as to the quality of life of the care recipient?
33. Support collaborative grants and initiatives of individual investigators?

---

*Responses were marked on a scale of 1–7.

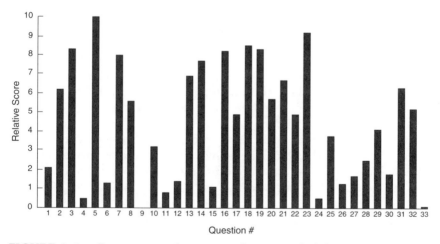

FIGURE A-2 Responses to the survey of private rehabilitation organizations: scores on a relative scale.

3. Identify and classify barriers to services with the goal of building better systems of services (Question 18; Score: 5.66)

4. Increase communication among the rehabilitation scientists and disability community (Question 19; Score: 5.63)

5. Determine the effectiveness of models that coordinate resources and use a community health orientation to support the health and functional needs identified by the person requesting services (Question 3; Score: 5.63)

Lowest Priority Concerns or Needs

1. Establish center grants to foster interdisciplinary studies (Question 9; Score: 4.56)

2. Support collaborative grants and initiatives of individual investigators (Question 33; Score: 4.57)

3. Increase the funding for qualitative and single case study designs (Question 24; Score: 4.62)

4. Determine the impact of rehabilitation science on the health of communities (Question 4; Score: 4.63)

5. Expand focus on studies of the environment and social participation (Question 11; Score: 4.76)

MISCELLANEOUS ACTIVITIES

The committee and staff also engaged in other activities to collect the pertinent information needed for this report. These activities ranged from obtaining necessary texts to conducting interviews with related agencies and programs. The Administration on Aging, for example, was contacted to discuss its methods and means for carrying out its charge. Former directors from pertinent agencies or programs were also contacted to collect other knowledgeable perspectives from people other than current government employees. Staff of committee members attended formal meetings conducted by such groups as the Subcommittee on Disability Statistics of the Interagency Committee on Disability Research and the NCMRR Advisory Panel. Finally, committee members or staff attended or made presentations to academic meetings and consumer groups, such as the Amputee Coalition. These activities put committee members and staff into contact with many different perspectives and ideas, all of which contributed to the whole of the report.

ACKNOWLEDGMENTS

Commissioned Papers and Other Written Contributions

"Participatory Action Research," "Demographics of Disability," and "Summary of Information Sources on Disability and Rehabilitation Research," contributions from **Christine Domzal**
Conwal Inc.

"Technology Transfer," contributions from **Betsy Phillips Tewey**
Conwal, Inc.

"Federal Administration of Rehabilitation Research: An Overview and Outline," contributions from **Jane West**
National Council on Disability

"The Role of Environment in Supporting Performance"
contributions from **Mary Corcoran, Ph.D., OTR**, and **Laura Gitling, Ph.D.**
Thomas Jefferson University

"Quality of Life" contributions from **Dorothy Edwards, Ph.D.**
Washington University

"Models of Service for People with Disabilities" contributions from
Mary Ann McColl, Ph.D., OTR/C
Queen's University

"The Relationship of Vision and Impairment" contributions from
Linda Hunt, M.S., OTR/C
Washington University

"The Relationship of Hearing and Impairment" contributions from
Gerald R. Popelka, Ph.D.
Washington University

Invited Participants and Guests

Judy Auerbach, Ph.D.
National Institutes of Health

Laura Baird, M.S.
Institute of Medicine

Praxedes Belandres, M.D.
Walter Reed Army Medical Center

Betty Jo Berland, Ph.D.
National Institute on Disability and Rehabilitation Research

David Beukelman, Ph.D.
University of Nebraska, Lincoln

John Bode
Sandia National Laboratories

Floyd Brown, Ph.D.
U.S. Department of Health and Human Services

Larry Burt
Centers for Disease Control and Prevention

Laura Cooper, J.D.
Attorney

Rory Cooper
Paralyzed Veterans of America

Francis V. Corrigan, EdD
National Institute on Disability and Rehabilitation Research

Dennis Chamot, Ph.D.
National Research Council

Gerben DeJong, Ph.D.
Medlantic Research Institute

Christine Domzal, Ph.D.
Conwal Incorporated

Pamela Duncan, Ph.D.
University of Kansas

Stephen Fawcett, Ph.D.
University of Kansas

Robert Felton
University of California at Los Angeles

Janie Fouke, Ph.D.
National Science Foundation

Marcus Fuhrer, Ph.D.
National Center for Medical Rehabilitation Research

Bruce Gans, M.D.
Wayne State University School of Medicine

Lynn Gerber, M.D.
National Institutes of Health

John Goldschmidt, M.D.
Department of Veterans Affairs

Dorothy Gordon, D.N.Sc., R.N., F.A.A.N.
The Johns Hopkins University School of Nursing

Margaret Gray
Personal Assistant

Mary Harahan
U.S. Department of Health and Human Services

Karen Hein, M.D.
Institute of Medicine

Jim Jenson
National Research Council

Petra Johnson
Interpreter

Bob Knouss, M.D.
U.S. Department of Health and Human Services

Philip Lee, M.D.
U.S. Department of Health and Human Services

James Lieberman, M.D.
College of Physicians and Surgeons of Columbia University

Phillip Marion, M.D.
Robert Wood Johnson Fellow

Maria Martino
U.S. Department of Health and Human Services

John Mather, M.D.
Social Security Administration

Lauren Meader
Institute of Medicine

John Melvin, M.D.
Mossrehab Hospital

Brian Millin
National Institute on Disability and Rehabilitation Research

Frank Morrone
Paralyzed Veterans of America

Larry Morton
National Institutes of Health

Jacques Normand, Ph.D.
National Research Council

James Reswick, Sc.D.
(retired) National Institute on Disability and Rehabilitation Research

Mark Rosenberg, M.D., M.P.P.
National Center for Injury Prevention and Control

Debbie Rothstein, Ph.D.
National Institute on Child Health and Human Development

Katherine Seelman, Ph.D.
National Institute on Disability and Rehabilitation Research

Valerie Setlow, Ph.D.
Institute of Medicine

Cynthia Shewan, Ph.D.
American Physical Therapy Association

Kenneth I. Shine, M.D.
Institute of Medicine

Joseph Sniezek, M.D., M.P.H.
National Center for Injury Prevention and Control

Suzanne Stoiber, Ph.D.
U.S. Department of Health and Human Services

R. Alexander Vachon, Ph.D.
U.S. Senate Committee on Finance

Richard Verville, Esq.
representing AAPM&R, AAP, ACRM

Richard Waxweiler, Ph.D.
National Center for Injury Prevention and Control

Alexandra Wigdor, Ph.D.
National Research Council

Dorrett Worrell
National Institutes of Health

Other Contributors

Jeanette Bair
American Occupational Therapy Association

Carol Kochhar
George Washington University

Keith Miller
Sandia National Laboratories

Don Wesenberg
Sandia National Laboratories

George Zitnay, Ph.D.
Brain Injury Association

B

Summary of Information Sources on Disability and Rehabilitation Research

Christine Domzal
Conwal Incorporated, McLean, Virginia

INTRODUCTION

The purpose of this summary is to present a brief description of federal agencies primarily involved in disability and rehabilitation research. It also provides brief descriptions of agencies that provide services and benefits, advise on policy, enforce compliance with federal statutes and regulations, and collect data on disability.

In February 1995, the 27 members of the Interagency Committee on Disability Research (ICDR) were invited to describe the information systems their agencies use to announce funding priorities, track the progress of funded research, and catalog and disseminate final reports of funded research. Not all members of the ICDR are funding agencies. Some agencies fund services, others are primarily responsible for enforcement of compliance with federal statutes and regulations, and some serve an advisory function. The 10 agencies that submitted information on their research programs represent the broad range of federal research activity in disability and rehabilitation.

This summary is organized by federal department. For each agency within the department, there is a brief description of its mission and the type of disability research it funds. Next, there is a description of the methods used to announce the availability of research funding, track in-progress research, and disseminate research reports.

ARCHITECTURAL AND TRANSPORTATION BARRIERS COMPLIANCE BOARD (ACCESS BOARD)

The Architectural and Transportation Barriers Compliance Board, also known as the Access Board, is an independent federal agency responsible for developing accessibility guidelines for buildings, facilities, and transit vehicles. Consequently, the Board's research program is focused on accessibility research pertaining to architecture and design, communication, and transportation. The Americans with Disabilities Act (ADA) of 1990 significantly broadened the Board's responsibility for developing design guidelines. Since passage of the ADA, the Board has given priority to research that supports the development of ADA design guidelines and of technical assistance materials.

Funding: $280,000 in fiscal year 1995.

Disability Research: Research projects are currently selected in the following order of priority:

1. research pertaining to issues or areas not currently covered by the Board's guidelines or scheduled for future rulemaking;
2. research addressing issues of compliance or clarity concerning specific provisions of the guidelines; and
3. research that reevaluates existing specifications that are long-standing and possibly dated.

The Board plans to continue to focus on design issues related to its ADA guidelines in fiscal years 1995 and 1996. Recent research projects undertaken by the Board include:

- **Technical requirements for ramps**. A study on existing specifications for ramps, including those for slope, landing, and length.
- **Detectable warnings.** A project to study the need for detectable warnings for persons with visual impairments at intersections and at hazardous vehicular areas.
- **Design requirements for persons using powered mobility aids.** Some of the provisions in ADA Accessibility Guidelines (ADAAG), such as those for clear floor space, maneuvering clearances, and reach ranges, are based on anthropometric data derived from studies involving persons using manual wheelchairs. This project investigated design specifications appropriate for persons using powered wheelchairs, scooters, and other motorized mobility aids.

- **ADAAG manual.** Development of a comprehensive manual on the ADAAG and recommendations on a distribution system for revisions and updates to the manual.
- **Recreation guidelines: regulatory impact analysis.** Impact assessment of proposed recreation guidelines.
- **Access to water transportation.** Additional funding for a project the Department of Transportation is undertaking to assess the feasibility and impact of making an established inventory of passenger vessels and related facilities accessible.
- **Swimming pool accessibility.** A project to develop guidance materials on the design options and products available for providing wheelchair access into swimming pools.

Announcing Funding Priorities: Announcements seeking public comment on priorities for the next two fiscal years are published in the *Federal Register*. Typically, a subsequent notice is published listing priorities as finalized by the Board. Priorities are also announced in the agency quarterly newsletter *Access America* and through direct mailing using an in-house mailing list.

Progress Reports on Funded Research: Under its current budget, the Board funds only one to three major research projects per year. Status reports on the progress of projects are prepared primarily for in-house use and briefing Board members. This information is available to the public upon request. The quarterly newsletter, *Access America*, also reports the status of projects and completion of tasks.

Final Reports on Funded Research: Final reports of funded research are available through *Access America*, and BBS. The Board also disseminates its research reports through the National Technical Information Service (NTIS). The Board may consider making research reports available through its electronic bulletin board enabling the public to download the information. Currently, only the notice of the availability of such reports is provided in BBS.

DEPARTMENT OF EDUCATION

National Institute on Disability and Rehabilitation Research

The National Institute on Disability and Rehabilitation Research (NIDRR) is part of the Office of Special Education and Rehabilitative Services (OSERS) in the U.S. Department of Education (ED). NIDRR's mission is to contribute to the independence of people with disabilities.

NIDRR accomplishes this mission by funding research, demonstration projects, training, and other related activities to maximize the full inclusion and integration of this population into society. Through grants, contracts, and cooperative agreements, NIDRR funds research designed to improve systems, products, and practices in the rehabilitation field. NIDRR is also charged with ensuring the widespread distribution of practical scientific and technological information in usable formats. This dissemination takes such forms as conferences, seminars, workshops, and publications.

The research funded by NIDRR covers every aspect of disability including brain injury, spinal cord injury, multiple sclerosis, back pain, and broader areas such as technology, accessibility, aging, service delivery, policy, ethics, recreation, and community integration.

Funding: $70 million in fiscal year 1995.

Disability Research:

- **Research and demonstration projects**. Rehabilitation priorities are identified by NIDRR and published in the *Federal Register*.
- **Rehabilitation research and training centers**. These centers:

— conduct research targeted toward the production of new knowledge which will improve rehabilitation methodology and service delivery systems, alleviate or stabilize disabling conditions, and promote maximum social and economic independence.

— institute related teaching and training programs to disseminate and promote the utilization of research findings thereby reducing the usual long intervening delay between the discovery of new knowledge and its wide application in practice.

- **Rehabilitation engineering research centers**. Provide support for advanced research of an engineering or technical nature.
- **Field-initiated research**. Designed to encourage eligible applicants to originate ideas for research and demonstrations.
- **Innovative Research**. Provides financial support to projects that test new concepts and innovative ideas; demonstrate research results of high potential benefits; purchase and evaluate prototype aids and devices; or conduct feasibility, planning, and evaluation studies and conferences, and other activities to disseminate specific research findings.
- **Small business innovative research**. To encourage new ideas and products useful to people with disabilities and the rehabilitation field.
- **State technology assistance.** This program, funded under the Tech-

nology-Related assistance for Individuals with Disabilities Act, supports consumer-driven plans for the delivery of assistive technology.

- **Technology-related projects of national significance**. Title II, Part C of the Technology-Related Assistance for Individuals with Disabilities Act funds training projects that: (a) educate people with disabilities and other relevant groups, in developing, demonstrating, disseminating and evaluating curricula, materials, and methods used to train people to provide technology-related assistance; and (b) prepare personnel to provide technical assistance and administer programs or to support the development and implementation of statewide programs in technology-related assistance.
- **Utilization projects**. This program supports activities that will ensure that rehabilitation knowledge generated from projects and centers funded by NIDRR and other sources is fully utilized.
- **ADA technical assistance programs**. NIDRR has funded 10 Regional Disability and Business Technical Assistance Centers which provide technical assistance training and resource referral on the ADA.
- **Model spinal cord injury systems**. Provides assistance to establish innovative projects for the delivery, demonstration, and evaluation of comprehensive medical, vocational, and other rehabilitation services to meet the needs of individuals with spinal cord injuries.
- **Research Training Grants**. Supports projects that provide advanced training in rehabilitation research.
- **Fellowships**.
- **International projects**.

Announcing Funding Priorities: NIDRR announces its funding priorities in the *Federal Register* and through electronic bulletin boards.

Progress Reports on Funded Research: Progress on projects is tracked by Project Officers.

Final Reports on Funded Research: Funded by NIDRR, the National Rehabilitation Information Center (NARIC) is a national disability and rehabilitation library and information center that collects and disseminates the results of NIDRR-funded research projects. Each NIDRR-funded project is required to provide NARIC with at least one copy of each of its publications—reports, monographs, journal articles, book chapters, training materials, and directories. The collection, which also includes commercially published books, journal articles, and audiovisuals, grows at a rate of 300 documents per month. NARIC currently has more than 44,000 documents on all aspects of disability and rehabilitation.

U.S. DEPARTMENT OF HEALTH AND HUMAN SERVICES

Agency for Health Care Policy and Research

The Agency for Health Care Policy and Research (AHCPR) was established in December 1989 under Public Law 101-239 (Omnibus Budget Reconciliation Act of 1989). AHCPR, a part of the U.S. Department of Health and Human Services, is the lead agency charged with supporting research designed to improve the quality of health care, reduce its cost, and broaden access to essential services. AHCPR's broad programs of research bring practical, science-based information to medical practitioners and to consumers and other health care purchasers. The Agency is comprised of 14 major functional components, with the Office of the Administrator directing the activities of the Agency to ensure that strategic objectives are achieved.

Funding: No special dollars are allocated to specific topics. Interest in vulnerable populations which includes disability.

Disability Research: The AHCPR research agenda includes eight topic areas:

1. **Patient outcomes research** evaluates the effectiveness of health care interventions to show how they affect results important to patients, including quality of life and functional status.
2. **Quality measurement and improvement** develops measurements and strategies to facilitate improved quality of care.
3. **Clinical practice guidelines.** AHCPR facilitates the development of clinical practice guidelines which are based on comprehensive reviews of the scientific literature. The guidelines help practitioners and consumers determine the best ways to prevent and treat diseases and other health conditions.
4. **Consumer choice** provides useful information on quality and value of health care.
5. **Cost and access** research is designed to understand trends occurring in health care and their implications for quality and consumer choice.
6. **Health care delivery** assesses and evaluates the health care marketplace.
7. **Technology assessments** provide information on the risks, benefits, and clinical effectiveness of new medical technologies.
8. **Data standards and health information systems development** contributes to the simplification of health care information systems.

Priorities include quality, effectiveness, and outcomes research; investigator initiated research; managed care and its effect on health care systems; and consumer decision making.

Announcing Funding Priorities: The *NIH Guide to Grants and Contracts*, *Commerce Business Daily*, and the AHCPR Web site at: **http://www.ahcpr.gov.**

Progress Reports on Funded Research: Grantees are required to prepare annual progress reports.

Final Reports on Funded Research *Research Activities* is a digest of research findings that have been produced with support from AHCPR and is published by AHCPR's Center for Health Information Dissemination. Information on funded research is also available on the AHCPR Web site.

Centers for Disease Control and Prevention: The Disabilities Prevention Program

The mission of the Centers for Disease Control and Prevention (CDC) is to promote health and quality of life by preventing and controlling disease, disability, and injury. To accomplish this mission, CDC works with partners throughout the United States and internationally to monitor health, detect and investigate health problems, conduct research to enhance prevention, develop and advocate sound public health policies, implement prevention strategies, promote healthy behaviors, foster safe and healthful environments, and provide leadership and training.

Funding: $9 million for disability prevention research in fiscal year 1995.

Disability Research: The Disabilities Prevention Program (DPP), located within the National Center for Environmental Health, has two major goals: (1) to reduce the incidence and severity of primary and secondary disabilities; and (2) to promote the independence and productivity of people with disabilities and to further their integration into the community. The DPP: provides states with technical and financial assistance to build disabilities prevention capacity, establishes surveillance systems for disabilities, identifies risk factors for disabilities, and identifies and develops appropriate interventions to prevent secondary disabilities.

• **Targeted disabilities.** During FY 1992, the DPP funded 28 capacity-building cooperative agreements with state agencies to help recipients develop their own state-level program for studying, preventing, or minimizing the effects of disabilities. The projects receiving awards focused on the following disabilities:

— Fetal alcohol syndrome.
— Mild mental retardation.
— Secondary conditions among children with cerebral palsy, spina bifida, or sickle cell disease.
— Traumatic head and spinal cord injuries.
— Secondary conditions among people with head and spinal cord injuries.

• **State disabilities prevention projects.** The Disabilities Prevention Program funds 28 capacity-building projects. Each project supports a state office of disability prevention, an advisory council, a disabilities surveillance system, and activities to develop, implement, and evaluate community intervention programs.

The following intervention programs, funded in part through DPP, show exceptional promise and could serve as models for other states and communities attempting to establish similar programs.

• A program that uses dramatizations to educate teenage students about ways of preventing disabilities. Dramatizations focus on (a) alcohol and other drug use during pregnancy, (b) drinking and driving, and (c) head and spinal cord injuries caused by improper seat belt use.
• A program that uses story, song, art, and dramatic play to encourage proper safety belt use among preschool and elementary school children.
• A program to promote health among persons with disabilities by awarding competitive minigrants to independent living centers.
• A comprehensive plan to develop a population-based fetal alcohol syndrome surveillance system.
• A statewide training program for professionals in a position to intervene with women at risk of having children with fetal alcohol syndrome or fetal alcohol effects.
• An intervention program to help parents at high risk for abusing or neglecting their children to recognize and address behaviors that may be precursors of child abuse and neglect.
• A comprehensive early-notification reporting system for spinal cord injuries. This system will allow public health officials to develop strategies for preventing secondary conditions.
• A model community program for promoting bicycle helmet use.
• A program of collaboration among the Governor's office, volunteers, and corporate sponsors to address childhood injury through peer education.

Announcing Funding Priorities: Program announcements are published in the *Federal Register*.

Progress Reports on Funded Research: Grantees are required to write semiannual progress reports. These reports are collected for internal use only.

Final Reports on Funded Research: Final reports are required of grantees upon completion of the project period. The grantee is responsible for the preparation and content of the final report. Grantees are also required to provide copies of any journal publications resulting from the research.

Centers for Disease Control and Prevention: National Center for Injury Prevention and Control

The Centers for Disease Control and Prevention (CDC) began studying home and recreational injuries in the early 1970s and violence prevention in 1983. From these early activities grew a national program to reduce injury, disability, death, and costs associated with injuries outside the workplace. In June 1992, CDC established the National Center for Injury Prevention and Control (NCIPC). As the lead federal agency for injury prevention, NCIPC works closely with other federal agencies; national, state, and local organizations; state and local health departments; and research institutions.

Funding: $16.2 million for injury prevention research grants in fiscal year 1996.

Disability Research: The National Center for Injury Prevention and Control conducts and monitors research on the causes, risks, and preventive measures for injuries outside the workplace including

• prevention of secondary conditions among people with disabilities.
• unintentional injuries related to falls, fires and burns, drowning, poisonings, motor vehicle crashes (including those with pedestrians), recreational activities, and playgrounds and daycare settings.
• intentional injuries related to suicide, youth violence, family violence, and firearms.

NCIPC also funds research by universities and other public and private groups studying the three phases of injury control (prevention, acute care, and rehabilitation) and the two major disciplines of injury control (epidemiology and biomechanics).

The **Division of Acute Care, Rehabilitation Research, and Disability** coordinates a national public health approach to reducing the impact of injuries by improving trauma care and rehabilitation systems. The program includes the prevention of injury-related disabilities and their secondary conditions. Current activities include:

- Development of guidelines for surveillance of injuries to the central nervous system (primarily traumatic brain and spinal cord injuries)
- Research on prevention of secondary conditions such as pressure sores
- Multistate surveillance system for traumatic brain and spinal cord injury.

The **Division of Unintentional Injury Prevention** monitors trends in unintentional injuries, conducts research to better understand risk factors, and evaluates interventions to prevent injuries due to motor vehicle crashes, fires, burns, falls, drowning, and poisonings.

The **Division of Violence Prevention** supports both intramural and extramural projects and activities to prevent violence. Extramural research includes studies on the relationship between exposure to violence, risk behavior, and psychological stress among children; risk and protective factors associated with interpersonal violence among adolescents and violence against women; the effects of psychological abuse, violence, and aggression on women's physical and mental health; the epidemiology of injuries to victims of domestic assault; intervention and evaluation research on suicide, intimate violence, and interpersonal violence among youth. Fourteen evaluation projects on preventing youth violence are currently under way in 11 cities. The Division also provides financial and technical support to state and local health departments in their efforts to prevent violence. These programs define and track injuries, develop interventions, mobilize coalitions for intervention and public education, and evaluate prevention effectiveness.

Announcing Funding Priorities: Program announcements are published in the *Federal Register* and also an the NCIPC Web site. The *Guide to Applying for Injury Research Grants,* available from the Office of Research Grants, provides members of the scientific community with guidance for applying to NCIPC for research grants.

Progress Reports on Funded Research: Grantees are required to write semiannual progress reports. These reports are collected for internal use only.

Final Reports on Funded Research: Final reports are required of grantees upon completion of the project period. The grantee is responsible for the preparation and content of the final report.

NIH/National Center for Medical Rehabilitation Research

The National Center for Medical Rehabilitation Research (NCMRR) was established within the National Institutes of Health (NIH) by legislation passed in 1990 (Public Law 101-613). The Center is a component of the National Institute of Child Health and Human Development (NICHD). The mission of NCMRR is to foster development of the scientific knowledge needed to enhance the health, productivity, independence and quality of life of persons with disabilities. This is accomplished by supporting research on enhancing the rehabilitation and healthcare of people with disabilities and on assisting them to achieve their functional capabilities of relevance in their daily lives. A primary goal of the Center is to bring the health related problems of people with disabilities to the attention of America's best scientists in order to capitalize upon the advances occurring in the biological, behavioral, and engineering sciences.

The Director of NIH was directed by P.L. 101-613 to establish the National Advisory Board on Medical Rehabilitation Research. The Advisory Board advises the directors of NIH, NICHD, and NCMRR on matters and policies relating to the Center's programs. The Advisory Board is comprised of 12 members representing health and scientific disciplines related to medical rehabilitation and 6 members representing people with disabilities.

Funding: $15 million in fiscal year 1995.

Disability Research: The *Research Plan for the National Center for Medical Rehabilitation Research* was based on a review of medical rehabilitation research being supported by various agencies, advice solicited from the scientific and consumer communities, and three field hearings at which public comment was obtained. The plan describes a framework for research to be supported by NCMRR and by other agencies that fund medical rehabilitation research. It focuses on the person with a disability and on how that person's functional limitations are affected by interacting biological, personal, and societal forces. Emphasis is placed on obtaining better information about the health-related factors that influence how persons with disabilities interrelate with their families, coworkers, and communities. Major issues in medical rehabilitation research are reviewed, including early and late onset of disability, traumatic injury, chronic and recurring disorders, and effects of aging.

The research initiatives and opportunities recommended in the *Re-*

search Plan for the National Center for Medical Rehabilitation Research are discussed in terms of seven cross-cutting areas in which increased research effort is needed. Those areas are:

- improving functional mobility;
- promoting behavioral adaptation to functional losses;
- assessing the efficacy and outcomes of medical rehabilitation therapies and practices;
- developing improved assistive technology;
- understanding whole body system responses to physical impairments and functional changes;
- developing more precise methods of measuring impairments, disabilities, and societal and functional limitations;
- training research scientists in the field of rehabilitation.

From FY 92 when NCMRR first began funding research projects until FY 95, 182 projects have been supported, including those funded by interagency agreements.

Announcing Funding Priorities: Research support has been provided primarily through research project grants, institutional training grants, and small business innovation research grants. The *NIH Guide to Grants and Contracts* is used to announce funding availability.

Progress Reports on Funded Research: Computer Retrieval of Information on Scientific Projects (CRISP) is a major scientific information system containing information on the research programs supported by the U.S. Public Health Service (PHS).

Final Reports on Funded Research: NCMRR does not publish results of funded research. Grantees are expected to publish their research findings in peer-reviewed journals.

Office of Disability, Aging, and Long-Term Care Policy

The Office of the Assistant Secretary for Planning and Evaluation (ASPE), in the Office of the Secretary for Health and Human Services, conducts research and policy analysis which is responsive to the needs of the Secretary and to the Department's policies and programs. ASPE includes the Office of Disability, Aging, and Long-Term Care (DALTCP) as well as offices of Health Policy and Human Services Policy.

DALTCP is responsible for the development, coordination, research and evaluation of DHHS policies and programs which support the independence, productivity, health and security of children, working age adults, and older persons with disabilities. The office is also responsible for policy coordination and research to promote the economic and social well-being of the elderly.

In particular, the Office is responsible for policies concerning: long-term care and personal assistance services including informal caregiving; linkages between the acute, postacute and long-term care systems; long-term rehabilitation services; children's disability; employment assistance; and the encouragement of mechanisms for coordinating the housing, health, income supports, and education, training and employment needs of people with disabilities. These responsibilities are carried out through policy planning, policy and budget analysis, regulatory reviews, formulation of legislative proposals, policy research, and evaluation.

Funding: $5 million for disability related projects in fiscal year 1995.

Disability Research: DALTCP has a mandate from the Assistant Secretary for an expanded program of disability-related research and policy analysis. In addition, the agendas of other offices within ASPE include projects relevant to disability. Recent disability-related projects of high priority in DALTCP include development of the program for long-term services included in proposed health reform legislation in the 103rd Congress. Experience with this proposed legislation has led to several new projects. DALTCP has also taken the lead in developing and funding the Disability Supplement to the 1994 and 1995 Health Interview Surveys.

Ongoing disability-related policy and evaluation research includes

- modeling use and costs of long-term services;
- client-directed personal assistance or home and community-based services;
- use and impact of managed care on persons with disabilities;
- subacute care and Medicare-funded home health services;
- residential options for persons with disabilities;
- database development; and
- international comparisons of long-term service systems.

Announcing Funding Priorities: Research funding availability is announced in the *Federal Register* and in the *Commerce Business Daily.*

Progress Reports on Funded Research: DALTCP periodically publishes Research Reports which summarize progress to date of current research projects as well as findings of completed projects (for example, see *Long-Term Care and Disability Research 1989–1992*, May 1992). In addition, progress reports may be available from the Policy Information Center (PIC), a component of ASPE. PIC is a centralized source of information on in-process, completed, and on-going health and human services evaluations; short-term evaluation research; and policy-oriented projects conducted by DHHS as well as by other federal departments and the private sector. PIC resources may be accessed in person, via the PIC on-line database query system, or via the Internet.

Final Reports on Funded Research: In addition to periodic Research Reports, DALTCP publishes and puts on-line a *List of Reports* which contains abstracts of all reports written by DALTCP staff and research projects funded through the DALTCP and ASPE.

DEPARTMENT OF HOUSING AND URBAN DEVELOPMENT

The Department of Housing and Urban Development (HUD) has a mission to help create cohesive, economically healthy communities—communities of opportunity—throughout America.

The Office of Policy Development and Research (PD&R) is responsible for providing advice and information to the Secretary to further the policy agenda; for maintaining current information to monitor housing needs, housing market conditions, and the operation of existing programs; and for conducting research on priority housing and community-development issues.

The primary mission of PD&R is to provide reliable and objective data and analysis to inform policy decision. It focuses on providing definitive answers to questions about what programs work and how they can be made to work better, through quick-turnaround studies and conferences as well as through long-term evaluations that systematically measures outcomes over an extended period. In addition, PD&R is committed to investing in the development of reliable databases describing housing market conditions and needs, as well as documenting how HUD programs work, how much they cost, and who they serve.

PD&R forms active partnerships with researchers, practitioners, advocates, industry groups, and foundations and is committed to involving a greater diversity of perspectives, methods, and researchers into HUD research.

Funding: $100,000 for disability-specific projects in fiscal year 1995.

Disability Research: Research priorities within PD&R have been developed to support and advance these Department policy priorities:

- Reduce the number of homeless Americans.
- Make public housing a source of pride to communities.
- Expand housing opportunities for low and moderate income people.
- Open housing markets to minorities.
- Empower communities.
- Bring excellence to HUD Management.

Within these policy priorities, PR&D supports research and information activities related to:

- Housing for special needs. Addresses housing and supportive service options for persons with physical or mental disabilities.
- Fair housing. Research, information, and evaluation on statutes and programs that protect the housing rights of persons with physical or mental disabilities.
- Building technology. Research on methods, materials, and trends affecting the construction and rehabilitation of housing; and improving housing safety and accessibility.
- Homeownership. Opportunities for persons with special needs.
- Regulatory barriers to affordable housing. Changes in state and local regulations that can foster development or accessory apartments, group homes, and other arrangements for community living.

Announcing Funding Priorities: Research is conducted through competitively procured contracts. PD&R announces and solicits proposals for large-scale research projects through the *Commerce Business Daily*. The procurement process is handled by the Office of Procurement and Contracts (OPC). Interested parties can request to be placed on a mailing list for notification of such procurements.

Progress Reports on Funded Research: Progress on projects is tracked by the HUD Project Managers using the HUD Project Management System.

Final Reports on Funded Research: Final reports of funded research are available through **HUD USER,** a research information service and clearinghouse sponsored by PD&R. **HUD USER** collects, develops, and distributes housing-related information and offers the following resources and services:

- Documents
- Audiovisual programs
- *Recent Research Results*

- The **HUD USER Database** is a bibliographic resource that contains over 5,000 reports, articles, case studies, and other research literature on topics related to housing and urban development.
- Resource guides
- *Directory of Information Resources in Housing and Urban Development, Third Edition.*
- Microfiche copies of noncopyrighted documents on the **HUD USER** database.
- Computer packages to address specialized needs for information on particular subject areas, including the Housing Discrimination Study Data Tape.

DEPARTMENT OF TRANSPORTATION

Transit Cooperative Research Project

Among its activities, the Department of Transportation (DOT) provides formula grants for state and local governments to buy new transit vehicles accessible to persons with disabilities; build accessible rail systems; modernize older rail car and stations, provide demand-response paratransit (van) service for those with disabilities unable to use the accessible fixed route services and fund eligible operating costs. It is also charged with ensuring accessibility of all modes of transportation under the ADA and the Air Carrier Access Act of 1986.

The Transit Cooperative Research Program (TCRP) was established in 1992 to provide a continuing program of applied research on transit issues. The program is sponsored by the Federal Transit Administration (FTA) and carried out under a three-way agreement among the National Academy of Sciences, acting through its Transportation Research Board (TRB); the Transit Development Corporation, an education and research arm of the American Public Transit Association (APTA); and the FTA.

The TCRP focuses on issues significant to the transit industry, with emphasis on developing near-term research solutions to a variety of transit problems involving facilities, service concepts, operations, policy, planning, human resources, maintenance, and administrative practices.

Funding: $1.7 million for disability-related projects from August 1992 through December 31, 1994.

Disability Research: In progress or recently completed disability-related projects include

- Computerized Paratransit Dispatching;

- Signs and Symbols in Transit Facilities;
- Transit Operations for Individuals with Disabilities;
- Attracting Paratransit Patrons to Fixed-Route Services
- Personal Mobility Aid Securement and Passenger Restraint on Transit Vehicles;
- Applicability of Low-Floor Light Rail Vehicles in North America;
- Measuring and Valuing Transit Benefits and Disbenefits;
- Quick Response for Special Needs;
- Wheelchair Restraint System;
- New Transit Bus;
- Customer Information at Bus Stops; and
- Low-Floor Transit Buses.

Announcing Funding Priorities: TCRP is intended to concentrate on low-risk, applied research projects with relatively quick turn-around. The program is directed at problems of an immediate, near-term nature that can be undertaken with moderate research funds. TCRP project-funding levels are typically less than $400,000. Research Project Statements (Requests for Proposals) are sent to the approximately 4,000 persons on the TCRP mailing list. TCRP program solicitations are also available through the Department of Transportation Information Center. In addition, the FTA will establish an FTA Home Page on the Internet to announce TCRP and other research project priorities and requests for proposals.

Progress Reports on Funded Research: Progress reports of funded research are available in *Transit Research Abstracts* and on UMTRIS, which provides on-line retrieval of abstracts and summaries of TCRP research projects in progress.

Transit Research Abstracts is an annual DOT publication of abstracts of completed and ongoing research projects on all public transit modes, including specialized ADA transit systems for access by persons with disabilities.

Final Reports on Funded Research: TRB provides a series of research reports, research results digests, legal research digests, syntheses of transit practice, and other supporting material developed by TCRP research. After publication, products are distributed widely through the TRB distribution system. Copies are sent directly to at least 2,000 TRB members who request transit publications as well as to about 100 libraries, 50 TRB transit representatives, and more than 150 university-liaison representatives. As a further means of disseminating the research reports, announcements of their availability are sent to the trade press. FTA personnel automatically receive a copy of each published report providing an additional conduit through which direct contact with possible users can be initiated. TRB also lists products annually in the TRB catalog. The FTA also publishes TCRP final report summaries in *Transit Research Abstracts*.

In 1994, the TRB published a *Research Results Digest* entitled *Transit Operations for Individuals with Disabilities*, which briefly summarizes the Phase I findings of the TCRP project of the same title.

Project ACTION

Project ACTION (Accessible Community Transportation in Our Nation) is a national research and demonstration project administered by the National Easter Seal Society under a cooperative agreement with the Federal Transit Administration of the U.S. Department of Transportation. Project ACTION is designed to facilitate cooperation between the transit industry and disability community in order to improve access to transportation for individuals with disabilities and assist transportation providers in implementing the Americans with Disabilities Act of 1990 (ADA). The Project ACTION Local Demonstration Program serves as a vehicle for developing and testing tools, techniques, and strategies to improve accessible transportation. Through annual solicitations since 1991, Project ACTION has funded 60 local demonstration projects.

Funding: $1 million in project year 1994.

Disability Research: Project ACTION funds transit accessibility demonstration projects that:

- identify persons with disabilities and their transportation needs;
- develop outreach and marketing activities to encourage public transportation use of persons with disabilities;
- provide training for transportation providers to increase their sensitivity to the needs of persons with disabilities;
- provide training for persons with disabilities regarding the use of public transportation; and
- encourage elimination of barriers to accessible services and facilities.

Complementing Project ACTION local demonstration efforts is the National Institute for Accessible Transportation (NIAT). The Institute disseminates information and resources developed under the Local Demonstration Program. NIAT conducts other activities which involve research, training, and technical assistance in the area of accessible transportation.

In project year 1994, Project ACTION funded $1 million in local demonstration programs in four categories:

- Develop and tests model procedures for determining ADA paratransit eligibility: $400,000.
- Develop and implement innovative methods of dissemination and replication: $400,000.
- Develop and apply technology to eliminate transportation barriers: $100,000.
- Develop model projects to address other accessibility issues: $100,000.

Announcing Funding Priorities: Project ACTION conducts its annual solicitation process through Requests for Proposals. Announcements are posted and advertised the *Federal Register,* the *Commerce Business Daily,* the *Project ACTION Update* (the quarterly newsletter), and *Project ACTION Request for Proposals.* Also used are trade publications, National Easter Seal Societies publications, and federal publications.

Progress Reports on Funded Research: Project ACTION tracks its local demonstration projects through quarterly reports submitted by contractors. Contractors produce articles detailing the progress of their projects in *Project ACTION Update* and other disability and transit trade magazines.

Project ACTION also has an on-line bulletin board system and e-mail which is used to maintain contact and sharing information with contractors and other agencies who are conducting research. The on-line system houses a copy of each *Project ACTION Update.* Abstracts are available via *Project ACTION Update* on the electronic bulletin board.

Final Reports on Funded Research: Project ACTION publishes its final reports through the National Institute for Accessible Transportation (NIAT). The Institute, the dissemination arm of Project ACTION, distributes all publications and deliverables developed through Project ACTION's local demonstration program. No changes are scheduled by Project ACTION for reports distribution, but the Federal Transit Administration plans to provide all ADA transit research reports on the Internet Website beginning in FY 1996.

DEPARTMENT OF VETERANS AFFAIRS

Research and Development (R&D) in the Department of Veterans Affairs (VA) advances the diagnosis and treatment of health problems prevalent among veteran patients by applying findings of VA medical research studies throughout the hospital system. VA is not a granting agency, but rather funds an intramural program for investigators at VA

Medical Centers. The VA program encompasses three areas of research and development: Biomedical, Health Services, and Rehabilitation.

Funding: $25 million for Rehabilitation R&D in fiscal year 1995.

Disability Research: The VA Rehabilitation R&D program integrates the multiple disciplines of science, engineering, and medicine to investigate and develop concepts, processes, and products that directly meet the special needs of impaired and disabled veterans. Scientific investigation is carried out in areas of physical orientation, mobility, and manual skills enhancement, prosthetics/amputation/orthotics, spinal cord injury, communication, cognition, auditory/visual sensory aids, vocational placement, and recreational opportunity. Priority emphasis is given to those investigator-initiated studies whose results benefit veterans with war-related injuries. Current special emphasis areas are

- Orthopedics: prosthetics, orthotics, amputation management;
- Neurology: spinal cord injury, traumatic brain injury, nerve injury;
- Communications, cognition and sensory aids: vision, audition, speech, deglutition; and
- Disabling conditions and associated aging: cardiorespiratory, metabolic, muscular, skeletal, stability.

VA investigators are further guided by letters of information stating current foci within these priority areas. Internal Letters of Information are developed through strategic planning workshops with the participation of rehabilitation clinicians and researchers, as well as users of rehabilitation technology.

Announcing Funding Priorities: Internal Letter of Information.

Progress Reports on Funded Research: Program monitors in each Rehab R&D special emphasis area track and monitor the orderly progress, resource use, and timely reporting of merit approved and funded projects. Funded investigators are required to submit annual Progress Reports for publication in *Rehabilitation R&D Progress Reports*. An internally developed database, Research and Development Information Service (RDIS), is primarily used to track funding.

Final Reports on Funded Research: Final reports on VA Rehab R&D are published annually in *Rehabilitation R&D Progress Reports* and quarterly in the *Journal of Rehabilitation Research and Development*. Abstracts from the

Journal and the *Progress Reports* are on an electronic bulletin board and VA Online.

NATIONAL SCIENCE FOUNDATION

The National Science Foundation is an independent federal agency created to promote and advance scientific progress in the United States. NSF is responsible for the overall health of science and engineering across all disciplines. In contrast, other federal agencies support research focused on specific missions, such as health or defense. NSF is also committed to ensuring the Nation's supply of scientists, engineers, and science educators. The Foundation is led by a presidentially appointed director and a National Science Board composed of 24 scientists, engineers, and educators from universities, colleges, industry, and other organizations involved in research and education.

Funding: $7 million for disability-related projects in fiscal year 1994.

Disability Research: All seven Directorates in NSF support individual projects related to disabilities. These are typically investigator-initiated projects that are recommended for funding during regular competitive review cycles. NSF operates two programs dedicated specifically to research for people with disabilities.

• The **Biomedical Engineering and Research Aiding Persons with Disabilities Program**, Division of Bioengineering and Environmental Systems, located in the Engineering Directorate, supports investigator-initiated research projects recommended for funding by expert panels. The projects relate to the application of biomedical engineering techniques to needs of people with disabilities. The Program also supports Student Engineering Design Projects to stimulate interest among engineering students in the needs of people with disabilities that may be addressed through the application of modern principles of engineering.

• The **Program for Persons with Disabilities** in the Directorate for Education and Human Resources is dedicated to achieving full inclusion and participation of students with disabilities in science and math studies and in career development opportunities in science, engineering, mathematics, and technology. Many of the projects focus on developing instructional materials, media, and educational technologies that are usable by all students:

• **Experimental Projects for Persons with Disabilities**. Provides support for the development and demonstration of exemplary strategies for the recruitment, education, and retention of students with disabilities in science, engineering, and mathematics.

- **Model Projects for Persons with Disabilities**. Designed to promote the development and dissemination of innovative intervention strategies that reduce the barriers that inhibit the interest, retention, and advancement of students with disabilities in science, engineering, and mathematics education and career tracks.

- **Information Dissemination Projects**. Funds proposals for the support of symposia, workshops, and the development of information on techniques, instructional materials, technologies, and adaptations that promote full inclusion and participation of students with disabilities in science, engineering, and mathematics curricula.

- **Facilitation Awards for Scientists and Engineers with Disabilities.** This Foundation-wide program provides funding for students and faculty with disabilities to obtain special equipment and services needed to reduce or remove barriers so they can participate in research and training activities supported by NSF.

Announcing Funding Priorities: Programs of funded research are publicized through program announcements and program guides.

Progress Reports on Funded Research: Periodic progress reports are required of researchers. These reports are collected for internal use only and are not available to the public.

Final Reports on Funded Research: Final reports are required of researchers upon completion of the grant period. The awardee is responsible for the preparation of the results for publication. The Foundation does not assume responsibility for the research findings or their interpretation.

OTHER RESEARCH PROGRAM ACTIVITIES

Department of Education

Office of Special Education Programs

OSEP currently supports research programs in all aspects of the education of individuals with disabilities. The research areas supported include early intervention, instructional methods, curriculum development, assessment, and teacher training. OSEP is in the process of consolidating its 14 program authorities into 5 authorities. Field-initiated research accounts for 60% of the research budget.

Department of Energy

DOE has a research budget of $6.5 billion and some of its research in hearing, visual modalities, and computer technology has applications for persons with disabilities.

Department of Health and Human Services

Administration on Developmental Disabilities

The ADD is responsible for planning and implementing programs that promote self-sufficiency and protect the rights of persons with developmental disabilities. The ADD accomplishes this primarily though the University Affiliated Program (UAP), a discretionary grant program. UAPs provide technical assistance, community service, dissemination, and interdisciplinary training to professionals. UAP research activities include empirical research on existing practices and developing models of practice and service delivery. The ADD funding provides operational and administrative support to UAPs so that they can attract research funding from various sources. UAP research topics include infancy, early intervention, educational inclusion, school-to-work transition, employment, and aging.

National Institute on Deafness and Other Communication Disorders

NIDCD conducts research in the normal and disordered processes of hearing, balance, smell, taste, voice, speech, and language. Its $22 million research budget supports research in disability-related areas such as hearing aids, cochlear implants, telecommunications relay services, and vestibular issues.

National Aeronautics and Space Administration

NASA funds no disability research. However, its work in engineering and space technology has had spinoffs in technology transfer to products for persons with disabilities.

SERVICES AND BENEFITS

Department of Education

Rehabilitation Services Administration

RSA has no research focus, but funds $300 million a year on demonstration projects and evaluation of service approaches.

Department of Health and Human Services

Indian Health Service

IHS provides health care to American Indian and Alaska Native people. Its past research budget has been $2 million, with expected reductions to less than $1 million in the next fiscal year. The research funded by IHS is oriented toward improving basic health care services. It does not fund disability research. However, some of its research activities concern prevention of disability in four areas: (1) fetal alcohol syndrome, (2) hearing loss due to childhood infections (3) amputation due to diabetes, and (4) motor vehicle accidents.

Department of the Interior Bureau of Indian Affairs

The Branch of Exceptional Education within BIA funds no research. It provides direct educational services.

Social Security Administration

SSA administers the Social Security Disability Insurance (SSDI) and Supplemental Security Income (SSI) programs. It conducts studies of its disability programs and supports intervention and service delivery models such as returning beneficiaries to work. SSA is in the process of redesigning its programs to include a functional assessment instrument and to identify rehabilitation needs. This redesign will probably result in a change in the definition of disability which SSA uses to determine eligibility for benefits.

ADVISORY PANELS

General Services Administration

The Center for IT Accommodation at GSA applies research findings in emerging technology to ensure that information technologies (e-mail, electronic documents, postal kiosks) are accessible to persons with disabilities.

President's Committee on Mental Retardation

The Committee funds no grants or research. It is responsible for reviewing federal policy in relation to research. Its 21 members review federal and state programs that have an impact on mental retardation. The Committee sponsors conferences and provides an annual report to the President.

President's Committee on Employment of Persons With Disabilities

The Committee works to advance the employment needs of persons with disabilities. It funds no direct research, but funds a grant to the Job Accommodation Network (JAN) which provides technical assistance on job accommodations from 60,000 contacts annually. It has developed a profile of savings in workers compensation and disability payments. It has a Disability Communication Network with 6,000 Advocates and a Business Leadership Network where employers speak to other employers about hiring and retaining workers with disabilities. It also has organized a minority initiative.

COMPLIANCE

Department of Justice, Office of Civil Rights

The Office of Civil Rights enforces civil rights laws, provides technical assistance, and comments on legislation. It provides grants to disseminate information on how to comply with disability rights laws.

Equal Employment Opportunity Commission

The EEOC funds no direct research, but it uses research. It interprets and enforces the employment provisions of the Americans with Disabilities Act (ADA) and the Rehabilitation Act of 1973. Because of the backlog of cases, the EEOC is actively developing alternative dispute resolution techniques. As a user of disability research, the EEOC is especially interested in research in the areas of reasonable accommodation, assistive technology, cost of accommodation, and the role of education, training, and rehabilitation in the employment for persons with disabilities.

United States Information Agency

USIA deals with all aspects of disability in student and scholar exchange programs. Congress has mandated a report on outreach and work with persons with disabilities.

STATISTICS AND DATA COLLECTION

Department of Commerce

Bureau of the Census

The Bureau of the Census does not fund disability research. However, it conducts three surveys which are a primary source of disability data: Current Population Survey (CPS), Survey of Income and Program Participation (SIPP), the Decennial Census.

Department of Health and Human Services

National Center for Health Statistics

NCHS conducts the National Health Interview Survey (NHIS) which is a source of disability data. In 1994 continuing through 1996, NCHS is sponsoring a Disability Supplement to the NHIS which will be a major source of data on all aspects of disability.

Department of Labor

Bureau of Labor Statistics

BLS funds no disability research. However, it has some limited data regarding disability through three programs: Current Population Survey (CPS), the National Longitudinal Survey of Youth (NLSY), and the Occupational Safety and Health Statistics Program.

C

Taxonomy

The following is based in part on the *International Classification of Impairments, Disabilities, and Handicaps (ICIDH) proposed by the World Health Organization*, as modified by the Institute of Medicine.[1] It is an example of the beginning of a taxonomy that identifies the consequences of disease and injury most often of concern to physical therapists, occupational therapists, physicians, and others working with physical disabilities. Measurement of these aspects of a person's status would be essential both for providing the basis for treatment planning, and for permitting objective evaluation of progress toward clearly defined therapeutic goals. This represents, therefore, a classification of both the problems addressed in physical rehabilitation and of the therapeutic outcomes sought through treatment of those problems.

A TAXONOMY OF CLINICAL MEASUREMENTS

I. IMPAIRMENTS—Abnormality or absence of structure or function at the organ level.
    A. *Musculoskeletal*
        1. joint mobility (including hyper and hypomobility and methods

---

[1]For a description and discussion of the original WHO taxonomy see: *International Classification of Impairments, Disabilities, and Handicaps: a Manual of Classification Relating to the Consequences of Disease*. Geneva: World Health Organization, 1980; see also: Pope AM, Tarlov AR (eds): *Disability in America: Toward a National Agenda for Prevention*, Washington, D.C.: National Academy Press, 1991.

for differentiating cause as well as describing extent of the impairment)
2. muscle performance (sometimes incorrectly called "strength")
   a.) force (ability to generate peak acceleration of a mass, or peak torque)
   b.) power (ability to develop power in a contraction, usually torque velocity)
   c.) endurance (ability to sustain or repeat a contraction)
3. postural alignment (includes spinal deviations such as scoliosis)

B. *Sensory/perceptual*
   1. pain
   2. superficial sensation (touch, temperature, etc.)
   3. deep sensation (includes vestibular, position sense and stereognosis)
   4. body schema (body image or percept)

C. *Neuromuscular*
   1. muscle innervation (includes root, spinal and peripheral nerve)
   2. central nervous system
      a.) spasm (associated with pain or tension)
      b.) spasticity
      c.) rigidity
      d.) tremor
      e.) clonus
   3. coordination
      a.) ataxia
      b.) athetosis
      c.) standing stability and postural reactions
      d.) associated movements (i.e., inability to individuate muscle action)

D. *Developmental*
   1. perceptual-motor
   2. musculoskeletal
   3. cognitive
   4. social

E. *Psychological*
   1. cognitive (includes memory, thinking, consciousness, attention)
   2. affective (includes motivation, anxiety and other factors which influence readiness to respond to and participate in treatment and to cope with illness and its consequences)

F. *Cardiovascular*
   1. cardiac function
   2. peripheral vascular function (includes autonomic)
   3. lymphatic (includes edema)

G. *Pulmonary*
　　1. ventilation (rate, volume, and pattern)
　　2. respiration (blood-gas exchange)
　　3. secretion clearance
H. *Skin and superficial soft tissues*
　　1. tissue breakdown and wound healing
　　2. scarring and contracture
　　3. cosmetic problems

II. FUNCTIONAL LIMITATIONS [DISABILITIES in ICIDH]—restriction or lack of ability, resulting primarily or secondarily from an impairment, to perform activities that are generally accepted as essential components of everyday life; disturbance of function at the level of the person.
　A. *locomotor*
　　1. ambulation (including stairs, rough terrain, etc.)
　　2. transfer (lying, sitting, standing, to and from floor, etc.)
　　3. transport (use of automobile, bus, etc.)
　B. *personal care*
　　1. hygiene
　　2. feeding
　　3. dressing and grooming
　C. *dexterity* (holding, manipulating, adjusting, etc.)
　D. *object transport* (lifting, carrying, pushing, reaching, balancing, etc.)[2]
　E. *work/stress tolerance*
　　1. physical (includes cardiac stress and metabolic costs of activity)
　　2. psychological (includes ability to tolerate such stress as change, criticism, uncertainty, need to cooperate, etc.)
　F. *environmental tolerance* (includes ability to tolerate temperature variations, noise, allergens, smoke, etc.)
　G. *psychological*
　　1. cognitive—ability to learn new ideas and techniques, to plan tasks, solve problems, etc.
　　2. affective—ability to take initiative, accept limitations, adapt, etc.

III. DISABILITIES [HANDICAPS in ICIDH]—person-in-context restriction due to conditions that interfere with one's productivity or quality of life; conditions that place the individual at a disadvantage relative to other members of society.

---

[2] Note: B, C, and D are often jointly called "instrumented or instrumental ADL."

A. *productivity: independence and integration*
   1. physical independence—ability to meet personal needs in an unmodified environment without use of special aids or assistance from others
   2. social integration—ability to establish and maintain social relationships customary for his/her age, sex, and culture
   3. occupational capacity—ability to carry out the employment, schooling, domestic, or recreational activities customary for his/her age, sex, and culture
B. *quality of life*—ability to find a degree of satisfaction in life equivalent to that of most others of his/her age, sex, and culture.

D

Committee and Staff Biographies

COMMITTEE

EDWARD N. BRANDT, JR., is Regents Professor and Director of the Center for Health Policy at the University of Oklahoma. He received his M.D. and Ph.D. from the University of Oklahoma Medical Center. Prior to assuming his current responsibilities in 1992, Dr. Brandt served as Executive Dean of the College of Medicine of the University of Oklahoma Health Sciences Center. From 1981 to 1984, Dr. Brandt was the Assistant Secretary for Health and U.S. Representative to the Executive Board of the World Health Organization (from 1982 to 1984). From 1985 to 1989, Dr. Brandt was President of the University of Maryland at Baltimore and Professor at the University of Maryland School of Medicine. Dr. Brandt has been a member of the Board of Regents of the National Library of Medicine (1985–1989), a member of the Council of the Institute of Medicine (1986–1991) and Vice-Chairman of the Governing Council (1987–1991), and Chairman of the Medical Schools Section of the American Medical Association (1979–1981).

SHARON BARNARTT has a Ph.D. from the University of Chicago and is currently Professor and Department Chair in the Department of Sociology at Gallaudet University, where she has taught for the past 16 years. Her primary research interest is the sociology of disability and deafness and focuses on three major areas: (1) the socioeconomic status of male and female deaf workers, (2) social movements in the deaf and disability communities, and (3) disability policy issues both in the United States and internationally. She coauthored the book *Deaf President Now: The 1988 Revolution at Gallaudet University*, and she has published a number of articles and made many professional presentations on her research topics of interest. She is on the editorial board of the *International Journal of Disability, Development, and Education*, and is a past president and board member of the Society for Disability Studies.

CAROLYN BAUM is the Elias Michael Director and Assistant Professor for Occupational Therapy and Neurology at Washington University School of Medicine. Dr. Baum has served as President of the American Occupational Therapy Association and as President of the American Occupational Therapy Certification Board, and she has recently completed a term at the National Center for Medical Rehabilitation Research at the National Institutes of Health and on the McDonnel Science Foundation Task Force for Improving Cognitive Rehabilitation. Her research is on the relationship of activity and function in persons with cognitive impairment and chronic disease. She heads an interdisciplinary faculty that is contributing knowledge and training clinicians and rehabilitation scientists in developmental neuroscience, work performance and occupational competency, and aging and performance to understand the personal and environmental factors that contribute to the performance of everyday life.

FAYE BELGRAVE is an Associate Professor of Psychology and Director of the Applied Social Psychology Program at George Washington University. Dr. Belgrave has conducted research in the area of psychosocial aspects of disability and chronic illness for over 12 years. Dr. Belgrave has been the Principal Investigator and Co-Investigator on several grants (National Institutes of Health, National Institute on Disability and Rehabilitation Research) on psychosocial aspects related to disability and rehabilitation among ethnic minorities. She has published extensively in this area. Dr. Belgrave received her Ph.D. in social psychology from the University of Maryland in 1982. Prior to coming to George Washington University, she was a Senior Research Associate at the National Rehabilitation Hospital in Washington, D.C. Before that, she worked as a research associate at Howard University's Center for Sickle Cell Disease. Dr. Belgrave teaches graduate and undergraduate courses in social psychology and health psychology. She currently is on the editorial board of the *Journal of Black Psychology* and is an editorial consultant to several journals in the areas of disability and health. She is completing a book entitled *Psychosocial Aspects of Disability and Chronic Illness Among African Americans*. Dr. Belgrave received the American Psychological Association's Minority Fellowship

Award for outstanding research on ethnic minorities (1993) and the Association of Black Psychologist's 1994 Distinguished Scholarship Award. In 1993, she was honored with a Distinguished Service Award for service to persons with disabilities by the Howard University Research and Training Center for Access to Rehabilitation and Economic Opportunity.

CLIFFORD BRUBAKER has been Professor and Dean of the School of Health and Rehabilitation Sciences and Professor of Industrial Engineering, Orthopedic Surgery, and Neurological Surgery at the University of Pittsburgh since 1991. Before coming to the University of Pittsburgh, Dr. Brubaker was Professor of Education and Biomedical Engineering at the University of Virginia and Director of the Rehabilitation Engineering Research Center on Wheeled Mobility. Dr. Brubaker has published more than 100 papers, chapters, and technical reports. He also has been awarded four U.S. patents. Most of his research and design efforts have been directed toward the improvement of wheelchairs and specialized seating for people with disabilities. Dr. Brubaker is a fellow of both the Rehabilitation Engineering and Assistive Technology Society of North America (RESNA) and the American Institute on Medical and Biological Engineering. He currently serves as the President of RESNA. He is also the Chairperson of the Steering Committee on Long-Range Planning for the National Institute on Disability and Rehabilitation Research of the U.S. Department of Education. Dr. Brubaker received the Isabelle and Leonard H. Goldensen Technology Award from the United Cerebral Palsy Research and Education Foundation in 1995.

DIANA CARDENAS is Professor in the Department of Rehabilitation at the University of Washington. She is also the Project Director and Principal Investigator of the Northwest Regional Spinal Cord Injury (SCI) System, one of 18 model SCI centers funded by NIDRR. She is also Clinical Director of the Spinal Cord Injury Service and Director of the Rehabilitation Medicine Clinic at the University of Washington Medical Center in Seattle. Dr. Cardenas has conducted research in the area of spinal cord injury for the last 15 years, focusing on the physiology of the neurogenic bladder. She has published over 65 articles, chapters, and books, many in the area of spinal cord injury. She received the 1996 New Jersey School of Medicine National Teaching Award in Physical Medicine and Rehabilitation. Currently, she is the Principal Investigator of a study (funded by the National Institute on Disability and Rehabilitation Research) on the prevention of urinary tract infection in people with spinal cord injuries and recently published a study on the urodynamic findings associated with age and aging with SCI. Dr. Cardenas received her B.A. in 1969 from the University of Texas in Austin and her M.D. in 1973 from the University of Texas Southwestern Medical

School in Dallas. She earned an M.S. in 1976 from the University of Washington, where she also completed her residency training in Physical Medicine and Rehabilitation in 1976. She is currently on the Editorial Board of the *Archives of Physical Medicine and Rehabilitation,* serves as a member of the Research Committee of the American Academy of Physical Medicine and Rehabilitation, and serves on the Board of Directors of the American Spinal Injury Association.

DUDLEY S. CHILDRESS received his B.S. and M.S. degrees in electrical engineering from the University of Missouri at Columbia. Following graduation, he worked with Westinghouse Electric Corporation, served in the U.S. Army, taught electrical engineering at the University of Missouri, and worked with an electrical firm in Austria. In 1967, he received his Ph.D. in electrical engineering from Northwestern University. His research concerned control and movement of the human eye; this work stimulated his interest in muscle mechanics, electromyography, and the human motor control system. In 1966, he joined the Orthopaedic Surgery Department at the Northwestern Medical School. He currently holds appointments as Professor of Orthopaedic Surgery and Professor of Biomedical Engineering. He directs the Prosthetics Research Laboratory (with the Lakeside VA Medical Center); the National Institute on Disability and Rehabilitation Research's Rehabilitation Engineering Research Center in Prosthetics and Orthotics; and the Prosthetics and Orthotics Education Program, all of which are connected with Northwestern University and located within the Rehabilitation Institute of Chicago. His current interests concern human movement, particularly human ambulation and aided ambulation, control mechanisms that permit subconscious control of multifunctional artificial arms, human mechanics measurement systems, and computer-aided engineering and manufacturing in prosthetics and orthotics.

DONALD L. CUSTIS is currently the Senior Medical Advisor to the Paralyzed Veterans of America. From 1980 to 1984, he served as Chief Medical Director for the Veterans Administration, having begun work there in 1976 as the Assistant Chief Medical Director for Academic Affairs. He had retired that year as the U.S. Navy's Surgeon General, with the rank of Vice Admiral. He earned his medical degree from Northwestern University Medical School in 1942 and interned at Presbyterian Hospital in Chicago before serving on board a U.S. Navy attack-transport in the South Pacific. Following World War II, he obtained his graduate surgical education at the Mason Clinic in Seattle and then resumed a navy medical career, first as surgeon in a series of naval hospitals and then, in 1969–1970, as commanding officer of the Naval Combat Hospital in

Danang, Vietnam, followed by command of the National Naval Medical Center in Bethesda, Maryland. He is certified by the American Board of Surgery and is a Fellow of the American College of Surgeons. His honors and awards include the Presidential Award of the Distinguished Service Medal, Legion of Merit with Combat V, the Veterans Administration Exceptional Service Award, the Citation for Meritorious Service from the American Hospital Association, the Silver Medal Award of the American College of Hospital Administrators, the American Medical Association's Nathan Smith Davis Award, the Alumni Award of Merit from Northwestern, and honorary degrees from Albany Medical College and Wabash College, his alma mater.

SUE K. DONALDSON is Dean and Professor of the School of Nursing and Professor of Physiology, School of Medicine at Johns Hopkins University. She received B.S.N. and M.S.N. degrees from Wayne State University and a Ph.D. in Physiology and Biophysics from the University of Washington. Before coming to Johns Hopkins, Dr. Donaldson was a Professor in the Department of Physiology at the School of Medicine and Professor and Chair of Nursing Research Center for Long-Term Care of the Elderly at the University of Minnesota. She continues to act as a consultant to the National Institute for Nursing Research and to universities around the country. Dr. Donaldson is a pioneer in nursing research and internationally known for her basic science research in cellular skeletal and cardiac muscle physiology. In 1992, Dr. Donaldson was inducted as a Fellow in the American Academy of Nursing. Dr. Donaldson is a member of the Institute of Medicine.

DAVID GRAY is Professor of Health Sciences in the Program in Occupational Therapy at Washington University. Prior to assuming his current responsibilities, Dr. Gray had a distinguished career in government, where he served in numerous positions including Director of the National Institute on Disability and Rehabilitation Research in the U.S. Department of Education from 1986 to 1987 and Deputy Director of the National Center for Medical Rehabilitation Research of the National Institute of Child Health and Human Development at the National Institutes of Health (NIH). He has received many awards including the NIH Directors Award, the Paralyzed Veterans of America Career Achievement Award, and the National Head Injury Foundation's Outstanding Service Award. Dr. Gray received his B.A. in psychology from Lawrence University. He received an M.A. in experimental psychology from Western Michigan University and his Ph.D. in psychology and behavioral genetics from the University of Minnesota.

DAVID E. KREBS is Professor of Physical Therapy and Clinical Investigation at the Massachusetts General Hospital's Institute of Health Professions in Boston, and Director of the hospital's Biomotion Laboratory. He also holds academic appointments in orthopaedics at Harvard Medical School and in mechanical engineering at the Massachusetts Institute of Technology. Dr. Krebs has more than one hundred publications and has been awarded more than $4 million as principal investigator on federal (National Institutes of Health, National Institute on Disability and Rehabilitation Research) and foundation research grants, primarily on the neural and biomechanical constraints of human locomotor control. He was the 12th Annual Eugene Michels Researcher's Forum Featured Speaker of the American Physical Therapy Association and received its 1994 Golden Pen Award for Distinguished Scientific Writing. He was the 1995 Steven J. Rose Visiting Professor at Washington University. Dr. Krebs received his B.S. in physical therapy and his M.A. in applied physiology from Columbia University, and his Ph.D. in pathokinesiology and physical therapy from New York University.

ELLEN J. MACKENZIE is Senior Associate Dean for Academic Affairs and Professor in the Department of Health Policy and Management of the Johns Hopkins School of Hygiene and Public Health. She also directs the Johns Hopkins Center for Injury Research and Policy. Dr. MacKenzie's research has focused on methodological and policy-relevant issues related to patient outcomes following traumatic injury. Her early work involved the development and evaluation of tools for reliably measuring the severity of injury. These tools have been applied in several major research initiatives to evaluate the organization, financing, and performance of regionalized systems of trauma care. More recently, Dr. MacKenzie has focused on the evaluation of long-term outcomes following traumatic injury. Of particular interest to her is the delineation of factors (both medical and nonmedical) that explain variations in outcome. Her work has contributed to our knowledge of the economic and social impact of injuries and to our understanding of the personal and environmental factors that influence recovery, especially the return to work.

MARGARET TURK is an Associate Professor of Physical Medicine and Rehabilitation at the State University of New York Health Science Center at Syracuse. She has a joint appointment in the Department of Pediatrics at the Health Science Center and is also Medical Director of St. Camillus' Brain Injury Rehabilitation Program. She serves as a physical medicine and rehabilitation consultant to Syracuse Development Center and EN-ABLE, the local United Cerebral Palsy Affiliate. She is a board member of ARISE, the Syracuse independent living center. In addition to her clinical responsibilities, Dr. Turk is involved in many facets of rehabilitation research. Currently, she is the Principal Investigator on a study of secondary conditions of cerebral palsy in adults, funded by the Centers for Disease Control and Prevention, as well as coauthor of monographs and curricula on secondary conditions and aging with a disability. Dr. Turk is very active in the education of professional and academic organizations as to the importance of secondary conditions of disabilities in their research and patient care. Mostly recently, Dr. Turk has focused her research interests on practice parameters and outcome measurement in rehabilitation. She belongs to numerous committees at the state and national levels that have spearheaded innovative research and training on these topics. Additionally, Dr. Turk assisted the Paralyzed Veterans Association in developing their practice parameters for spinal cord injury rehabilitation. In the publication sphere, Dr. Turk sits on the editorial board for *Muscle and Nerve*. She is awaiting the release of *The Health of Women with Physical Disabilities: Setting the Research Agenda for the 90s*, a book that she edited with Drs. Krotoski and Nosek, and a chapter on outcome measurement in *Outcome Measurement Research in Rehabilitation: Setting the Agenda*, edited by Marcus Fuhrer.

GLEN WHITE has been involved in the rehabilitation and independent living field for over 25 years. As Codirector and Director of Research at the Research and Training Center on Independent Living (for underserved populations), Dr. White has conducted research in the areas of housing, advocacy, developing community support for independent living centers, and prevention of secondary conditions. He has recently served under Presidents Bush and Clinton as a Board Member on the Corporation for National Service. Dr. White is currently First Vice-President of the American Disability Prevention and Wellness Association and President-Elect of the National Association of Rehabilitation Research and Training Centers. He also serves as a Board Member on the Paralyzed Veterans of America's Education and Training Foundation. Dr. White currently has a appointment as an Assistant Professor in the Department of Human Development and Family Life at the University of Kansas, where he teaches in the areas of behavioral and community psychology and disability studies.

SAVIO L.-Y. WOO is the A.B. Ferguson Professor and Vice Chairman for Research, and Director of the Musculoskeletal Research Center in the Department of Orthopaedic Surgery, University of Pittsburgh Medical Center. He also holds concurrent positions as Professor in the Department of Mechanical Engineering, the Department of Civil and Environmental Engineering, and in the Department of Rehabilitation Science and

Technology. Prior to joining the faculty at the University of Pittsburgh, Dr. Woo was Professor of Surgery and Bioengineering at the University of California at San Diego and Director of Orthopaedic Bioengineering Laboratory at the San Diego Veterans Affairs Medical Center. Dr. Woo's research interests include solid mechanics and biomechanics; experimental, theoretical, and numerical analyses of the nonlinear material properties of biological tissues; healing and repair of tendon, ligament, articular cartilage, and meniscus; and joint kinematics and the use of robotics technology. He has published extensively and has received many awards and distinctions for his research. He has served as President for the Orthopaedic Research Society, the American Society of Biomechanics, and the International Society for Fracture Repair and as Chairman for the Bioengineering Division of the American Society of Mechanical Engineers, the United States National Committee on Biomechanics, and the College of Fellows of the American Institute for Medical and Biological Engineering. Dr. Woo is a member of the Institute of Medicine and the National Academy of Engineering.

EDWARD YELIN is Codirector of the Education, Epidemiology, and Health Services Research Component of the Multipurpose Arthritis Center at the University of California at San Francisco (UCSF) and of the Disability Statistics Rehabilitation and Research Training Center. He is also a member of the Division of Occupational and Environmental Medicine and the Institute for Health Policy Studies, and Professor of Medicine in the Department of Medicine, all at UCSF. His research has emphasized the causes and consequences of disability, especially the impact of chronic disease on employment. He is the author of *Disability and the Displaced Worker* and numerous research articles. He received his A.B. in public affairs from the University of Chicago and his M.C.P. and Ph.D. in city and regional planning from the University of California at Berkeley. He is an active member of the Arthritis Foundation and the American College of Rheumatology. Dr. Yelin recently received both the Clarke Award for Outstanding Research from the Arthritis Foundation and the Outstanding Scholar Award from the American College of Rheumatology.

WISE YOUNG is Director of the Neurosurgery Research Laboratories at New York University (NYU) and Bellevue Medical Center, and Professor of Neurosurgery, Physiology, and Biophysics at NYU Medical Center. He received his B.A. from Reed College, where he majored in biology and chemistry, was a member of Phi Beta Kappa National Honor Society, and received the Award for Excellence in Mathematics and Science. He received his Ph.D. in physiology and biophysics from the University of Iowa and his M.D. from Stanford University. Dr. Young has authored over 100 journal articles. He is recipient of the Jacob Javits Neuroscience Award from the National Institute of Neurological Disorder and Stroke, the Wakeman Award for Research in the Neurosciences, and the Neurotrauma Society Service Award.

IOM STAFF

ANDREW M. POPE is a Senior Staff Officer and Study Director in the Institute of Medicine's Division of Health Sciences Policy. With expertise in physiology, toxicology, and epidemiology, his primary interests focus on disability and the environmental and occupational influences on human health. As a Research Fellow in the Division of Pharmacology and Toxicology at the U.S. Food and Drug Administration, Dr. Pope's research focused on the biochemical, neuroendocrine, and reproductive effects of various environmental substances on food-producing animals. During his tenure at the National Academy of Sciences, and since 1989 at the Institute of Medicine, Dr. Pope has directed and edited numerous reports on environmental and occupational issues; topics include injury control, disability prevention, biologic markers, neurotoxicology, indoor allergens, and the inclusion of environmental health content in medical and nursing school curricula.

THELMA L. COX is a project assistant in the Division of Health Sciences Policy. During her 7 years at the Institute of Medicine, she has also provided assistance to the Division of Health Care Services and the Division of Biobehavioral Sciences and Mental Disorders. Ms. Cox has worked on several IOM projects, including Designing a Strategy for Quality Review and Assurance in Medicare; Evaluating the Artificial Heart Program of the National Heart, Lung, and Blood Institute; Federal Regulation of Methadone Treatment; Legal and Ethical Issues Relating to the Inclusion of Women in Clinical Studies; and Review of the Fialuridine (FIAU/FIAC) Clinical Trials. In 1995, she received the National Research Council Recognition Award and, in 1994, an IOM Staff Achievement Award.

GEOFF FRENCH is a Research Assistant in the Division of Health Sciences Policy; he has been with the Institute of Medicine for 2 years. His undergraduate degree is in history and anthropology, and he has completed his M.A. in national security studies at Georgetown University.

VALERIE PETIT SETLOW is the Director of the Division of Health Sciences Policy. In this capacity, she is responsible for the development of public policy activities related to (a) biomedical research, including fundamental science and clinical research; (b) infrastructure to support research; (c) drug development and regulation; (d) education, training, and mentoring of health professionals; and (e) the ethical, legal, and social implications of biomedical advances. Dr. Setlow received her B.S. in chemistry from Xavier University and her Ph.D. in molecular biology from Johns Hopkins University. She has conducted research in molecular hematology and virology and has had a distinguished career in government, serving in numerous positions including as Director of the Cystic Fibrosis Research programs at the National Institutes of Health, and in her last position, as Acting Director of the National AIDS Program Office. Her expertise includes molecular biology and genetics, health science program management, health policy analysis, and program development. She also holds an adjunct appointment at Howard University in the Department of Community and Family Medicine.

Index